HELPING COUPLES AND FAMILIES NAVIGATE ILLNESS AND DISABILITY

Helping Couples and Families Navigate Illness and Disability

An Integrated Approach

John S. Rolland

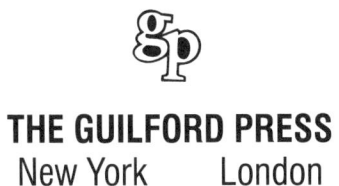

THE GUILFORD PRESS
New York   London

Copyright © 2018 The Guilford Press
A Division of Guilford Publications, Inc.
370 Seventh Avenue, Suite 1200, New York, NY 10001
www.guilford.com

All rights reserved

No part of this book may be reproduced, translated, stored in a retrieval system, or transmitted, in any form or by any means, electronic, mechanical, photocopying, microfilming, recording, or otherwise, without written permission from the publisher.

Printed in the United States of America

This book is printed on acid-free paper.

Last digit is print number: 9   8   7   6   5   4   3   2   1

The author has checked with sources believed to be reliable in his efforts to provide information that is complete and generally in accord with the standards of practice that are accepted at the time of publication. However, in view of the possibility of human error or changes in behavioral, mental health, or medical sciences, neither the author, nor the editor and publisher, nor any other party who has been involved in the preparation or publication of this work warrants that the information contained herein is in every respect accurate or complete, and they are not responsible for any errors or omissions or the results obtained from the use of such information. Readers are encouraged to confirm the information contained in this book with other sources.

Library of Congress Cataloging-in-Publication Data
Names: Rolland, John S., 1948– author.
Title: Helping couples and families navigate illness and disability :
   an integrated approach / John S. Rolland.
Other titles: Complemented by (work): Families, illness, and disability.
Description: New York : The Guilford Press, [2018] | Includes bibliographical
   references and index.
Identifiers: LCCN 2018002802 | ISBN 9781462534951 (hardback)
Subjects: | MESH: Family Health | Family Therapy—methods | Couples
   Therapy—methods | Chronic Disease | Disabled Persons
Classification: LCC RC455.4.F3 | NLM WA 308 | DDC 616.89/156—dc23
LC record available at *https://lccn.loc.gov/2018002802*

About the Author

John S. Rolland, MD, MPH, is Professor of Psychiatry and Behavioral Sciences at Northwestern University Feinberg School of Medicine. He is also Co-Founder and Executive Co-Director of the Chicago Center for Family Health and Director of its Families, Illness, and Collaborative Healthcare Program. Internationally recognized for his integrated conceptual model, clinical work, and research on couple and family psychosocial challenges with serious health conditions, Dr. Rolland is coeditor of *Individuals, Families, and the New Era of Genetics*. He is past president of the American Family Therapy Academy (AFTA); Distinguished Life Fellow of the American Psychiatric Association; Senior Fellow of the Group for the Advancement of Psychiatry, Family Committee; past board member of the Collaborative Family Healthcare Association; and former Fellow of the Yale University Institute for Social and Policy Studies. Dr. Rolland is a recipient of the Innovative Contributions to Family Therapy Award from AFTA and the Blanche F. Ittleson Award from the American Orthopsychiatric Association (now the Global Alliance for Behavioral Health and Social Justice). He is an active speaker and consultant on family-oriented systemic approaches to illness and disability challenges.

Preface

Over half of Americans over age 18 live with a chronic health condition, leaving virtually no family untouched. This book was inspired by the profound unmet needs of couples and families living with illness and disability. Family members' personal struggles and suffering often remain hidden from those outside the family, sometimes even from one another.

As a young adult, I became acutely aware of these challenges when illness struck in my own life. I had completed medical school and begun my psychiatry residency at Yale University. I was exposed to hundreds of patients and their families, but I did not appreciate the many dilemmas and strains for families with serious health problems until my own marriage and family life were directly affected. Within a year, my mother had a disabling stroke, and my first wife, Essie, at age 27, was diagnosed with an incurable form of cancer. Although I was a young physician and came from a highly educated, financially secure, and close-knit family, I was wholly unprepared for the strains of coping with their life-threatening conditions. No one in my immediate family had ever been seriously ill. There were stories of tragedy and loss related to my parents' experience as Jewish refugees from Nazi Germany, but there were no family stories about how to cope with long-term illness or disability.

Over the next 5 years, as my loved ones' conditions worsened and they ultimately died, I learned through trial and error many of the excruciating illness-related challenges that commonly confront couples and families over time. It was an eye-opening, painful, and humbling experience. I became aware of how little my own professional discipline offered people in my family's predicament. The tendency to focus almost exclusively on individual issues of the patient or caregiver did not suit the many challenges in couple and family relationships or the reverberations for the extended family network. Individual colleagues were supportive of me, but traditional psychotherapeutic models seemed both too narrowly focused on the individual patient and based too much on theories of psychopathology rather than on the normative strains of families coping with adversity. Caregiver strains were not addressed within the rich network of family or community relationships. There were scattered accounts of personal resilience in the face of major illness, but little in terms of how couples and families can adapt well—and even grow stronger.

In situations of illness, caregivers and other family members tend to highlight their shortcomings in a self-critical way: "I should have been able to do more." I was no exception. However, I started to ask myself a different question: What would have been useful information or support for me and my family members at different phases of the illness that could have made a difference in our ability to cope and adapt? This question provided a new and empowering lens through which to view my personal experience, but also motivated me to think about a model that would help all couples and families challenged by illness or disability. The most immediate and simple answer was, "I wish at the time of diagnosis that a professional had suggested that the whole family meet to discuss the illness and its implications for our lives." At the time, I was working in a mental health center connected to a community-based hospital in a predominantly working-class region. As a provider of psychiatric consultations for the hospital medical units, I noticed that family members were often present or available in the evenings during visiting hours, and I began to routinely respond to consultation requests by meeting with patients and their families. To my initial surprise, the referring physicians were highly supportive and, since this was a community hospital, they often had some direct knowledge of the families. I found that I could address the problems of the patient more effectively and efficiently, and simultaneously could deal with the concerns of other family members. And spouses and family members were appreciative.

From this simple beginning, my life's work emerged. I developed the Family Systems Illness (FSI) model for psychoeducation, consultation, assessment, and intervention with couples and families challenged by chronic and life-threatening conditions. I cofounded two centers based on this model dedicated to training, clinical services, and collaborative health care program development. In 1985, working with a multidisciplinary team of colleagues, I started the Center for Illness in Families in New Haven, Connecticut. Its mission was to provide a collaborative, strengths-based, family-centered clinical approach to the psychosocial needs of families dealing with a range of major health conditions in children and adults.

In 1991, Froma Walsh and I cofounded the Chicago Center for Family Health (CCFH), a nonprofit independent affiliate of the University of Chicago, that brought together a faculty of talented colleagues with varied areas of expertise and approaches in couple and family therapy. We shared a collaborative, resilience-oriented meta-framework in family systems training and practice, community-based partnerships, and a commitment to serving diverse families and underserved populations. The Center's internationally recognized Families, Illness and Collaborative Healthcare (FICH) programs provide state-of-the-art clinical training; services to couples and families; and research that promotes healthy family functioning, life cycle development, and adaptation to serious illness, disability, and loss. Over the years, the Center has trained clinicians across professional disciplines and diverse work settings through continuing education seminars, workshops, intensive institutes, and extensive training in a 2-year certificate program and full-time doctoral fellowships in family systems approaches to health care.

Over the past 26 years, the integrated practice approach presented in this book was further elaborated and enriched through our Center's collaborations with both primary and specialty care health care delivery systems and services. Applying the FSI model as a conceptual base for behavioral health care collaboration, our involvement has included program design and implementation; staff, family, and community outreach education; and clinical services. We have partnered with two primary care family medicine programs providing integrated care at the University of Chicago–affiliated MacNeal Hospital and at Advocate Illinois Masonic Family Practice Center, through the on-site placement of full-time FICH doctoral fellows. Within specialty care, I have worked with many diverse programs, such as those in diabetes, oncology, heart disease, multiple sclerosis, genetic risk screening, dementia, HIV, dialysis, rehabilitation medicine, and palliative care and hospice. This volume describes and illustrates the useful application of my FSI model to this broad range of conditions in primary and specialty care settings.

A guiding conviction of this approach is that any couple and family facing illness and disability should routinely be offered a family prevention-oriented consultation near the time of a condition's onset, as well as continued access to such services over the course of the condition. This affirms a partnership with families, especially caregiving members, seeing them as a valuable resource in collaborative care. It engages them in a biopsychosocial model of care from the outset. And it identifies couples and families at high risk of maladaptation to the challenges ahead. The "health-related family unit" is considered the psychosocial hub for effective coping and adaptation. This approach is resilience oriented, normative, and preventive. A variety of consultations and brief and more intensive interventions are offered for individuals, couples, families, and multifamily groups. Collaborative behavioral health care is essential as patients and their family members experience a variety of contexts, including stays at hospitals and extended care facilities and outpatient, home, and hospice care. One particularly striking statistic is that approximately two-thirds of the families served over the years have never previously seen a mental health professional. With the growth of integrated health care, biomedically focused providers increasingly collaborate with mental health providers more preventively, involving them as valued team members in the overall treatment plan for their patients with chronic conditions. Psychotherapists in practice need to be proactively included in the health care team.

This book presents an integrative practice guide that synthesizes my professional and personal experiences over the past 40 years. The FSI model offers a comprehensive way of organizing our thinking about the multiple interactions related to a chronic condition among a patient, his or her family, and health care professionals. This model is distinctive in addressing their dynamic interplay over the course of the illness and the evolving phases of the life cycle. The clinical applications of the FSI model, informed by research in the field, are described and illustrated to be clinically relevant and useful to the many real-life family situations with illness and disability that clinicians are likely to encounter in a range of health care and counseling practice settings. In this book, the FSI-informed practice approach is applied to a full range of adult- and childhood-onset illnesses and disabilities, including neurocognitive and genomic disorders.

Throughout this book, we will see how illness challenges and strains family functioning, affecting all members and their relationships, and how, in turn, family processes can influence the well-being of all members, their relationships, and the management and course of the illness or disability. A major health crisis can shake the foundation of the family, and it can also awaken family members to opportunities for more satisfying, fulfilling bonds and life pursuits. The FSI practice approach addresses the challenges and emphasizes the possibilities for both patient and family positive adaptation and growth.

In brief, Part I provides an overview of the FSI model and describes the psychosocial typology and time phases of illness; Part II highlights family organizational and communication processes in illness; multigenerational themes; the interaction over time between illness and individual and family development; and the role of health belief systems. Part III features applications of the FSI model and offers practical guidelines for illness-phase-related challenges for specific populations including children, adolescents, and parents, and for later-life conditions, couples relationships, genomic and neurocognitive conditions, and the challenges of threatened loss and terminal phase issues. Part IV focuses on the clinician's personal experience and collaborative practice.

This book is designed to serve the varied needs of a broad range of health and mental health professionals from the disciplines of psychiatry, social work, psychology, nursing, marriage and family therapy, pastoral care, and other medical specialties and allied health fields. Its guiding principles can be usefully adapted to fit clinicians' varied roles, settings, and intervention approaches.

In all my work with couples and families, I continue to be amazed at their potential to live well in the face of serious illness and disability. And I have seen countless times how we as health care providers can make a remarkable difference in their quality of life.

Acknowledgments

Foremost, I want to acknowledge the many exceptional families I have been privileged to work with and learn from in their quest to live well despite illness and disability—among my loved ones, my mother, my first wife, Essie, and my sister-in-law, Wendy, who lived well in the face of death, and my father, who lived well until almost 101—and Froma and Claire and the rest of my family, whose continued love and support are so important to my life.

 I would like to thank a number of people for their help, support, wisdom, and friendship in bringing this book to fruition. I owe a special debt of gratitude to my wife, Froma Walsh, for her tireless love and support, for the many important conversations that helped shape and refine the ideas presented in this book, and for her invaluable help in reviewing all stages of the manuscript. I would especially like to thank some of my colleagues at the Chicago Center for Family Health, who reviewed different chapters in progress: Hernan Barenboim, Gene Combs, Limor Gildenblatt, Miriam Klevan, Laura Lynch Christensen, Peter Rainey, Alexandra Zaikova, Max Zubatsky, and Stevan Zuckerman. I also want to express my appreciation to Susan Lanier for her administrative assistance in preparation of the manuscript. Finally, at The Guilford Press, I would like to thank Senior Editor Jim Nageotte and Assistant Editor Jane Keislar, for their patience and first-rate guidance, as well as Senior Production Editor Anna Nelson, and Barbara Watkins and Louise Farkas for their expert editing.

Contents

PART I. THE FAMILY SYSTEMS ILLNESS MODEL: THE EXPERIENCE OF ILLNESS AND DISABILITY

1. **A Family Psychosocial Map with Chronic Conditions**   3
   The Social Context of Illness and Disabilities   4
   Aims of This Book   5
   The Core Concepts and Components of the Family Systems Illness Model   9
   The Organization of This Book   16

2. **The Psychosocial Typology of Illness**   19
   A Psychosocial Typology of Illness   20
   A Psychosocial Typology Matrix   29
   Psychosocial Perspective   36

3. **The Time Phases of Illness**   37
   The Initial Crisis Phase   38
   The Chronic Phase   44
   The Terminal Phase   44
   Transition Periods   45
   A Psychosocial Developmental Model   48
   Implications for Clinical Assessment and Intervention   50
   Clinical Applications: The Therapeutic Triangles   51
   Service Delivery Applications   53

PART II. THE FSI MODEL: WORKING WITH COUPLES AND FAMILIES

4. An Integrated Practice Approach with Couples and Families — 57
   Levels of Systems-Based Involvement with Families 57
   Basic Principles of Intervention 60
   Timing of Consultations 66
   Treatment Modalities 67

5. Facilitating Family Organizational and Communication Processes — 76
   A Normative Perspective 76
   Family Organization and Communication 77
   Conclusion 88

6. Understanding Multigenerational Experiences — 89
   Different Disciplines and Settings 90
   Uses of the Family Genogram 90
   The Basic Family Genogram 91
   Time Line 93
   The Family Health Genogram 93
   Psychosocial Typology and Time Phases 93
   Life-Cycle Coincidences across Generations 95
   Family Processes 96
   General Experiences with Crisis and Adversity 98
   Case Examples 99

7. Addressing Life-Cycle Issues with Chronic Conditions — 108
   Core Life-Cycle Concepts 109
   Integrating Individual, Family, and Illness Development in Clinical Practice 112
   Case Illustration 120
   General Clinical Discussion 124

8. Tapping the Power of Family Belief Systems — 128
   Overview 128
   The Experience of Illness: Levels of Meaning and Influence 129
   Assessment of Health Beliefs 131
   Integrative Medicine and Healing Practices 154

Contents

PART III. PHASE-RELATED ISSUES AND SPECIFIC POPULATIONS: PRACTICE GUIDELINES

9. Helping Families with Anticipatory Loss and Suffering — 159
  Illness Type and Time-Phase Issues 162
  The Family Life Cycle 168
  Belief Systems 175

10. Helping Families in the Terminal Phase — 177
  Living during the Terminal Phase 178
  Three Terminal-Phase Periods 186
  Ethical and Legal Issues at Life's End 194
  Clinician Self-Care 199

11. Chronic Conditions in Childhood and Adolescence — 200
  Crisis-Phase Issues 201
  Communication 204
  Developmental Issues 206
  Challenges for Siblings 213
  Developmental Disabilities: Challenges in Adulthood 217

12. Parental Illness and Later Life Challenges — 221
  Parental Illness and Disability 221
  Aging Parents and Caregiving 228

13. Intimacy Issues for Couples — 240
  Conjoint and Individual Sessions 241
  Intimacy in Illness and Disability 242
  LGBTQ Couples 256
  Inclusion of Clinicians in the Couple's Relationship 256

14. Rebalancing the Couple's Relationship — 258
  Establishing Healthy Boundaries 258
  Keeping the Roles of Patient and Caregiver within Bounds 261
  Togetherness and Separateness 265
  Recovery and Adaptation Imbalances 266
  Belief System Imbalances 267
  Life-Cycle Imbalances 268

15. Individual and Family Challenges in the New Era of Genetics   272

*The FSGI Model: Psychosocial Typology and Time Phases
    of Genomic Disorders   274
Cultural Meanings and Beliefs   289
Additional Life-Cycle Issues   291
Combining the FSGI and FSI Models   293
Integrated Collaborative Practice   295
Ethical and Legal Considerations   296
Conclusion   300*

16. Neurocognitive Impairment: Mastering Challenges over Time   301

*Neurocognitive Conditions: Symptoms, Prevalence, and Etiology   302
Psychosocial Typology Issues   303
Time Phase-Related Issues   307
Life-Cycle-Related Issues   316
General Family Challenges   318
Challenges for Couples   321*

PART IV. THE CLINICIAN'S EXPERIENCE AND COLLABORATIVE PRACTICE

17. Personal Themes for Clinicians: The Shared Experience of Illness   325

*Facing Loss and Personal Limits   325
Clinicians' Multigenerational Legacies with Illness and Loss   330
Life-Cycle Timing   332
Health Professionals' Belief Systems   332
Issues Generated in the Clinician's Own Family   333
General Guidelines for Meeting Clinician Needs   336
Case Illustration   339*

18. Collaborative Health Care: Linking Families with Systems of Care   347

*Overview   347
Collaboration in Different Health Care Settings and Contexts   351
Beliefs and Expectations: Fit among Clinicians, Health Care Systems,
    and Families   362
Principles for Family-Oriented Programs and Policies   367*

References   369

Index   387

PART I

THE FAMILY SYSTEMS ILLNESS MODEL

THE EXPERIENCE OF ILLNESS AND DISABILITY

CHAPTER 1

A Family Psychosocial Map with Chronic Conditions

Miriam, a young married woman with two small children, received the most up-to-date medical treatment and expert surgical interventions during her 4-year bout with cancer. Eight months after her physician pronounced her cured, Miriam and her husband, Dave, separated. Behind the scenes and unknown to the health care team, serious family difficulties had developed over this stressful period. A previously stable marriage had become increasingly conflictual and distant. Dave had developed a serious drinking problem and became verbally abusive toward his wife. A prolonged emotional and financially draining divorce and custody battle followed. Both children developed behavioral problems that required crisis intervention, bringing this struggling family to therapy for the first time.

In a twist on the popular aphorism "the treatment was successful, but the patient died," conventional treatments of serious illness may save the patient, but the family may suffer irreparable harm from the accumulation of psychosocial strains. Chronic or life-threatening conditions confront families with profound challenges. The diagnosis, or recurrence, of cancer or the ongoing challenges of a serious disability reverberate throughout the family system leaving no one untouched. For some families the quality of life deteriorates, whereas others forge ahead with resilience and thrive.

Illness and disability strike all families. The questions are when in our lives they will occur, under what conditions, how serious they will be, and how long they will last. Perhaps most important is how the experience will affect couple and family bonds and shared hopes and dreams. With major advances in medical technology and with improved standards of living for many segments of society, people with access to health care are living much longer and better with conditions such as cancer, heart disease, diabetes, and HIV/AIDS. Many children with chronic illnesses that previously were fatal or necessitated institutional care are surviving into adulthood, often needing extensive family support to integrate into mainstream life.

Longer life spans have heightened strains on sons and daughters and their families, who are increasingly geographically dispersed and contending with the competing demands of elder care, child rearing, and job responsibilities. Ever-growing numbers of families are living with chronic disorders over an increasingly long time period and are coping with multiple challenges simultaneously.

In acute health crises that are resolved within weeks or months, a focus on good biomedical care takes priority. Psychosocial demands on families may be intense, but they are time limited. Like sleep-deprived parents with an infant, a predictable time frame helps families endure the inevitable hardships and maintain a positive outlook. With chronic conditions, however, uncertainties and ambiguities can extend into the distant future, frequently with the expectation that the illness will worsen and eventually result in death. Over time, cumulative strains on the family unit are unavoidable.

THE SOCIAL CONTEXT OF ILLNESS AND DISABILITIES

Families' experiences of illness and disability are enormously influenced by the dominant culture and the health systems embedded in it. In the United States, a major illness often means financial ruin, with almost two-thirds of bankruptcies linked to illness and medical bills (Himmelstein, Thorne, Warren, & Woolhandler, 2009). Millions with disabilities cannot obtain the assistance that would enable independent living. Tens of thousands die each year needlessly because they lack health care coverage for necessary treatments and medications (Wilper et al., 2009).

A lack of access to adequate basic health care has serious ramifications in terms of the incidence of illness, disease course, survival, quality of life, and varied forms of suffering caused by discrimination. For racial and ethnic minority and low-income groups, chronic diseases are more prevalent, tend to occur earlier in the life cycle, and have a worse course and prognosis because of inadequate medical care and limited access to resources. They are disproportionately represented among the approximately 33 million uninsured (U.S. Census Bureau, 2015) and the tens of millions underinsured (Collins, Rasmussen, Beutel, & Doty, 2015). Recent data, showing that black male life expectancy is almost 5 years less than that of white males, give a glaring example of these larger societal issues (Kochanek, Arias, & Anderson, 2013).

As populations age worldwide, the number of people with chronic conditions will vastly increase over coming decades. Over half of the U.S. adult population lives with at least one chronic condition (U.S. Census Bureau, 2015), a number that is climbing rapidly. With advances in technology and extended survival with chronic illnesses, the strain on families to provide adequate caregiving is unprecedented. For example, in the United States in 1970, there were 21 potential family caregivers for each elderly person. By 2010, there were only 7 potential caregivers, and this caregiver support ratio is projected to decline further to 4 to 1 by 2030 and to 3 to 1 by 2050 (Redfoot, Feinberg, & Houser, 2013). Many factors are involved, including decreasing birthrates, family networks that are becoming smaller and more top-heavy, with more older than younger family members, and geographic distance among members. Most women are in the workforce, juggling job and child-rearing demands, and are unable to fill traditional female role expectations to serve as unpaid family caregivers.

AIMS OF THIS BOOK

This book describes the Family Systems Illness (FSI) model for psychoeducation, consultation, assessment, and intervention with couples and families challenged by chronic and life-threatening conditions. It extends my earlier framework (Rolland, 1984, 1987a, 1990, 1994a, 2012, 2013) to include in-depth coverage of a wide range of practice applications. The FSI model offers a comprehensive way of organizing our thinking about the multiple interactions involving a patient, his or her family, and health care professionals during the course of dealing with a chronic condition. It considers the complexities and diversity of contemporary family life in a social context and in relation to health care systems. It can be used to address the breadth of clinical issues faced by couples and families, where one or more members suffer a serious illness or disability. This model is distinctive in addressing the changing interactions among these parts of the system over the course of the illness and the evolving phases of the life cycle.

FSI is a family-focused, resilience-based, and prevention-oriented clinical model that fosters healthy psychosocial adaptation. Intended for a broad range of health and mental health care practitioners across disciplines in varied health care and counseling settings, this book provides core knowledge and skills to work effectively with families facing illness and disability. It offers both families and clinicians a useful approach that promotes a sense of mastery and empowerment over a complex and uncertain long-term process.

The Need for an Integrated Family Systems Illness Model

Over the past 30 years, family-centered, collaborative, and biopsychosocial models of health care have grown and evolved (Doherty & Baird, 1983; Engel, 1977; Kissane & Parnes, 2014; McDaniel, Doherty, & Hepworth, 2014; Miller, McDaniel, Rolland, & Feetham, 2006; Peek, 2015; Rolland, 1994a; Seaburn, Gunn, Mauksch, Gawinski, & Lorenz, 1996; Talen & Burke Valeras, 2013; Wood et al., 2008, Wright & Bell, 2009). There is substantial evidence for the mutual influence of family functioning, health, and physical illness (Carr & Springer, 2010; D'Onofrio & Lahey, 2010; Proulx & Snyder, 2009; Weihs, Fisher, & Baird, 2002) and for the usefulness of family-centered interventions with chronic health conditions (Campbell, 2003; Hartmann, Bazner, Wild, Eisler, & Herzog, 2010; Kazak, 2006; Law & Crane, 2007; Martire, Lustig, Schultz, Miller, & Helgeson, 2004; Martire, Schulz, Helgeson, Small, & Saghafi, 2010; Shields, Finley, Chawla, & Meadors, 2012). Highly regarded texts describe applications in various health care settings and across different disciplines (Gelhert & Browne, 2018; Heru, 2013; Hodgson, Lamson, Mendenhall, & Crane, 2014). The multidisciplinary journal *Families, Systems, and Health* has been a crucial voice advocating theoretical and clinical research and provider training in family-oriented collaborative health care. The many advances in specific areas will be interwoven throughout the book.

The vast majority of research and clinical publications address a particular illness or disability (Shields et al., 2012). For instance, family therapy interventions with diabetes are the most intensively researched and have included Multisystemic Therapy (MST) (Ellis et al., 2008) and Behavioral Family Systems Therapy (BFST-D) (Wysocki et al., 2007) models. Other investigators have included a combination of cognitive and behavioral interventions with childhood cancer (Kazak, 2005, 2006) and the bio-behavioral family model with pediatric asthma (Wood et al., 2008). While this research provides valuable insights about a specific disorder using specific interventions, the interventions may be applied either too narrowly or too broadly to conditions with markedly different psychosocial demands. The application of a particular psychosocial intervention can become overgeneralized, with insufficient stock taken of the complexities of different conditions over time. The Family Systems Illness model described in this book addresses this issue, providing a conceptual framework that can be applied to a full range of adult- and child-onset illnesses and disabilities, including neurocognitive and genomic disorders.

Promoting Family Resilience

Nearly two-thirds of patients and families referred to me and my colleagues at the Chicago Center for Family Health over the past three decades have never before seen a mental health professional. This has profound clinical implications: Any comprehensive model needs to be useful for typical families coping with common illness-related strains, not just for those with serious dysfunction more often seen in mental health settings.

Our thinking has advanced past stereotypical definitions of "the family." Research has amply documented that a broad range of diverse, multicultural family forms and styles of functioning are compatible with normal, healthy individual and family development (Walsh, 2012). Countering the myth of normal family life as "problem-free," we know that all families are challenged by adversity. When serious illness strikes, we need to reject an outdated, rigid, or romanticized ideal of coping. This family-centered model views a broad range of family forms and processes as normative. Supported by a growing body of research on resilience, it describes how families can adapt successfully to illness and disability along many varied pathways (Walsh, 2016b).

Families with problematic relational patterns may well have more difficulty handling the stresses of a chronic illness. Yet, clinicians need to be careful not to reflexively append the label "pathological" or "dysfunctional" to families beset by serious conditions. In fact, components of family functioning, such as cohesion, exist on a continuum, and cultural norms vary widely. Different types or phases of illness may need varying levels of family cohesion for optimal coping and adaptation. High versus low family cohesion is not viewed as inherently healthy or unhealthy. Rather, the organizing principle becomes relative: What degree of family cohesion tends to work optimally with this illness at this time, and how might that change in future phases of the condition? Very high levels of cohesion should not be presumed to be dysfunctional. Studies have found high cohesion in positive close, caregiving bonds to be adaptive with a major health condition (Green & Werner, 1996). And, I have seen families with enmeshment function very well when faced with a rapidly progressive, fatal illness, such as metastatic cancer, where high cohesion is needed.

Family Systems-Oriented Unit of Care

The FSI model broadens the unit of care from the medical model's narrow focus on the ill individual to the family or caregiving system ("health-related family unit") (McDaniel et al., 2014), including all members and relationships affected by the illness-related challenges and those who could be helpful allies in care. The model considers the impact for siblings of an ill child or for the couple bond of a spouse who is providing elder care. Systemically, an effective biopsychosocial model attends to the impact of the illness on the family network of relationships, which, in turn, can influence the course of an illness and the well-being of the affected person. By using a broad definition of family as the cornerstone of the caregiving system, as suggested by the Institute of Medicine report (Weihs et al., 2002), the model describes successful coping and adaptation based on supporting family system strengths and addressing its vulnerabilities.

This model is a sharp contrast to the narrow focus on the patient by most current models of intervention in behavioral medicine, consultation-liaison psychiatry, and psychotherapy. At worst, families are relegated to the background; it is recognized that they affect the patient's psychosocial adjustment, but they are not considered to need help with their own stressful challenges. Early intervention acknowledges the importance and concerns of all family members, prevents them from being marginalized, and draws on their potential as vital partners and resources in the treatment process. Further, I view collaboration as a mindful way of resisting pressures to dehumanize the experience of illness and reduce the ill person and a living family system to a diseased patient or disorder.

From Psychosomatic to Holistic and Interactive

The literature describing the impact of chronic disorders on individuals and families is extensive. However, the influence of individual and family processes on disease has historically been defined in terms of psychosomatic processes and almost invariably in pathological terms. The designation of a condition as "psychosomatic" is a shame-laden label associated with pejorative cultural meanings that imply family dysfunction and negative influences that exacerbate symptoms and suffering. This designation tends to overpathologize families and to label them pejoratively as "psychosomatic families." Further, a skewed focus on dysfunction distorts our understanding of typical or optimal family coping and adaptation to illness. More recent investigators have shifted attention toward the influences of social support and key family processes that promote adaptation. A growing literature examines the positive impact of individual and family functioning on health and well-being and, in the context of illness, the quality of life for all family members as well as the disease course and outcome (Carr & Springer, 2010; D'Onofrio & Lahey, 2010; Weihs et al., 2002).

The FSI model describes psychosomatic processes in more holistic, interactive, and normative terms. All illnesses can be viewed as having a psychosomatic interplay, in which the relative influence of biological and psychosocial factors varies over a range of disorders and illness phases. Even with regard to highly virulent diseases such as HIV/AIDS, there is compelling evidence that family and community support affects the patient's quality of life and the course of the illness. In a psychosomatic interplay, psychosocial factors, not just biomedical interventions, can be important influences in well-being and disease course. With this approach, professionals can undercut pathologizing family and cultural beliefs and help families approach biopsychosocial interaction as an opportunity to make a positive difference. This mindset increases their sense of control and overall quality of life.

Rigid, gender-based standards for couples and families define a narrow range of roles and expectations for coping with illness and disability. Traditional models of patient and caregiver roles can shackle families—especially the designated female caregiver—in the face of the protracted strains of illness and threatened loss. The FSI model expands views of role functioning for men and women and views the family network as a caregiving team.

To summarize, the FSI model gives clinicians a useful way of describing the complex mutual interactions among the illness, the ill family member, and the family system within a normative framework attuned to the diversity in contemporary families. It provides a framework for addressing the challenges families confront and for expanding their possibilities for adaptation and growth. Throughout this book, we will see how illness challenges and strains family functioning, affecting all members and their relationships; and how, in turn, family processes can influence the well-being of all members, their relationships, and the management and course of the condition. A serious health crisis can shake the foundation of the family, and it can awaken family members to opportunities for more satisfying, fulfilling bonds and life pursuits. This useful clinical model addresses these challenges and emphasizes the possibilities for patient and family positive adaptation and growth.

THE CORE CONCEPTS AND COMPONENTS OF THE FAMILY SYSTEMS ILLNESS MODEL

Family Systems Theory

The Family Systems Illness (FSI) model is grounded in systems theory. Family systems theory emphasizes interaction and context; individual behavior is viewed within the context in which it occurs. From this perspective, function and dysfunction are defined by the fit between the individual and the family and their social context, the psychosocial demands of the health condition, and other stressors in family life.

A family systems orientation is distinguished by its view of the family as a transactional system. The ongoing interactive patterns within the family and between a family and other systems (for example, health institutions) are considered central in influencing individual behavior. Stressful events and the problems of an individual member, such as a major health crisis, affect the whole family as a functional unit and have ripple effects for all members and their relationships. In turn, the family response to problems and major life challenges, such as serious illness, contributes significantly to positive adaptation or to individual and relational dysfunction. Family members are interrelated such that each individual affects all the others and the group as a whole, in turn, affecting the first member in an ongoing chain of mutual influence. Thus, individual challenges, such as a serious health condition, need to be assessed and treated in the context of the family system and its social and developmental location. Overall, *the family is regarded as an essential resource and partner in treatment, with the potential of fostering optimal adaptation.*

In a systemic model of human development, individual and family development are seen to coevolve over the life course and across the generations. Therefore, a broad multigenerational and multicultural conception of the family evolving over the life cycle is essential (McGoldrick, Garcia Preto, & Carter, 2016). Relationships grow and change, boundaries shift, roles are redefined, and adaptation is needed when a new child is born or a member dies.

Each developmental phase presents salient challenges; distress often occurs around major transitions, such as the birth of the first child or later-life caregiving needs.

For clinicians and researchers alike, transactional patterns are at the heart of all systems-oriented biopsychosocial inquiry. In physical illness, particularly chronic and life-endangering disorders, the primary focus is systemic—which means a condition, individual and family processes, and other biopsychosocial systems mutually influence one another (Engel, 1977). The FSI model views the family as its central unit because in clinical assessment and intervention it may provide the best system through which to understand these multilevel systems. This choice is made with the recognition of biological influences and ongoing family transactions with larger environmental factors. The impact of chronic disorders is affected by economic resources, extended kin and social support, and the health care system, particularly through access, availability, and the quality of services.

The FSI model is based on the concept of systemic interaction between an illness and family that evolves over time. The FSI model has three dimensions: (1) a psychosocial typology of illness, (2) major time phases in an illness's evolution, and (3) key family systems components.

A Psychosocial Typology of Chronic Conditions

The landscape of chronic conditions is diverse and complex, presenting a vast range of symptoms and trajectories, accompanied by a variety of psychosocial demands over the evolution of the disorders. Although there are elegant and detailed descriptions of the physical demands of particular conditions, these accounts do not consider the pattern of psychosocial demands of the illness over time or the systemic ramifications in the relational network. This book presents a psychosocial typology of illness that organizes the diversity and the commonalities of chronic disorders in a way that can be useful to both clinicians and families and serves as a bridge between the biomedical and the psychosocial worlds. As shown in Figure 1.1, illnesses can be typed by their pattern of onset, course, outcome, degree of disability, and level of uncertainty.

Illness Time Phases

A longitudinal perspective is essential with chronic conditions. We need a multigenerational developmental model that coherently integrates legacies and themes related to the illness with three interwoven threads—the illness, individual family members, and family development—in a manner useful for assessment and intervention.

By their nature, chronic conditions evolve over many years. The model presented here is useful in combining illness and disability in a schema that

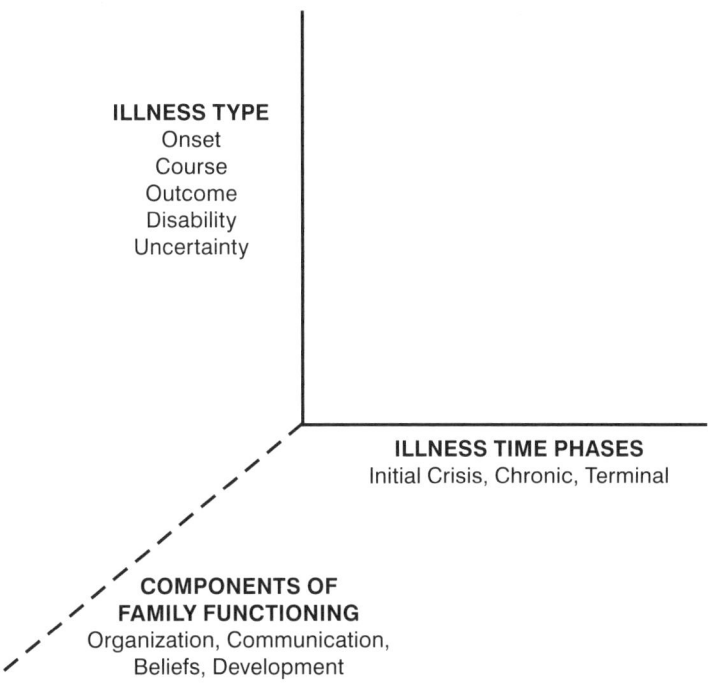

FIGURE 1.1. FSI model: Three dimensions.

links the past, present, and future. The literature has generally focused on a specific phase of what I refer to as the "illness life course" (e.g., disease onset, terminal phase, or bereavement). There are three illness time phases in the FSI model: the initial crisis phase, including the initial diagnosis and adjustment; the chronic phase; and the terminal phase. It is crucial to consider the evolution of illness-related developmental challenges over the entire course of a disorder.

Components of Family Functioning

The framework of family assessment in the FSI model is based on an evaluation of four basic domains of family functioning, drawing from Walsh's family resilience framework and advances in research on normal family processes (Walsh, 2012, 2016b).

- Organizational/structural patterns
- Communication processes
- Belief systems
- Development: multigenerational patterns and family life course

12 THE FSI MODEL: THE EXPERIENCE OF ILLNESS AND DISABILITY

At its core, the FSI model attends to the expected psychosocial demands of a disorder through its various time phases in relation to these domains of family functioning. The model emphasizes family and individual life-course development, multigenerational patterns, and belief systems. It includes the influences of culture, ethnicity, race, spirituality, gender, and socioeconomic level, along with related forms of discrimination. Figure 1.2 represents one way to conceptualize the relationship between these different levels of influence.

Interaction with Individual and Family Development

It is vital to attend to illness-associated developmental issues of other key family members and the family as a functional unit. Too often, if developmental issues are addressed, they tend to be restricted to a particular person, usually the patient. The impact of chronic conditions differs for the patient, for a child in cases of parental or sibling illness, and for key caregivers, and depends on when an illness strikes in family development and in each member's individual life course. Because the course of different conditions varies greatly over time, developmental implications for the family unit and all members need to be highlighted. Developmental skews among family members become inevitable during the course of an illness or disability. Thus, the FSI model coherently integrates individual and family life-cycle passage in relation to the evolving disorder over time.

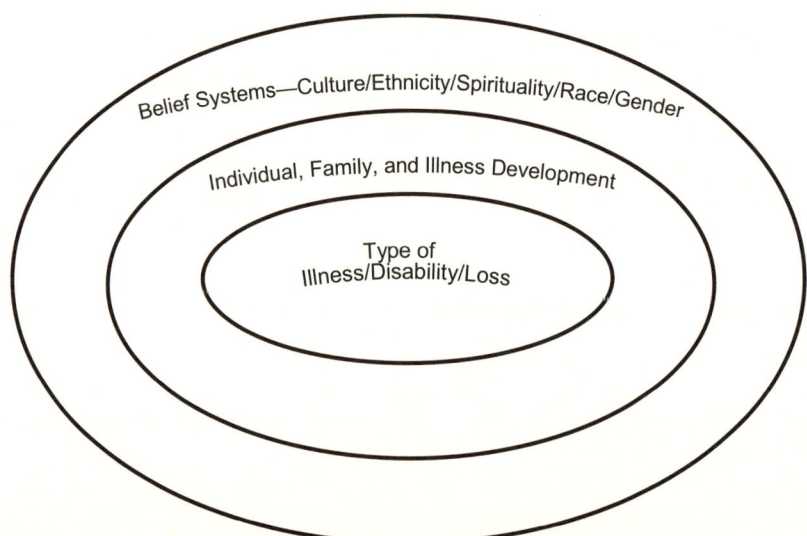

FIGURE 1.2. FSI model: Levels of influence.

Multigenerational Influences

Systems thinkers have stressed that a family's present behavior cannot be adequately understood apart from its history (e.g., Bowen, 2004; Byng-Hall, 2004; McGoldrick et al., 2016). Multigenerational legacies and patterns of adaptation shape beliefs and expectations that strongly influence how families perceive a current health crisis and guide its modes of dealing with adversity. Attention to these legacies is part of the FSI model.

Family Belief Systems

Belief systems play a central role in family coping and adaptation with chronic disorders. Vivid descriptions from medical anthropology highlight the kinds of explanations and meanings people attach to health problems (Groleau, Young, & Kirmayer, 2006; Kirmayer, Guzder, & Rousseau, 2014; Kleinman, 1988, 2009). In the area of cognitive psychology, attribution theory and social construction theory have examined the ways in which people develop narratives and meanings about how things happen, especially significant personal events (e.g., Beck & Haigh, 2014; Niemeyer, 2001). Meaning-making occurs through the narratives individuals and families develop to make sense of their experiences, their social context, and their place in it (Freedman & Combs, 1996). With a serious health condition, efforts in meaning-making come to the fore as individuals and families strive to integrate its significance into their life passage.

There have been important contributions to our understanding of family-shared meaning systems and the evolution and significance of family belief systems (Antonovsky, 1998; Hansson & Cederblad, 2004; Reiss, 1981; Walsh, 2009, 2016b). This includes understanding the ongoing systemic processes in families relative to meaning systems with illness and loss (Nadeau, 2008; Wright & Bell, 2009).

In situations of chronic disorders, a basic task for families is to make meaning for a health condition that promotes the family's sense of active agency and mastery. At the extremes, competing ideologies can leave families divided between a biological explanation of an illness and one that holds the individual family member responsible (e.g., illness as retribution for wrongdoing). Also, families desperately need guidance and reassurance that they are handling illnesses as best they can (and that bad things do happen to good people). Thus, belief systems are included in the FSI.

The FSI model emphasizes the *quality of fit* between the psychosocial demands of the chronic condition over time and the family style of functioning and resources. This is a prime determinant of successful versus dysfunctional coping and adaptation. The systemic interaction between an illness and the family is shown schematically in the diagram in Figure 1.3. From this perspective, no single family pattern is regarded as inherently healthy or

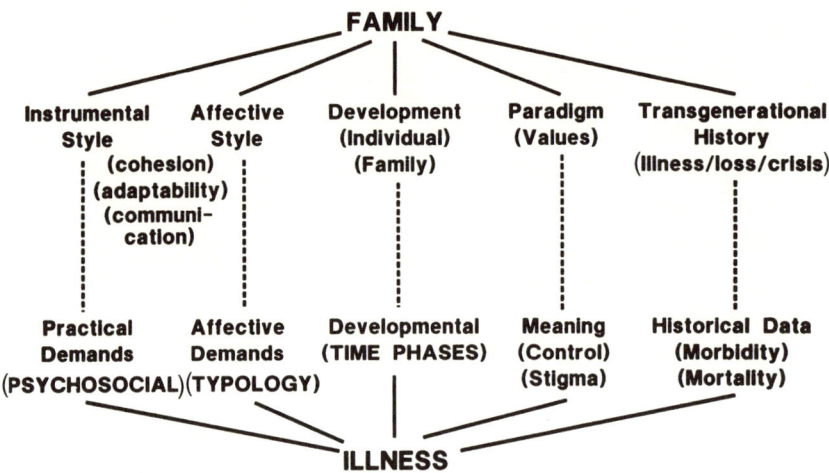

FIGURE 1.3. Interface of chronic illness and the family. From Rolland (1987b). Reprinted by permission.

unhealthy. Rather, the organizing principle becomes relative: What degree of family cohesion or kind of communication is optimal for adaptation in diverse families, with different kinds of conditions, and in different phases of chronic disorders?

A Psychosocial Map for the Experience of Illness and Disability

Families encounter the world of illness and disability without a psychosocial map. Often they desperately need a psychosocial guide that can provide information, support, and reassurance that they are handling an illness well. Many families, particularly those with untimely disorders, find themselves in unfamiliar territory without a map. A preventive, psychoeducational approach helps families anticipate normative illness-related developmental tasks in a fashion that maximizes their sense of active agency, mastery, and acceptance in dealing with the condition. To create a normative context for their illness experience, families need to understand the following:

1. *Understand themselves as a systemic functional unit.*
2. *Have a psychosocial understanding of the condition in systems terms.* This means learning the expected pattern of practical and affective demands of a disorder and its treatment over the course of the condition. This includes a time frame for disease-related developmental tasks associated with different phases of an unfolding condition.

3. *Appreciate individual and family life-cycle patterns and transitions.* This facilitates incorporation of changing developmental priorities for the family unit and individual members in relation to evolving challenges of a chronic disorder.
4. *Understand the cultural, ethnic, spiritual, and gender-based beliefs that inform the type of caregiving system they construct.* This includes guiding principles that delineate roles, rules of communication, meaning-making, definitions of success or mastery, and the fit with the beliefs of the health care providers.

Family understanding in these areas facilitates a more holistic integration of their illness experience and the family as a functional family-health/illness system evolving over time.

Application to Diverse Health Care Disciplines and Settings

The FSI model provides a conceptual base for approaching clinical practice and research regarding illness and disability from a family systems perspective. The emphasis is on the initial consultation and assessment process and the common issues and challenges faced by families as they experience a condition. This model and practice guidelines are useful for clinicians who may use varied intervention approaches. The model can be applied across disciplines by both health and mental health care providers. It has been designed with an awareness that the level of psychosocial intervention will vary considerably depending on the context and the professional training and role of the clinician. Throughout this book, using the FSI model, I will underscore different levels of psychosocial involvement with families, beginning with minimal provision of biomedical information and psychoeducation, consultation and a systemic assessment, brief interventions, periodic "family checkups," and more intensive family-oriented therapy (Doherty, McDaniel, & Baird, 1996; McDaniel, Campbell, Hepworth, & Lorenz, 2005). (See Chapter 18.) The FSI model should be helpful at every level of intervention.

Each chapter provides enough detail to be useful for more comprehensive assessments or intensive interventions. I will discuss a range of important issues and dilemmas and offer sample questions, so that clinicians can get a feel for how I might elicit information about various areas of family life. Naturally, I never cover all questions or all issues in detail with any one family. Those clinicians who function under enormous time pressures and have limited opportunities with families can adapt this approach to make best use of their time. For instance, instead of doing a detailed multigenerational history, asking a few well-chosen questions can serve as a "screening scan." If a critical issue is identified, clinicians can decide whether to pursue it further or refer the family to an appropriate colleague.

THE ORGANIZATION OF THIS BOOK

This volume is organized into four parts. The rest of Part I (Chapters 2 and 3) focuses on the illness aspects of the FSI model by describing the psychosocial typology and illness time phases.

Part II (Chapters 4–8) describe the family aspect of the model, providing case vignettes and clinical guidelines to work with families. Chapter 4 describes basic principles of effective systemic interventions for practitioners, and I provide guidelines for family-oriented consultations for both an initial session and timely follow-up sessions. Flexible use of individual, couple, family, and multifamily discussion group interventions and psychoeducation are described. Chapter 5 discusses family organizational and communication processes in chronic disorders. Chapter 6 describes the importance of multigenerational themes related to illness and loss, and offers case examples. It covers family legacies, including toxic issues, catastrophic expectations, strengths, and learned differences between family members. Using concepts from contemporary individual and family life-course models, Chapter 7 discusses the mutual interactions between the course of an illness and the development of the family and its individual members. Timing of onset and future nodal transition points are highlighted.

Chapter 8 describes the role of belief systems in chronic disorders. The discussion includes key elements of families' health belief systems and the influences that shape them over the course of a condition. Special consideration is given to beliefs about normative illness experiences; biopsychosocial–spiritual influences in health and illness; mastery, control, and acceptance; cultural and ethnic meanings attached to symptoms and illnesses; gender issues; assumptions about influences in the cause, course, or outcome of a disorder; the fit of beliefs among family members; and the role of integrative medicine. The chapter examines beliefs that induce blame, shame, and guilt and the interventions that foster more adaptive beliefs and promote competency and mastery.

Part III (Chapters 9–16) discusses applications of the FSI model and offers practice guidelines for phase-related and specific populations. Chapter 9 addresses anticipatory loss issues for families over the entire course of a chronic or life-threatening condition. Beyond the concept of anticipatory grief, in the terminal phase of an illness, the concept of anticipatory loss recognizes that families often live for years with painful ambiguities and the uncertainties of threatened loss. This includes living with genetic risk information. Considered here are specific issues such as distinguishing among anticipation of disability, cognitive impairment, suffering, and death and the different strains for families dealing with possible versus probable or inevitable loss. The chapter highlights ways to help families think about anticipated loss in relation to future nodal points in their personal and family life course.

Facing our own mortality or the death of a loved one is profoundly challenging. The way we approach life's end and painful losses can yield unexpected personal relational growth and transformation. Chapter 10 provides guidelines that address key clinical and ethical challenges in the terminal phase such as meaning-making; handling dilemmas related to end-of-life decisions; opening blocked communication; secrecy and denial; facilitating reconciliation and healing of intergenerational conflicts and estrangement; integrating medical treatment with palliative care and hospice; dignity and control in the dying process; and conflicts in values of health care professionals, patients, and families.

Chapter 11 addresses assessment and treatment issues for chronic conditions in childhood and adolescence. Guidelines are provided for such issues as communication, control, determining reasonable medical management goals that support normative development, transition to adulthood, and meeting the challenges for siblings. Chapter 12 explores family challenges with parental illness and disability, and with later life conditions. It includes caregiving issues related to gender, negotiating shared responsibilities among family members, balancing caregiving of parents/elders with child rearing, inclusion of professional caregivers, and skilled facility placement planning.

Chronic disorders often wreak havoc on a couple's relationship. Chapters 13 and 14 address the challenges in maintaining a viable mutual relationship, coping with uncertainties, and achieving developmental goals in the face of threatened loss. The FSI model provides a basis for discussing common challenges regarding intimacy, sexuality, communication issues, patient–caregiver and other relationship imbalances, gender roles, coparenting, and the use of individual and conjoint consultations.

Chapter 15 addresses the impact of advances in genomics, which pose unprecedented clinical and ethical challenges for families and health care professionals. Expanding on my Family Systems Genetic Illness (FSGI) model (Rolland & Williams, 2005), this chapter examines core clinical issues and sociocultural influences in decision making about genetic testing, communication with partners and family members, and living with risk information across the life cycle. The areas discussed include belief conflicts, ethical issues and decisions (e.g., privacy vs. right to know by others at risk, fetal information), couples and childbearing, multigenerational patterns, and behavioral genetics.

Chapter 16 employs the FSI model to address some key family challenges with mild and advanced dementia and traumatic brain injury. Conditions involving neurocognitive impairment are among the most difficult for couples and families. Although there are a number of approaches to help individual caregivers, a broad family systems approach, now underutilized, can be effective.

Part IV (Chapters 17 and 18) focuses on the clinician's experience and collaborative practice. Chapter 17 addresses the vital importance for clinicians to understand how our own belief systems, personal experiences, and multi-generational and life-cycle issues related to illness and loss affect our professional engagement with patients and their families and our practice effectiveness. The chapter examines health care professional challenges related to facing loss and personal limits in the context of work demands, while striving to maintain a satisfying personal and family life. I describe an in-depth case example involving a personal illness story and its relational ramifications for a couple coping with cancer.

The concluding Chapter 18 uses the FSI model to look at larger systems and the ways in which families can be connected to systems of care. The chapter provides an overview of integrated family-oriented care and describes innovative examples of family-based programs of collaborative care in specialty care services and with consumer-based organizations. In this context, I prefer the word *consumer* because it connotes a more balanced, less hierarchical relationship to health care professionals than *patient* or *patient's family*. As is common in health care settings, I will use the word "patient" throughout the book, yet with the respect due to the "consumer of care." The chapter discusses clinical challenges (e.g., belief systems) at the interface between the patient and family, health care providers, and systems of care, over the illness course. Finally, key principles and policies for advancing family-oriented health care are provided.

CHAPTER 2

The Psychosocial Typology of Illness

In order to think in a mutually interactive manner about a chronic condition and a family, we need a way to describe the condition in systems terms. The myriad biological diseases also need to be recast in psychosocial terms. This chapter and Chapter 3 describe a psychosocial typology and time-phases framework that facilitate a fluid interplay between the illness and the family in the illness–family system. Such a framework must be relevant to the interactions of the psychosocial and biological worlds and provide a common meta-language that transforms or reclassifies the usual biological language. Also, for such a systems framework to be useful, it needs to facilitate thinking about the interaction between chronic disorders and the health-care provider team and systems of care, as well as with other relevant systems.

There have been two major impediments to progress in this area. First, insufficient attention has been given to the areas of diversity and commonality inherent in different chronic disorders. Second, there has been a glossing over of the qualitative and quantitative differences in how various chronic diseases evolve over time. This great variability has challenged investigators who have attempted to identify the most salient psychosocial variables relevant to disease course or treatment adherence. The standard disease classification used in medical settings is based on purely biological criteria clustered in ways to establish a medical diagnosis and treatment plan, rather than on the psychosocial demands for patients and their families.

Clinical practice and psychosocial research in physical illness are significantly hampered by a singular use of this biologically based disease classification. The FSI model that I have developed provides a better link between the biological and psychosocial worlds and thereby clarifies the relationship between chronic illness and disability and the family.

Historically, the specific illness orientation has tended to push clinicians' and researchers' views of the relationship between psychosocial factors and physical illness toward dichotomous thinking about either each specific disease or "illness" in general. At one extreme, individual and family coping with a particular disorder are approached narrowly, without highlighting general aspects of adaptation they share with other conditions. At the other extreme, research findings and clinical wisdom regarding a particular disease are overgeneralized to all illnesses. Both of these extremes hamper clinicians, who lack guidelines in balancing unifying principles and useful distinctions with the wide range and varied trajectory of chronic conditions. Either a monolithic psychosocial approach is applied to all chronic illnesses, or findings or experiences with one type of disorder may be inappropriately transposed to other conditions that pose quite different challenges.

The psychosocial typology, described in this chapter, and the illness time phases covered in Chapter 3 allow tracking of psychosocial demands for all chronic conditions. Illness variability and time phases are addressed on two separate dimensions: (1) key biological similarities and differences that present significant and distinct psychosocial demands for patients and their families and (2) prime developmental time phases in the evolution of chronic disease.

A PSYCHOSOCIAL TYPOLOGY OF ILLNESS

A typology is a subjectively constructed map for orienting one to a territory (Bateson, 1979). The goal of a psychosocial typology is to define meaningful and useful categories with similar psychosocial demands for a wide array of chronic disorders affecting individuals throughout the lifespan. It is designed not for traditional medical treatment or prognostic purposes, but for examining the relationship between family or individual processes and chronic disease.

This typology conceptualizes five broad variables with distinct patterns of (1) onset, (2) course, (3) outcome, (4) type and degree of disability, and (5) level of uncertainty (see Figure 2.1). I have found these variables to be the most psychosocially significant for a wide range of illnesses and disabilities. Also, these variables were chosen because they strongly influence the nature of the developmental tasks associated with each of the time phases of the illness—initial crisis, chronic, and terminal—described in Chapter 3. For example, the type of onset significantly affects the nature of the developmental tasks normally associated with the initial crisis phase. Although each variable actually exists on a continuum, it will be described here in a categorical manner by selecting key anchor points along the continuum. Consider these anchor points as guideposts that can clarify the many shades of gray.

The Psychosocial Typology of Illness

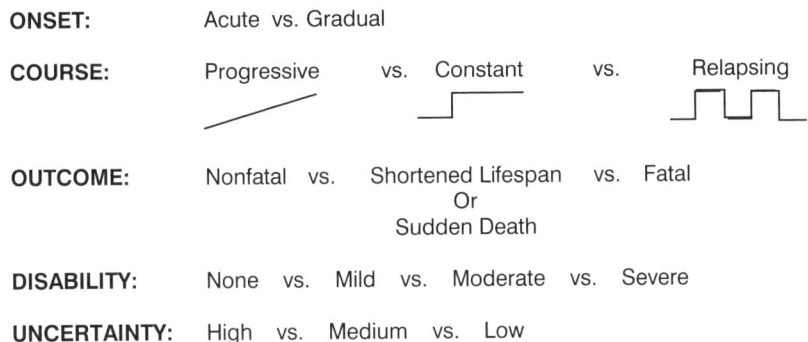

FIGURE 2.1. Psychosocial illness types.

Onset

Illnesses can be divided into those that have either an *acute* or a *gradual* onset. This division is not meant to differentiate types of biological development, but to highlight the kinds of symptomatic presentation that can be experienced by the patient or noted by other people. Strokes, heart attacks, traumatic brain injury (TBI), and meningitis are examples of conditions with sudden clinical presentation, although they may have long periods of biological development that led to a marker event. Examples of illnesses with a gradual onset include arthritis, chronic lung disease, and Alzheimer's disease. For a gradual-onset illness, the diagnosis serves as a somewhat arbitrary confirmation point after clinical symptoms have appeared.

A gradual-onset condition presents a different form of patient–family stressor than a sudden crisis does. The total amount of readjustment of family organization, roles, problem solving skills, and affective coping may be the same for both types of illness. However, for those families experiencing an acute-onset condition the emotional and practical changes are compressed into a short time and require more rapid family mobilization of crisis management skills.

Some families are better equipped than others to cope with rapid change. Families able to tolerate highly charged emotional situations, exchange roles flexibly, problem-solve efficiently, and utilize outside resources effectively will have an advantage in managing acute-onset conditions. Other families' style of coping may be more suited to gradual change: like the tortoise versus the hare, they take a slow and steady approach. Given enough time, they will achieve their goal. Such families adjust well to gradual-onset disorders such as Parkinson's disease, but may be initially overwhelmed by conditions such as stroke. The problem of fit between this family style and the initial demands of an acute illness calls for a brief, early intervention to support family members through this vulnerable phase and help avert long-term dysfunction. Once "in gear," the family very well may have the resources to manage the complexities of a long-term disorder, particularly one without repeated, acute changes or new and unfamiliar symptoms.

The slower rate of family change required to cope with gradual-onset diseases, such as arthritis or Parkinson's disease, allows for a more protracted period of adjustment, but can generate more anxiety because establishing an accurate diagnosis may take longer. For acute-onset diseases, there is a relatively greater immediate strain on the family in simultaneously trying to prevent further loss and death and cope with a new challenge.

Course

The course of chronic disorders can take three general forms: *progressive, constant,* or *relapsing or episodic.* Varying levels of uncertainty overlay these forms, each posing differing psychosocial challenges.

Progressive Conditions

With a progressive disease, the family is often faced with a perpetually symptomatic member whose disability worsens in a stepwise or gradual way. Such diseases include incurable cancers, Alzheimer's disease, arthritis, and emphysema. Periods of relief from illness demands tend to be minimal. Families need to be prepared for continual adaptation and role changes.

At each stage of a progressive illness, the family needs to organize itself to deal with a particular level of disability and degree of uncertainty. Yet, the family cannot really "settle in" at any particular stage because progression looms ahead, and it must be prepared to keep reforming its system to keep pace with the changing picture of the illness. The increasing strain on family caregivers is caused by both the risks of exhaustion and the continual addition of new caregiving tasks as the disease progresses. Family flexibility in terms of both role functions and willingness to use outside resources is crucial.

In progressive disorders clinicians need to be aware that, like a marathon runner, any family can "hit the wall"—literally come to the end of its physical, emotional, or financial stamina and/or its ability to adapt its system. At this point, a family may need to radically restructure its way of handling necessary changes. In systems terms, this family needs to make more fundamental second-order versus first-order change. Second-order change has to do with altering aspects of one's worldview and the basic rules that go with it, a transformation that is more discontinuous with the past. For example, one elderly couple governed by traditional gender roles made it through the initial phases of the wife's progressive respiratory condition by giving added effort in performing their traditional, gender-defined roles; but as the condition worsened, the couple finally reached a stage at which they could carry on only by redefining their basic roles so that daily tasks could be shared. When families lack the resources or flexibility to make fundamental changes, they may have to allow professional caregivers into their home or consider institutional placement for the ill member.

Early family consultation and assessment can help a clinician judge when a family has reached its limits. Evaluative discussions are particularly important when dealing with progressive disabling disorders, in which caretaking demands alone can eventually result in a family increasingly defining its life mission and source of mastery in terms of successful caregiving. Such families may be on a collision course because of the incompatibility between their caregiving ideal and the exhaustion inherent in many progressive illnesses. And, as discussed in Chapter 7, a collapse or perceived "failure" of the caregiving mission can have serious negative consequences that reverberate throughout the family. Clinicians can help a family avert a crisis by laying the groundwork for basic change that will improve their staying power. It is also valuable to explore family attitudes about such choices as extended, home-based, professional caregiving.

It is useful to distinguish further between illnesses that progress rapidly or slowly. The demands on a family of a rapidly progressive illness, such as metastatic lung cancer or acute leukemia, are different from those illnesses with a much longer and unpredictable course, such as arthritis, chronic lung disease like emphysema, or type 2 diabetes. The pace of adaptation required for coping with the continual changes and ever-new demands of a rapidly progressive disease mount as the time shortens. A slowly progressive illness may place a higher premium on stamina over a long period rather than on continual adaptation and change. With a rapidly progressive illness, such as a fast-growing brain tumor, the pileup of psychosocial demands can easily outstrip a family's ability to adapt (much like the body's inability to keep up with the tumor). In such situations families with limited resources may have to prioritize the challenges confronting them. This can involve making a daunting and agonizing decision, especially if the consequences are great. One lower-income family trying to manage a grandmother's advancing dementia felt torn between overwhelming financial pressures and a commitment to keep the grandmother alive and in the family home. Clinicians can help a family decide what, within its limits, is most important. This is particularly useful when working with families that have an ethos of mastering a situation themselves, no matter how great the challenge.

Constant Course

With a constant-course condition, the occurrence of an initial event, such as a one-time heart attack, a spinal cord injury, or a TBI, is followed by a stable biological course. Typically, after an initial period of recovery, the condition is characterized by some clear-cut deficit such as paraplegia, speech loss, or cognitive impairment. There may be residual functional limitations, including a diminished tolerance of physical stress or a restriction of previous activities. Recurrences are possible, but the individual or family is faced with a semipermanent change that is stable and predictable over a considerable time span. The potential for family and patient exhaustion exists, but without the strain of new role demands over time that characterize progressive disorders.

It is easier for families in this situation, in a relative sense, to resume normal living than it is with a progressive condition. Once the patient and family learn how to manage the disability, they can plan for the future without the continual uncertainties inherent in a progressive illness. In family consultations with me and the rehabilitation team, a man with a spinal cord injury who was paralyzed from the waist down was able to devise a slow, methodical plan to return to work within 2 years. This plan, which depended largely on a predictable trajectory of the illness, required the family to establish and follow a realistic program. The predictability of the man's condition was also essential in assuring his employer's willingness and ability to accommodate to the employee's physical limitations.

Relapsing or Episodic Course

Relapsing or episodic course conditions, such as spinal disc disorders, inflammatory bowel disease, asthma, migraine headaches, multiple sclerosis (MS), and forms of cancer in remission (e.g., those that are resectable or chemotherapy responsive), are distinguished by the alternation of stable low-symptom periods with periods of flare-up or exacerbation. Often family members can adhere to a normal routine, though the specter of a recurrence looms (see Chapter 8).

Compared with progressive or constant-course illnesses, relapsing conditions may require less continuous caretaking or role change. Families, however, are strained by both the frequency of transition between crisis and noncrisis situations and the ongoing uncertainty of *when* a recurrence will occur. This unpredictability requires flexibility in alternating between two forms of family organization. In a sense, the family is always on call to cope with crises and handle exacerbations of the illness. The wide psychological discrepancy between low-symptom versus flare-up periods is a particularly taxing feature unique to relapsing diseases. These disorders may not be as biologically severe as those with a progressive or constant course, yet over the course of an illness, they can be the most psychosocially challenging.

For instance, in one family the father had had a chronic disc problem that had been asymptomatic for several years. Family members, including Dad, had almost forgotten about his problem. One Saturday morning he went outside to do some light yard work, unthinkingly lifted something slightly too heavy, and threw his back out, becoming instantly disabled and suffering severe pain. He then had to be confined to his bed for 2 weeks. In a matter of hours, the family, rudely reawakened to the fact that the father had a chronic disorder, had to rapidly shift roles and expectations to accommodate to his disability. Flare-ups of relapsing disorders often coincide with periods of great family or other stress, which affect physical health. In this case, the father had been subjected to recent stressors at work that had tightened up his back muscles and perhaps made him more vulnerable to reactivating his disc problem.

It is important to understand a family's expectations about the course of a disorder, and the following questions can be helpful in eliciting this information.

- What information has the medical team or particular providers given you about the expected course of your or your family member's condition?
- What were you told about how uncertain the course could be?
- Does this information differ in any way from the family's or patient's expectations about the course and its degree of uncertainty?

These questions help determine what, specifically, has been said to the family and to which members directly. They help clarify whether, despite what health care providers have said, family members have their own ideas based on previous experience or other sources of information. Clinicians may learn about discrepant viewpoints within the family that can help explain conflicts between members about how the condition should be handled. They can assess who is knowledgeable and who is uninformed, and why. Did the physician choose to communicate with only certain family members? Did key family members decide who should get information directly from the primary source? Were different family members, for instance, the patient or children, given different information, and for what reasons, for instance, age-appropriate distinctions versus overprotection? Such questions reveal whether the medical team has provided consistent information. Divergent viewpoints about the expected course from "the experts" can create tremendous turmoil within a family. Often health care providers are unaware that colleagues have communicated significantly different information to a family or particular family members. Addressing these sorts of issues early on helps avert long-term dysfunctional patterns within the family and with providers.

Outcome

The extent to which a chronic illness is a likely cause of death or shortens one's life expectancy has profound psychosocial impact. The most crucial factor is the *initial expectation* of whether a disease is likely to cause death. On one end of the continuum are illnesses that do not typically affect the lifespan, such as disc disease, blindness, arthritis, spinal cord injury, or seizure disorders. At the other extreme are progressive and fatal conditions, such as widespread metastatic cancer and Huntington's disease. An intermediate, more unpredictable category includes illnesses that can shorten the lifespan, such as cystic fibrosis, type 1 diabetes, and cardiovascular disease, and those with the possibility of sudden death, such as hemophilia or recurrences of heart attack or stroke.

A major difference between these kinds of outcomes is the degree to which the family experiences anticipatory loss and its pervasive effects on family life (Rolland, 1990, 2004, 2006a). All chronic illnesses potentially involve a loss of bodily control, key aspects of one's identity, and intimate relationships. In a life-threatening illness, the loss entails greater consequences—death and the permanent loss of relationships. In developmental terms for conditions with an untimely onset, the ill member can fear dying before his or her life plans have been realized. The family can fear surviving alone in the future. For all involved there is an undercurrent of anticipatory grief and separation that can permeate every phase of adaptation. The future expectation of loss can make it extremely difficult for a family to maintain a balanced perspective. These topics will be discussed fully in Chapter 8.

A torrent of emotions can distract a family from the myriad practical tasks and problem solving that maintain family integrity. With fatal conditions, a tendency to see the ill family member as practically in the coffin can set in motion maladaptive responses that divest him or her of important responsibilities. The result can be the structural and emotional isolation of the ill member from family life, which has been associated with poor medical outcome in a life-threatening illness (Campbell, 2003; Weihs et al., 2002).

When loss is less certain, illnesses that may shorten life or cause sudden death provide a fertile ground for varied family perspectives. The "it could happen" nature of these illnesses creates a nidus for both overprotection by the family and powerful secondary gains for the ill member. This is particularly relevant to childhood illnesses such as hemophilia, type 1 diabetes, and asthma.

It is vitally important for clinicians to be informed about the prognosis, particularly about the probability and timing of loss; for this to happen, direct contact with the primary physician is often essential. Family members frequently organize themselves and set priorities concerning major life issues in direct relation to their ideas about the prognosis. Clinicians can inquire about each family member's perceptions in this regard. Significant differences about the life-threatening potential of an illness among family members or between the family and health providers are critical and often are a source of major conflict. Inquiry about and awareness of cultural or spiritual norms are crucial.

To assess family perceptions about outcome, I ask several questions, such as the following.

- What has your physician told you about your family member's (or your) prognosis?
- Do you think your family member's illness can or will shorten his or her life? If so, when do you think this could happen?
- Do your views differ from what you have been told by your doctor(s)? If so, how is this difference managed?

- Who has been included or excluded in family discussions? Are any members excluded? If so, why?
- What cultural or spiritual beliefs guide your viewpoint and ways of handling these issues?
- Is there agreement about the prognosis within the family? If not, who disagrees with whom, and how are differences of opinion handled?
- If the illness can be fatal, how does this knowledge affect the emotional climate, members' roles, family communication, and priorities that are part of day-to-day family life? Who talks with whom about it? Are certain family members, for example, children and aged grandparents, excluded? If so, why?

This line of inquiry allows the clinician to identify coping strategies, areas of misinformation that can be corrected, areas of denial, patterns of communication about threatened loss, and differences in perception that a clinician should address.

Typically, disregarding these issues increases the odds of dysfunctional family patterns, risking a family's overall ability to adapt. I believe that these risks far outweigh any immediate concern about approaching sensitive and painful subjects with the family. Keeping cultural norms in mind, it is valuable that all family members be given an opportunity to answer these questions. I prefer to do this, when possible, with everyone present, including the patient. Sometimes, I may begin by meeting separately with each family member or with the adults and children separately. The overall goal is to facilitate the family's ability to have a timely open discussion about sensitive issues when appropriate over the course of the condition.

To assess a family's preparedness to face a downhill course, particularly in high-risk illnesses, I suggest that clinicians ask the following kinds of questions:

- Although we are all very hopeful for a good response to treatments, if things do not go well, at what point or on the basis of what symptoms or information from the health care team will you begin to focus on possible loss?
- What would you, as a family, envision doing differently from what you do now?
- Can you imagine any information that would be useful to your family now to relieve specific worries, such as concerns about pain control?

Posing these questions gives families an opportunity to express their fears and, at the same time, to distinguish the current situation from a later possibility. This is like an insurance policy that, once drawn up, can be put on the shelf with the hope that it will never be needed. Generally, families find that this process increases their sense of control.

Disability

Disability can involve impairment of cognition (e.g., Alzheimer's disease), sensation (e.g., blindness), movement (e.g., stroke with paralysis or MS), stamina (e.g., heart or respiratory diseases), disfigurement (e.g., mastectomy), or conditions associated with social stigma, such as HIV or chronic mental disorders (Olkin, 1999).

Social stigma is an important cause of disability in many disorders. For example, cerebral palsy, severe burns, or psoriasis are cosmetically disabling and distorting of body image to the extent that the attendant social stigma interferes with normal social interaction. Often treatment procedures produce psychosocial difficulties because of disfiguration resulting from a mastectomy or side effects, such as the typical hair loss from chemotherapy. HIV remains potentially socially disabling because of the combined effects of its perceived risk of contagion, its potentially long asymptomatic period, its ongoing status as incurable, and its links with groups in our society that experience discrimination—LGBTQ and users of intravenous drugs. Even during asymptomatic periods, people with HIV still contend with challenges related to stigma: they may lose their jobs, family, and friends, and general sense of self-worth. Labeling a difficult-to-diagnose patient who has confusing symptoms of persistent tiredness with chronic fatigue syndrome can be socially incapacitating because of ambiguities surrounding its cause and its continued association with underlying mental disorders, such as depression.

The extent, kind, and timing of disability involve sharp differences in the degree of family stress. For instance, the combined cognitive and motor deficits often caused by a stroke necessitate greater family role reallocation than that needed for a spinal cord injury in which cognitive abilities are unaffected. Some chronic diseases, such as hypertension, gastroesophageal reflux disease, many endocrine disorders, or migraine headache cause mild or only intermittent disability or none at all. These differences are very significant in moderating the degree of stress facing a family.

For some illnesses, such as stroke, disability is often worst at the beginning. Physical incapacity at this point magnifies family coping related to onset, expected course, and outcome. In progressive diseases, such as Alzheimer's, disability looms as an increasing problem in later phases of the illness, allowing a family more time to prepare for anticipated changes and an opportunity for the ill member to participate in disease-related family planning while still cognitively able (Boss, 2011).

Family expectations of a member with disabilities are important. An expectation that the ill member can continue to have responsible roles and autonomy has been associated with both a better rehabilitation response and successful long-term family integration. Typically, families have the greatest difficulty deciding realistic role expectations both in mildly disabling illnesses, where demands are very ambiguous, and in the most severely incapacitating ones, because of the sheer amount of role change required. Early psychoeducation-oriented consultations help families develop realistic expectations and guide family organization and planning.

To summarize, the net effect of disability on a particular individual or family depends on how the type of disability interacts with the premorbid role of the affected member and a family's overall organization, belief system, flexibility, and emotional and financial resources. Conceptually, the presence or absence of any significant disability can provide a useful psychosocial dividing line to construct a psychosocial illness typology.

A PSYCHOSOCIAL TYPOLOGY MATRIX

By combining the kinds of onset (acute or gradual), course (progressive, constant, or relapsing/episodic), outcome (fatal, shortened life span, or nonfatal), and disability (present or absent) into a grid format, we generate a typology that clusters illnesses according to similarities and differences in inherent biological features that pose differing psychosocial demands (see Table 2.1). For instance, a stroke has an acute onset and a constant course after the initial recovery; it can also shorten life and is disabling. The psychosocial demands of stroke are largely related to the combined effects of those four qualities. A TBI, which also is characterized by sudden onset, a constant course, and disability, is different in that it does not involve the psychosocial strain of being a life-threatening illness.

Using this information, a clinician can think about the psychosocial demands of a condition both independently and in relation to others. According to clinician or researcher needs, the number of illness types can be reduced by combining or eliminating specific variables. The decision to do so would depend on the relative need for specificity in a particular situation.

Level of Uncertainty

The predictability of a disorder and the degree of uncertainty about the specific way or rate at which it unfolds is vitally important, but has not been included in Table 2.1. Because of its overarching importance, the degree of uncertainty should be seen as a meta-characteristic of all conditions that overlays and colors the variables of onset, course, outcome, and disability. Families coping with highly unpredictable diseases, such as MS, often state that these ambiguities are the hardest aspects to accept and master. The more uncertain the course and outcome, the more a family must make decisions with flexible contingencies built into their planning. Normally complicated life decisions are always layered with a myriad of illness-related ambiguities. This process requires a kind of ongoing, strategic problem solving that can exhaust even the most resilient and adaptive families (see Chapter 6 for a detailed case example).

TABLE 2.1. Categorization of Chronic Illnesses by Psychosocial Type

		Disabling		Nondisabling	
		Acute	Gradual	Acute	Gradual
Fatal	Progressive	Pancreatic cancer Metastatic cancer (e.g,. breast, liver, lung)	Lung cancer with CNS metastases Bone marrow failure Amyotrophic lateral sclerosis Huntington's disease		
	Relapsing			Incurable cancers in remission	
Possibly Fatal/Shortened Lifespan	Progressive		Parkinson's disease Emphysema Alzheimer's disease Multi-infarct dementia Multiple sclerosis (advanced) Chronic alcoholism Cystic fibrosis		Type 1 diabetes (early) Poorly controlled hypertension Insulin-dependent Type 2 diabetes
	Relapsing	Angina	Early multiple sclerosis Episodic alcoholism	Sickle cell disease (early) Hemophilia (early)	Systemic lupus (early) Inflammatory bowel disease
	Constant	Stroke Moderate/severe myocardial infarction	PKU and other congenital errors of metabolism	Mild myocardial infarction Cardiac arrhythmia	Dialysis-treated renal failure Hodgkin's disease

(continued)

TABLE 2.1. *(continued)*

		Disabling		Nondisabling	
		Acute	Gradual	Acute	Gradual
Nonfatal	Progressive		Rheumatoid arthritis Osteoarthritis		Non-insulin-dependent Type 2 diabetes
	Relapsing	Lumbosacral disc disorder	Refractory recurrent depression	Kidney stones Gout Migraine Seasonal allergy Asthma Epilepsy	Peptic ulcer Ulcerative colitis (controlled) Chronic bronchitis Irritable bowel syndrome Psoriasis
	Constant	Traumatic brain injury (TBI) Congenital malformations Spinal cord injury Acute blindness Acute deafness Survived severe trauma and burns Posthypoxic syndrome	Nonprogressive intellectual disabilities Cerebral palsy Fibromyalgia	Benign arrhythmia Congenital heart disease (mild)	Malabsorption syndromes (controlled) Hyper/hypothyroidism Pernicious anemia Controlled hypertension Controlled glaucoma Controlled bipolar disorder

Note. Revised from Rolland, J. S. (1984). Reprinted with permission of *Family, Systems, and Health*.

There are two distinct ways in which illnesses can be unpredictable: They can be more or less uncertain in terms of the actual nature of their onset, course, outcome, or disability, and they can vary in the rate at which changes will occur. Some conditions, such as spinal cord injury, have a highly predictable course. Alzheimer's disease has a clear end point, but the timetable for getting there is very unpredictable. The course and outcome of other illnesses, such as MS, stroke, heart attack, hypertension, or lung cancer, are rather unpredictable. In these kinds of disease, the initial prediction of type may change. For instance, if a second episode occurs, a stroke or heart attack can be considered relapsing or progressive. Lung cancer can become incapacitating if brain metastases occur. Some cases of lung cancer progress rapidly, and others advance slowly, with a long remission or none at all. Other illnesses, such as arthritis or migraine headaches, tend to have a predictable, long-range course, but can be highly variable from day to day, which can interfere more with daily rather than with long-term planning. This illness typology cannot predict these changes. In a particular case, if important changes occur during the course of a disease, a clinician should take note that the patient has switched from one illness type to another. The family may need help in reorienting to a new set of psychosocial demands and expectations.

The experience of uncertainty is affected by a number of factors, including the degree to which the pattern of symptoms is consistent and predictable (Mishel, 2014; Stewart & Mishel, 2000). Families dealing with diabetes eventually begin to recognize the early warning signs and subtleties of an insulin reaction. In one case in which a grandmother had mild cognitive deficits from a stroke, the patient and her family learned with time to detect subtle cues of "wooly thinking" in the morning that alerted family members that she would have difficulty coping with her usual daily routines. Disorders in which the cues are more complex or in which progression means encountering novel and unfamiliar symptoms or treatments can heighten anxieties for families. In these instances, clinicians need to achieve a balance between overloading a family with information about possible future crises and allaying anxieties by providing useful information concerning uncertainties. Also, it is valuable to distinguish between helping families reduce uncertainty through knowledge and helping them learn to tolerate living with it. For optimal long-term adaptation to highly uncertain disorders, such as multiple sclerosis, families need a blend of minimization/positive illusions and incorporation of illness uncertainty into daily life and life-cycle planning (see Chapters 7 and 8).

Other Illness Characteristics

Several other important attributes differentiate conditions beyond the basic components of the illness typology and should also be considered, where appropriate, in a thorough assessment. The visibility, frequency, and intensity of symptoms; the likelihood and severity of medical crises; and the role of genetics (see Chapter 15) are other disease characteristics with important psychosocial significance. Also, the complexity, frequency, and efficacy of a treatment regimen and the amount of home- versus hospital-based care required by a condition vary widely among disorders. These factors have important implications for individual and family adaptation, including their demands on family financial resources.

Symptom Visibility

A number of investigators have described the vicissitudes of having a visible versus an invisible disorder. Some symptoms, including paralysis, disfigurement, and rash, for example, are visible. Other signs of a disease, such as high blood pressure, are invisible, but can be easily measured. Yet others, pain being the primary example, are invisible and much more subjective in terms of measuring their severity. A physician sympathized with the plight of a woman with chronic migraine headaches: because her appearance did not reveal her condition, people were insensitive to her distress. The physician and patient joked that her family and colleagues would be more responsive if only she had a bandage wrapped around her head!

Although visible signs of an illness or disability have the potential disadvantage of stigma and shame, they do permit others to gauge their interactions with the patient in a relatively more objective way than is the case with invisible disorders. Invisible signs of disease foster ambiguities in several ways. For some patients and family members, denial or minimization is more possible on a day-to-day basis—in other words, "out of sight, out of mind." For others, this ambiguity becomes a constant source of rumination and rehearsal of worst-case scenarios. This is particularly true for invisible disorders, such as cancers in remission, which are potentially life threatening. Invisible symptoms are more likely to invite different family perceptions and positions: Families can be split in their mixed feelings, with one family member expressing minimization of risk, while another worries for the entire family.

Invisible symptoms that can fluctuate, like pain, become an important currency in family interactions. They can fuel preexisting dysfunctional relationship problems. Patients can use such symptoms to control family interactions or the power balance in a conflictual relationship. These possible sources of secondary gain can engender a distrust of the patient by other family members. The fact that various treatments for pain are only partially successful adds to the ambiguities that reverberate through the family's interactions.

These inherent ambiguities of invisible disorders or symptoms can powerfully influence narratives and metaphors that become ascribed to pain. The distinction between the literal or physical and the metaphorical is blurred. For families this blurring enhances the possibility that family legacies and beliefs transform physiological pain into a mirror reflecting core family issues. The patient with pain who says to her spouse on one occasion, "I am in pain" and on another, "You are a pain" is extending the meanings of her pain to include the idea that her spouse is a source of her pain, and therefore influences her overall physical condition. We will explore the power of belief systems in Chapter 8.

Likelihood and Severity of Crises

It is important to consider the likelihood and severity of disease-related crises. Fears about illness-related crises are often a major source of a family's undercurrent of anxiety.

A clinician can gauge the family's understanding of the possibility, frequency, and severity of a medical crisis. How congruent is the family's understanding with that of the health care team? Do family members expect a catastrophe? Do they minimize real dangers? Insulin reactions for persons with diabetes are one example. Many families worry that a member who has such a reaction while sleeping could die, which causes parents or a spouse to lie anxiously awake at night. In fact, this is quite rare. Are there clear warning signs that the patient or family can recognize? People with diabetes may perspire, become tremulous, lose their concentration, or act confused or irritable. Conversely, the increasing blood pressure that may precede a fatal stroke can be completely silent. Can a medical crisis be prevented or mitigated by the detection of early warning signs and the institution of prompt treatment? When a patient or family heeds the early warning signs of a diabetes insulin reaction or an asthma attack, a full-blown crisis can usually be averted. How complex are the rescue operations? Do they require simple measures carried out at home, such as medication or bed rest, or do they necessitate outside assistance or hospitalization? How long can crises persist before a family can resume day-to-day functioning?

It is valuable to ask a family about its planning for such crises. In particular, the extent and accuracy of the family's medical knowledge are of paramount importance. Has the family thought through who will be in charge, who will offer emotional support, and how will resources outside the family be used? Who in the family has been trained to give Mom an injection of a glucose formula in an emergency? Frequently, children capable of doing this have not been instructed and live in terror that they will be alone with Mom and helpless to render aid. If an illness has begun with an acute crisis such as with a stroke, then assessment of that event gives the clinician useful information on how the family handles unexpected crises. Evaluating the overall viability of the family's crisis planning is key. Offering clear information and guidelines is crucial in helping families construct viable and flexible planning for possible crises.

Treatment Regimens

Some treatment procedures, for example, home kidney dialysis, involve significant expenditures of time and/or energy or require another person to carry them out, as with postural lung drainage required in children with cystic fibrosis. Treatments for other diseases, even severe ones such as advanced hypertension, may involve taking medication and regular checkups that the patient can handle alone. These factors illustrate the salience of the fit between the demands of the illness and the family pattern of functioning. A relatively disengaged family has far more trouble with disorders requiring regular teamwork than with those, such as hypertension, that demand a minimum of collaboration. Although they reduce time-consuming dependence on medical centers, treatments that are given at home place a greater responsibility on the patient or family. Therefore, the degree of family emotional support, role flexibility, effective problem solving, and communication in relation to these treatment factors will be crucial predictors of long-term treatment adherence and the appropriateness of home-based care. For home dialysis, a more disengaged family may not be a good fit with the requirements for effective medical care.

Clinicians need to familiarize themselves with a client's treatments. For instance, how complex and frequent are the interventions? Are treatments on a fixed schedule or on a more unpredictable one dictated by symptoms? What are the possible side effects, such as discomfort or fatigue? How much energy is needed to administer treatments, and are other people required to be involved? These considerations have important implications in terms of the level of disruption to family life and the degree of family involvement and teamwork required for successful disease management. Sometimes a fixed treatment schedule can be more disruptive than a flexible one. If a daughter's brittle diabetes requires a controlled diet with dinner at 5:00 P.M., it may necessitate separate dinner sittings and multiple meal preparations, add considerable strain to family life, and potentially turn a previously pleasant family ritual into an ordeal.

Treatments that have a considerable impact on a person's lifestyle, are difficult to accomplish, and have minimal effects on the level of symptoms or prognosis are those least likely to be adhered to. Also, interventions that are visible and possibly stigmatizing can interfere with adherence. This is particularly true for children and adolescents. Cancer chemotherapy that results in hair loss is a good example.

The degree to which couple or family functioning can have an impact on disease course varies among different kinds of conditions. To what extent can the patient's health and functional capacities and the course and outcome be influenced by the effectiveness and persistence of couples' or families' coping efforts? For example, heart disease is highly responsive to these efforts, in contrast to many forms of cancer or advanced congestive heart failure in which the relationship between coping efforts and medical outcome is less clear. We need to be mindful of these significant distinctions, particularly in situations in which family efforts clearly can affect the disease course. Yet it is important to recognize the limits of our knowledge and interventions in this area. We return to this topic later in relation to family efforts to sustain hope (see Chapter 8 on family belief systems).

Age at Onset

Finally, the age at onset of an illness, in relation to child, adult, and family phases of development, is a critical factor. The psychosocial demands of any disorder can be understood only in relation to other developmental challenges for each family member and the family as a whole (see Chapter 7 on life-cycle issues).

PSYCHOSOCIAL PERSPECTIVE

Gaining a psychosocial understanding of illness is one of the basic tasks of families entering the world of living with chronic disorders. For each of the typology variables that has been described, I am particularly interested in how family members' expectations are in sync with, or differ from, one another and from those of the involved health care providers. I ask members about the sources of their information so that I may begin to understand whether differences are due to contradictory information or to processing the same information through different historical, ethnic, or cultural lenses (see Chapters 6 and 8). Routinely, I ask families to discuss these issues either in an initial consultation or as a homework assignment. This exercise is an excellent way to achieve rapport with families that are unaccustomed to dealing with health/mental health professionals or to sitting together as a family to discuss sensitive issues. We begin by talking about what is foremost on their minds—a significant health problem. Then, they are guided to consider their overall understanding of the condition and to begin building a bridge from the technological to the psychosocial world of illness and disability.

Family members are frequently astonished to learn that they have very different ideas about the anticipated illness course and outcome. This process of revealing differences allows potential areas of conflict to be discussed preventively at an early stage of a long-term endeavor before maladaptive patterns are set in motion. When misinformation is an issue, I advise both the family and the physician that a meeting be arranged to discuss the illness and its treatment. To the busy physician, I reframe this extra meeting as "a stitch in time" that will "save nine." I emphasize that it will help avert frequent phone calls and adherence issues and promote family cooperation during times when much technical biomedical care is required. If appropriate, I offer to be present at the meeting, to facilitate a dialogue that will include recasting information in psychosocial terms.

In one case, a young physical therapist had developed severe asthma. She and her husband were referred because of increased marital conflict following her diagnosis. They fought mostly about what symptoms were really due to the illness and what were not. Because the symptoms seemed to crop up precipitously, the husband felt that his wife was using her illness as an excuse for anything she did not want to do. In this case, each partner had different levels of comprehension about asthma. The husband clearly did not understand much about the condition and, since the diagnosis, had left all asthma-related discussions to his therapist wife and her physician. A consultation that involved both partners had been missed at the time of diagnosis and was now needed to better clarify the condition and encourage more family-oriented care going forward.

CHAPTER 3

The Time Phases of Illness

To complete a meaningful psychosocial schema of chronic disorders, the developmental time phases of an illness need to be included as a second dimension. Too often, discussions of "coping with cancer," "managing disability," or "dealing with life-threatening illness" approach illness and disability as a static state and fail to appreciate the evolution of illness processes over time. The concept of time phases provides a way for clinicians and families to think longitudinally and to understand chronic illness as an ongoing process with normative landmarks, transitions, and changing demands. Each phase of a chronic disorder poses its own psychosocial challenges and developmental tasks that may require significantly different capabilities, attitudes, or changes in order for families to adapt.

The natural history of chronic disease can be described as having three major phases: (1) initial crisis, (2) chronic, and (3) terminal. A more detailed chronic disease time line in relation to the three broad time phases is shown in Figure 3.1.

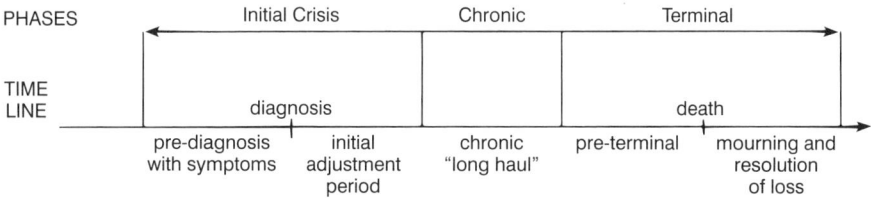

FIGURE 3.1. Time line and phases of illness. From Rolland (1984). Copyright 1984 by the American Psychological Association. Reprinted by permission.

THE INITIAL CRISIS PHASE

The initial crisis phase includes any symptomatic period before diagnosis when the individual or family has a sense that something is wrong, but the exact nature and scope of the condition are not clear. For some people, the physician's suspicions on a routine examination mark the beginning of the initial crisis phase. This phase also includes the initial period of readjustment and coping after a diagnosis is made and an initial treatment plan is created. For an acute injury or a sudden-onset illness, such as stroke or heart attack, the initial crisis phase may extend through a protracted rehabilitation period.

However the journey begins, families have a strong need for reassurance that they are handling things normatively. They have only a vague psychosocial map, or none at all. This initial period is often a time of excruciating vulnerability and uncertainty, in which all experiences seem heightened in intensity and family members grope for ways to reassert control. A time line for accomplishing illness-related developmental tasks can be of enormous help in stabilizing a family: It helps avert feelings of being overwhelmed that are inevitable when all the challenges over the years of an illness are viewed as compressed into a two-dimensional picture. If we experienced all of life's hurdles that way, most of us would feel crushed by the weight of reality.

The immediate challenge for many families is deciding which tasks belong where in the sequence. Some families immediately tackle issues that can be shelved for 6 months, when the long-term picture will be clearer. One woman put her house up for sale, started giving her valuable possessions away, and discussed funeral arrangements with her adult children during her initial treatment for breast cancer when, in reality, she had a small tumor and an excellent prognosis. She had not discussed the prognosis with her physician; and her children, who lived in another part of the country, accepted her portrayal of the situation as true.

The initial crisis phase entails a number of key tasks for the ill member and his or her family. From the perspective of the FSI model, two tasks are most important. First, a systems perspective helps families to better understand themselves as a functional unit. Viewing themselves and the health challenge confronting them through a systems-oriented lens provides an organizing framework that fosters empowerment and effectiveness. In my own work, I need to remind myself that this perspective is usually a novel one for families. I can remember how unfamiliar these ideas were to me when my mother had a stroke during the first year of my psychiatric training. We, as a family, grappled with all the variables, such as role reallocation, communication issues, and threatened loss; but we did so in a piecemeal and somewhat random fashion, without a family-oriented systemic framework for effectively approaching the situation.

Second, family members need to gain a psychosocial understanding of the disorder in systems terms. They need to be introduced to the notion of an illness course that has developmental tasks associated with each phase. Their grasp of themselves as a functional unit within the context of the pattern of practical and emotional demands of the illness over time provides the groundwork for a viable family–illness system.

In addition, families need to address certain universal, practical, and illness-related tasks, including: (1) learning to cope with any symptoms or disability; (2) adapting to different health care settings (e.g., hospital, clinic) and treatment procedures; and (3) establishing and maintaining workable collaborative relationships with the health care team. Last, there are more general and existential tasks that are crucial in helping families to optimize their well-being, including the following:

1. Define the challenge of a chronic condition as a shared one in "WE" terms. This is fundamental to optimal individual and family coping and adaptation over the illness course. A belief that illness is a shared challenge helps avert many of the dysfunctional patterns and relationship imbalances that can eventually develop.
2. Create a meaning for the illness experience that maximizes a sense of mastery and competency (see Chapter 7).
3. Pull together to cope with the immediate crisis.
4. Grieve for the losses incurred by the illness.
5. Gradually accept the illness as long term, while maintaining a sense of continuity between their past and future. Although life will be different, families need help in affirming positive values and those parts of family life that can remain intact. During the initial crisis phase, a family gathering at the bedside or participation in a ritual to promote healing can be extremely beneficial. Recalling other crises the family has weathered in the past can help establish a sense of continuity. For example, one family recounted its escape from Nazi terrorism and coming to the United States as refugees during the Depression and eventually succeeding as a family.
6. In the face of uncertainty, develop flexibility about future goals (see Chapter 8).

Framing Events

During this initial crisis period, health professionals have enormous influence over a family's sense of competence and the strategies they use to accomplish these developmental challenges. Initial meetings and advice given at the time of diagnosis can be thought of as "framing events." Discussions with health care providers about the nature of the disorder, its prognosis, and prescriptions for management are all part of the framing event.

Because families are so vulnerable at this point, clinicians need to be extremely sensitive in how they interact with them and be aware of messages conveyed by their behavior. What clinicians actually say or leave unsaid or unclear about the nature of the illness and its prognosis is critical. Who is included or excluded from initial discussions can be interpreted by the family as a message about how they should plan their illness-related communication going forward. For instance, if a clinician meets the parents separately from adolescents to give them information about a cancer diagnosis and prognosis, they may assume they are being instructed implicitly to protect the adolescent from any discussion of the illness. Meeting only with a spouse or primary caregiver may fuel anxiety about whether and how to share information with children or other members. Clinicians can ask patients for their preferences about who they would like to include in important discussions. Clinicians also need to be careful not to undercut a family's attempt to sustain a sense of mastery by implicitly blaming the patient or the family for an illness because of a delay in seeking an appointment, negligence by the parents, or poor health habits, or by distancing themselves from the family.

As part of every assessment, I suggest that clinicians inquire about families' initial experiences with health care providers, particularly at the time of diagnosis. What did these experiences mean to them, and how did they shape the patient's and the family's views and behaviors about how to live with symptoms and treatments? How did these experiences affect the formative stage of their relationship with the health care providers?

Framing events can go awry for many reasons. A major source of mistrust between a family and a health care provider arises when there has been an insufficient attempt by the health care team to include all relevant family members in discussions about the patient. Neglecting this critical step can be considered noncompliance on the part of the health care team. The family often experiences such an omission as being dismissive of its importance in the overall treatment plan. Disregarding the family only heightens an imbalance inherent in the relationship because of the technological nature of the initial crisis phase when the medical team generally is in charge. Families often express their dissatisfaction as "Our doctor doesn't understand us."

In one family, a young woman was admitted to the hospital for a diagnostic workup for suspected cancer. At the evaluation's conclusion, the oncologist came to the patient's room where her husband and close family members were gathered. He asked the family to come into the hallway outside the patient's room. Because of intense anxiety at that moment, no one objected. He then gave the family the dire diagnosis and prognosis.

This is a framing event. To communicate this critical information, the physician separated the patient and her family, as well as the husband and wife. He could be considered to have modeled a form of illness-related communication that the family and couple could adopt going forward, likely dysfunctionally. It took several days for the family to realize and process together how this choice was a violation of their usual way of communicating—hearing good or bad news

The Time Phases of Illness

together without excluding anyone. The patient and her family never told the oncologist how angry they were, but it damaged their relationship with him, the health care team leader, irreparably. He was no longer considered a healer, someone who could provide a full range of biopsychosocial support. He was now reduced to a technical expert in biomedical cancer care that the family needed to reluctantly accept, despite harboring considerable anger toward him. The consequences were a profound and damaging loss for the patient, her family, and the health care provider. This difficulty was compounded by the physician's interpreting the family's anger as arising solely from their difficulty in accepting the diagnosis, rather than from the family recognizing that he disregarded their style of communication.

Often, physicians, burdened by relentless demands on their time, can confuse the family's need for information and for being included in decisions with a desire for lengthy discussions. Although other members of the health care team can address many details about illness management, an initial meeting between the health care team leader and the family promotes the mutual understanding necessary for optimal relationship development. Sometimes a provider fears an emotional conversation with the patient and family that will go beyond his or her comfort zone (see Chapter 17 on clinicians' personal themes).

A provider should lay the groundwork for such a moment by inquiring earlier about each family's preferred way of receiving important information, particularly the results of a medical workup. This can be communicated by saying to the family, "I will need to share important information with you over the next few days. Generally I find it best to talk with everyone together. Does this fit your way of getting important news, or do you like to handle things differently?" Asking this question conveys respect for the family. It helps clarify normative multicultural differences among family members and serves to identify family patterns of communication that are potentially problematic, such as avoiding sensitive subjects related to loss with the patient, children, or emotionally vulnerable family members.

It is valuable to ask about family preferences and cultural norms about receiving information from providers, even when a family says it does not want to hear or share certain information. At a minimum, it provides the clinician with an opportunity to share with a family the possible risks of remaining in the dark or to protect certain family members, typically children or aging, frail parents, from receiving information. Rather than heightening resistance this approach permits families to often rethink their norms about communication in light of such discussions with a professional. It allows a clinician to anticipate possible crossroads in a progressive disorder in which initial family decisions about the dissemination of information among all concerned might create a crisis, for example, upon entering a terminal phase.

Determining Chronicity

The question of permanency is pivotal. The issue is whether a patient and family need to make the transition to a chronic phase and everything that goes with that reality, or whether it can resume life with no mandate for basic change. In many acute illnesses, chronicity is ambiguous at the beginning. The physician may propose a moratorium on this question while trying various interventions. For problems such as trauma, infections, or some surgical procedures, a certain amount of time is needed for natural healing to occur. The physician may inform the patient and family members that there may be residual difficulties or that in a certain percentage of cases the condition becomes chronic. During this period, the need to accept a long-term condition is still uncertain, but preparation for that possibility is a different story and should be addressed directly.

It is helpful to inquire whether family members have decided that the patient's condition is chronic. How did they arrive at that conclusion? Was the physician or someone else their source of information? If the source was not someone on the health care team, it is important to know whether the decision emerged from something in the family's history or culture or from a particular family member or other significant person in the family's network. One family, whose inclination was always to assume the worst, decided early in the recovery phase that the father's mild heart attack was totally and permanently disabling, and family members started to reorganize accordingly. The oldest son had already developed plans to drop out of school and take a job to help support the family. In this case, the physician expected a nearly complete recovery that would require only minor lifestyle modifications.

Clinicians can ask if there is any disagreement about chronicity within the family or between the family and health care team and how these different viewpoints are being handled. Such disagreements are significant since they may signal that the family is not accepting the physician's perspective or that conflicts exist among the members. Silent but potentially life-threatening conditions, such as hypertension, often create the biggest challenges for families. After hypertension is diagnosed, a husband may ignore medical advice and stubbornly continue to eat salty foods, while other family members nag him and fret about his health. One man said, "My father ate whatever he wanted until he died at 85. I feel fine. I plan to live the same way he did." It is extremely difficult for a family to move on to the next phase of adaptation if its members have different views about chronicity since they will be at cross-purposes. This may be a juncture at which family consensus will be necessary for healthy, long-term coping and adaptation.

If the prognosis is still unclear, the patient and his or her family are entitled to know when and how it will be clarified. Frequently, the physician has at least a rough estimate that has not been communicated to the patient or family. Raising this question early allows a family, on the basis of the best information available at that time, to plan and pace itself through a period of uncertainty. In this regard, family members often put plans on hold to help their ill member through this initial crisis phase. It is useful to inquire when the time will come for the patient and other family members to make decisions about the patient's condition in relation to short- and longer-range individual and family plans. What significant issues will the family and individual members face at that time? Such questions acknowledge the family's transitional crisis organization and that much is in limbo; they also imply that this kind of organization is useful in only a time-limited way and would not be appropriate with either a cure or a long-term illness.

Other questions raise more specific issues about permanency. Asking the family how it would see the patient and other members functioning differently with a permanent condition as related to family organization and communication helps assess different aspects of family functioning (see Chapter 5). If the condition is chronic, who would provide caregiving? How would such a caregiving relationship affect the rest of the family? How would the caregiver be identified? Is the caregiving role a shared, flexible one (an important consideration in progressive illness and long-term disability)? Or is it assigned to one member based on cultural norms, gender, or sibling-position expectations? Frequently an oldest daughter is expected to assume the caregiver role with respect to an ailing parent. Sometimes a son or daughter who never has felt validated and still seeks affirmation from a parent may volunteer to be the sole caregiver for that parent. Early identification of such issues offers an opportunity to address them when options are often more fluid, and potentially dysfunctional illness-related family patterns are less entrenched.

Questions such as the following can facilitate accepting chronicity: If you were to think of your disability as permanent, what about it would be hardest to accept? Who in the family would have the easiest and the most difficult time accepting that fact? For many patients and their families the most intense grieving occurs at the time of accepting permanency, because loss must then be definitively acknowledged. Years ago, I developed what turned out to be a chronic back condition after I had a bad fall while skiing. Initially, I was told by my primary physician to rest for several months before resuming strenuous physical activities. The pain subsided, but when I resumed strenuous yard work, the pain recurred. Next, he advised 4 months of recovery time. Again, it reappeared, this time while running. Then 6 months after the initial accident, he said, "You will always know you have a back." He was telling me that it was a chronic condition with limitations. This was when the permanency struck me, and I grieved.

A critical issue for patients and their families is relinquishing hope for a cure, yet remaining optimistic and sustaining reasonable hope (Weingarten, 2012). Asking family members what would be their new version of hope if a full recovery is not possible opens a discussion of this issue. In my modest personal example, I took up bicycling. Finally, if the illness is chronic, clinicians can explore whether any family members, including the patient, feel that they failed or are blamed by others (see Chapter 8).

THE CHRONIC PHASE

The chronic phase, whether it is long or short, is the time span after the initial diagnosis and readjustment period and before issues related to death and dying predominate. It is sometimes referred to as "the long haul" or "the day-to-day living with chronic illness" phase. This phase can be marked by constancy, recurrence (e.g., heart attack), progression, or episodic flare-ups. Its meaning can be grasped not by simply knowing the biological behavior of an illness, but by understanding it in a psychosocial context. Often the patient and the family have come to grips, psychologically and organizationally, with long-term changes and have devised an ongoing coping strategy. At the extremes, the chronic phase can last for decades as a stable, nonfatal, chronic illness, or it may be nonexistent, as in an acute-onset, rapidly progressive, fatal disorder in which the initial crisis phase is contiguous with the terminal phase.

The ability to maintain the semblance of a normal life with a chronic condition and heightened uncertainty is a key family task in this phase. If the illness is fatal, this is a time of living in limbo. For certain highly debilitating but not clearly fatal illnesses, such as a massive stroke or dementia, a family can feel saddled with an exhausting, unending problem. Paradoxically, a family may feel its hope to resume a so-called "normal" life can only be realized after the death of its ill member. The maintenance of maximum autonomy for all family members in the face of protracted adversity helps offset these trapped, helpless feelings. Clinicians can help families develop new priorities and realize opportunities for relationship growth within a "new normal." Many of the clinical issues in the chronic phase for families, couples, and clinicians are addressed in Chapters 11 through 14.

THE TERMINAL PHASE

In the terminal phase of an illness, the inevitability of death becomes apparent and dominates family life (see Chapter 10). It encompasses the periods of mourning and bereavement. At this point the family must cope with issues of separation, death, mourning, and resumption of family life beyond the loss (Walsh & McGoldrick, 2004, 2013).

As families enter this phase, one of the key tasks is shifting from the possibility of a terminal phase to its probability and, finally, to its inevitability. Hopes for a cure and long-term survival must be relinquished. Clinicians should expect feelings that range from intense grief to relief related to giving up the often-protracted struggle to overcome or control an illness. Families adapt best when they are able to transfer their feelings of hope and mastery from controlling the illness to a successful process of "letting go." Optimal coping involves emotional openness as well as dealing with the myriad practical tasks at hand. It includes seeing this phase as an opportunity to share precious time together, to acknowledge the impending loss, to deal with unfinished business, to say good-byes, and to begin the family reorganization process.

In the terminal phase, as in the initial crisis phase, families generally need to accept more intense involvement from health care providers. However, the role of providers and of medical intervention is geared more toward palliative care and providing physical and emotional comfort, than toward medical stabilization and improvement. In this sense, families may need increased contact with health care providers but will need to perceive the latter's role differently. This change in roles can be more challenging for the health care team than for the family, because of strong beliefs that equate professional success with life, not death.

Families face a number of practical tasks in the terminal phase. They have to decide when and whom to inform about the transition. If they have not done so beforehand, the patient and key family members need to decide about issues such as a living will; the extent of medical heroics desired; who will serve as a legal proxy if the patient's competency to make sound decisions is compromised; preferences about dying at home, in the hospital, or at hospice; and wishes about a funeral or memorial service and burial or cremation. Chapter 10 addresses the common clinical and ethical issues for families in this phase.

TRANSITION PERIODS

Critical transition periods link the three time phases. The importance of transition periods has been emphasized in the literature on family and individual life-cycle development (McGoldrick et al., 2016; Levinson, 1986). Similarly, the transitions between phases in the disease course are crucial for individual and family adaptation. Transitions in the illness course are times when families reevaluate the appropriateness of their previous life structure in the face of new illness and disability-related demands. Helping families address unfinished business from the previous phase can facilitate handling these transitions. Families or individual members can become permanently frozen in a structure that has outlived its utility (Penn, 1983). For example, the usefulness of pulling together in the crisis phase can become maladaptive and stifling for family members through the initial chronic phase.

Table 3.1 outlines the developmental tasks associated with each illness phase.

TABLE 3.1. Phases of Illness Developmental Tasks

Initial Crisis Phase

1. Understand the family as a systemic functional unit.
2. Develop a psychosocial understanding of illness.
   a. In practical and emotional terms.
   b. In longitudinal and developmental terms.
3. Appreciate a developmental perspective (individual, family, illness).
4. Begin crisis reorganization.
5. Define challenge as a shared one in "WE" terms.
6. Create meaning that promotes family mastery and competency.
7. Accept permanence of illness/disability.
8. Grieve loss of "normal life" before chronic disorder.
9. Acknowledge possibilities of further loss while sustaining hope.
10. In the face of uncertainty, develop flexibility to future goals and ongoing psychosocial demands of illness.
11. Learn to live with symptoms.
12. Adapt to treatments and health care settings.
13. Establish functional collaborative relationship with health care providers.

Chronic Phase

1. Maximize autonomy for all family members given the constraints of illness.
2. Balance connectedness and separateness.
3. Minimize relationship imbalances.
4. Be mindful of the possible impact on current and future phases of family and individual life cycles.

Terminal Phase

1. Complete the process of anticipatory grief and unresolved family issues.
2. Support the terminally ill member.
3. Help survivors and the dying member live as fully as possible in the time remaining.
4. Begin the family reorganization process.

Illness phase transitions are major turning points at which a family's basic organization for coping and adaptation needs reevaluation. The transition between the crisis and the chronic phases is perhaps the most significant: it marks the beginning of the long haul and the time at which to draw up a viable family plan for living with a chronic condition. Families can be encouraged to consider midcourse corrections, based on their experiences in the early phase of the illness, before they inadvertently settle into rigid patterns.

In one case, a 42-year-old single woman presented with a major depression. She had, for the past 20 years, been the primary caregiver of her mother, who was disabled by crippling arthritis. At the beginning, being the oldest of six siblings in an Italian family, she had taken a leave of absence from school to help her father with her mother and siblings. Twenty years later, her siblings had all moved on in life, but she remained the primary caregiver, having sacrificed her career plans and an independent life of her own. Because she had been so effective as the caregiver during the initial crisis, certain rehabilitation possibilities for the mother had been overlooked. The successful crisis organization assumed a life of its own and became permanent. As the loyal oldest daughter, she had never openly discussed the sacrifice she made. When the initial crisis phase ended, the family never reevaluated its understanding of the situation and developed more flexibility in the chronic phase so that the developmental possibilities of all the family members might be maximally realized.

At the other end of the illness course, the transition from the chronic to the terminal phase presents families with a different set of challenges. A family that is adept at handling the day-to-day practical tasks of a long-term, stable illness but is limited in emotional coping skills may encounter difficulty if their family member's disease becomes terminal. The relatively greater demand for emotional coping skills in the terminal compared with the chronic phase of an illness may create a crisis for a family navigating this transition.

A family with three children, ages 18, 12, and 9, had seemingly coped with the mother's breast cancer for 5 years; they had steadfastly believed in their ability to conquer the disease. Mom had become disease free, and the family never mentioned her illness. In general, the family seldom talked about their feelings, and when metastatic spread was discovered, the family became emotionally paralyzed. During the time when new treatments were tried and failed, no one could discuss the next phase. The children, particularly the two younger ones, were emotionally shielded and not prepared for Mom's impending death. The 9-year-old was excluded from the funeral; she became severely withdrawn and depressed within a year. The 18-year-old moved away and limited her contact with the family. The 12-year-old became overfunctioning and watched over Dad and her younger sister. Dad, the family wage earner, was ill prepared to provide the nurturing side of family life, especially under such emotionally difficult circumstances.

This family's somewhat rigid style and lack of communication about emotional issues made them vulnerable to a terminal illness. They could live with a chronic condition in which the threat of loss was in the background. When a recurrence of the cancer heralded the next phase, they were not prepared to adapt to the wrenching emotional demands.

Families characterized by extreme high cohesion, because of their often fused and rigid nature, can have particular difficulties in negotiating delicate transitions. Appreciating the wide range of cultural diversity regarding norms, high cohesion is mostly very helpful during the initial crisis phase. Some relaxation of personal and generational boundaries for the sake of the family group effort is adaptive and strengthens family bonds. "We-ness" is at a premium during this time. However, when issues of forging autonomy within the constraints of chronicity become salient, overly cohesive families can encounter their Achilles heel. Negotiating autonomy and separateness is often a source of conflict in such families. Chronic disorders, especially disabling ones, may present ongoing tension between autonomy and dependence that challenges such families' vulnerabilities.

A PSYCHOSOCIAL DEVELOPMENTAL MODEL

The interaction between the time phases and the illness typology provides a framework for a normative psychosocial developmental model for chronic disease and disability that resembles models for human development. The crisis, chronic, and terminal phases can be considered broad developmental periods in the unfolding of chronic disease. Each period has certain basic tasks independent of the type of illness. Each "type" of illness has specific supplementary tasks. This model is analogous to the relationship between certain universal life tasks and a particular individual's development. For example, the initial crisis phase is similar in certain fundamental ways to the period of childhood and adolescence. Parents often temper other developmental plans, such as a career, to allow time for rearing children. Similarly, the initial crisis phase is a period of learning the basics of living with a chronic disorder during which the family frequently puts other life plans on hold to accommodate socialization to the illness demands.

While there is wide cultural diversity, themes of autonomy and individuation are often important in the transition from adolescence to adulthood. In a similar fashion, the transition to the chronic phase emphasizes autonomy and the creation of a viable, ongoing life structure in light of illness realities. In this transition, families need to reevaluate any moratorium on other developmental tasks that were necessary during the initial period of adaptation to life with a chronic condition. The separate developmental challenges of living with a chronic condition and living the other parts of one's life must be taken into account and forged into one coherent life structure. In Chapter 7, I address issues related to the interaction of illness, family, and individual member development.

Psychosocial typology and phases of illness can be combined in a two-dimensional matrix, as shown in Figure 3.2. In the matrix, illnesses are grouped and differentiated according to important similarities and differences. It subdivides the types of illness and disability according to three time phases, which allows examination of a long-term illness in a more detailed way. Each disorder can be typed according to a general pattern of psychosocial demands that will change as a family experiences the condition's time phases. For instance, the psychosocial demands of a gradual-onset, progressive, fatal, disabling illness (GPF+) such as amyotrophic lateral sclerosis (ALS), or Lou Gehrig's disease, can be thought about in relation to each of the three phases of illness—crisis, chronic, and terminal.

The Time Phases of Illness 49

ONSET
A = acute
G = gradual

COURSE
P = progressive
C = constant
R = relapsing

OUTCOME
F = fatal or shortened lifespan
NF = nonfatal

DISABILITY
Yes = (+)
No = (−)

ILLNESS TYPE	PHASE		
	I CRISIS	II CHRONIC	III TERMINAL
A P F +			
A P F −			
A P NF +			
A P NF −			
A C F +			
A C F −			
A C NF +			
A C NF −			
A R F +			
A R F −			
A R NF +			
A R NF −			
G P F +			
G P F −			
G P NF +			
G P NF −			
G C F +			
G C F −			
G C NF +			
G C NF −			
G R F +			
G R F −			
G R NF +			
G R NF −			

FIGURE 3.2. Matrix of illness types and time phases.

In the three-dimensional FSI model (see Figure 1.1), the dimensions of "psychosocial types" of illness and the illness time phases both interact with each other and with the third dimension, the broader family system and family processes (organization, communication, beliefs, multigenerational patterns, and life-cycle development) (see Chapters 5–8). This way of depicting the FSI model allows some flexibility between aspects of the family–illness system. It facilitates a consideration of clinical issues and the generation of research hypotheses about the importance of strengths and vulnerabilities in various components of family functioning, such as cohesion or affective communication, in relation to different types of conditions at different illness phases.

IMPLICATIONS FOR CLINICAL ASSESSMENT AND INTERVENTION

The psychosocial typology and time-phases parts of the FSI model have important implications for clinical practice. At their core, the typology components offer a means of grasping the nature of a chronic illness in psychosocial terms. They form a bridge for the clinician between the biological and the psychosocial. Most significantly, they constitute a framework for assessment and intervention that enables clinicians to think and plan with greater clarity and focus. Attention to features of onset, course, outcome, disability, and the degree of uncertainty guide clinical assessment and intervention. For instance, acute-onset illnesses demand high levels of adaptability, problem solving, role reallocation, and balanced cohesion. In such circumstances, helping families to maximize flexibility enables them to adapt more successfully.

The concept of time phases provides a way for the clinician to think longitudinally and better appreciate chronic illness as an ongoing process with landmarks, transition points, and changing demands. An illness time line delineates psychosocial developmental phases of an illness, each phase with its own salient developmental challenges. As in human development, it is important for family members to address phase-related tasks during each particular phase. In particular, mastering the initial crisis-phase related tasks provides a foundation for successful adaptation as the illness progresses. Attention to time phases allows the clinician to assess a family's strengths and vulnerabilities in relation to the present and future phases of the illness.

The typology and time phases inform other aspects of a comprehensive assessment, which includes a range of general and illness-specific family processes. Other important components of an illness-oriented family assessment include the family's illness belief system and process of meaning-making (see Chapter 8); developmental phase in relation to illness and individual member development (see Chapter 7); multigenerational history of coping with illness, loss, and crisis (see Chapter 6); medical crisis planning; capacity to perform home-based medical care; illness-oriented communication, problem solving, and role functions (see Chapter 5); social support; and availability and use of community resources. Subsequent chapters of this book consider these issues in detail.

Foremost, the FSI model clarifies treatment planning. Goal setting is guided by an awareness of the aspects of family functioning most relevant to the particular type or phase of an illness. Sharing this information with the family and deciding on specific goals offer them a better sense of control and a more realistic sense of hope. This process empowers families in their journey of living with a chronic disorder. A more laissez-faire family that is not accustomed to rigorous and timely problem solving may benefit from additional guidance in mastering the precise, day-to-day decision making needed for effective management of diabetes, for example. Such knowledge educates family members about warning signs that alert them to seek help at appropriate times for brief, goal-oriented behavioral health care. The framework is useful for timing family psychosocial checkups to coincide with key transition points in the illness. In short, the psychosocial typology and illness time phases promote an understanding of and the ability to predict the relative need for family and health care team involvement and provide a way to optimize the quality of relationships.

CLINICAL APPLICATIONS: THE THERAPEUTIC TRIANGLES

It is well established that clinicians need to be included in the conceptualization of any family interventions. The application of this idea to health care has led to various descriptions of an essential functional triangle (Doherty & Baird, 1983), wherein the patient, his or her family, and the health care provider team are considered as a system.

The inclusion of psychosocial illness types and time phases in this schema creates an expanded system composed of four interlocking triangles as shown in Figure 3.3. One can conceptualize the illness and time phases as a fourth member of the system, having a personality (based on the pattern of onset, course, outcome, disability, and predictability) and a developmental life course (the illness time phases).

The inclusion of health care providers also elevates their position within the system. Before the diagnosis, the primary care physician may have resembled a distant relative seen occasionally; a chronic illness often transforms this distant relative into a central figure in family life. His or her centrality in the life of both patient and family will vary according to the level of technological care required. In life-threatening conditions, such as acute leukemia, the physician and the illness can easily become omnipresent in all significant family interactions and decisions. This relationship can ebb and flow with the illness phases. During health crises, the centrality of the health care team reemerges, and the family may need to relinquish significant control to health professionals at such times.

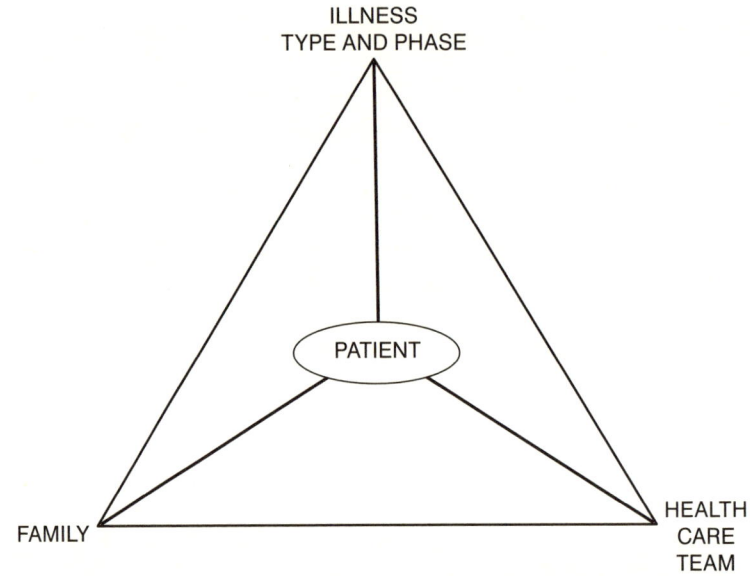

FIGURE 3.3. Therapeutic triangles with chronic conditions.

The psychosocial typology and time phases help clarify the personality of the illness and the timing and degree of importance the physician or other members of the health care team will have within the family. In many disorders, such as incurable forms of cancer, the initial crisis, periods of flare-up, and the terminal phase would be natural points in the illness at which primary and specialty care providers become more important. This is particularly true if the patient requires hospitalization or regular treatment at a health facility. With progressive or disabling diseases, the team involvement may increase gradually over time, without intermissions.

The impact of these various forces on a family and its relationship with the health care team depends on (1) the type and phase of the illness and its relative demand for professional medical care (it is important to remember that some illnesses, such as spinal cord injury, are severely disabling, but may require little medical input after the initial rehabilitation phase); (2) the location of medical care (if in the home, the family may retain a greater sense of control); and (3) the meaning the family ascribes to this relationship (see Chapter 18).

The typology and time-phase framework allow a clinician to think about the impact of an illness on a specific family, based on an understanding of cultural norms, family processes, and the psychosocial type of illness. Sometimes, the illness can function as a third leg in dysfunctional family triangles (see Chapter 5). For instance, a husband's heart attack can serve him in being a powerful ally against his wife: he can blame his heart attack on her incessant nagging. And because heart attacks can recur and be fatal, he may use this life-threatening aspect, along with blaming her for the first attack, as a weapon in assuming control of conflictual aspects of their relationship.

This framework can be used to understand the differences that emerge in the health beliefs of the patient, family, and health care team (see Chapters 8 and 18). Consider beliefs about the ability to control the course and outcome of an illness. A certain level of agreement concerning this kind of health belief is critical to establishing and maintaining a viable collaborative relationship among the patient, his or her family, and the health care team. The degree of consensus concerning beliefs about biological control can vary dramatically for this triad, depending on the type or phase of a condition. One particular family physician had a good working relationship with a family that had consulted him over the years for minor health problems. When the father suffered a serious heart attack, differences in beliefs about healing and control surfaced in relation to this life-threatening and possibly disabling illness. The stability of the long-standing, healthy, collaborative relationship became seriously threatened. In this case, the physician, aware of increased tensions with the patient and family, thought about his own beliefs regarding serious heart disease and questioned the family about theirs, thus averting a potentially serious rift in their previously excellent working relationship.

SERVICE DELIVERY APPLICATIONS

In terms of organization of services, the FSI model allows for a periodic reevaluation of the family in relation to the illness/disability course. The time phases and transition points suggest the timing of the consultation. Strengths and weaknesses in various components of family functioning can be addressed, taking into account all the factors relevant to the psychosocial type of the illness. Scheduling timely, preventive "psychosocial checkups" is inherently appealing to most families. For example, I consulted several times with a family whose members were anxious about the possibility of life-threatening bleeding episodes in their son, who had just been diagnosed as having hemophilia. A year later, anticipating possible heightened separation fears within the context of these illness-related risks, I offered the family a consultation as a preventive measure several months before the child's scheduled start of preschool.

The concept of psychosocial checkups is a useful way to normalize and operationalize a psychosocial component of care that, analogous to a medical checkup, is not tied into medical crises. It encourages a nonpathologizing, prevention-oriented psychosocial mindset, which normalizes a behavioral health provider's role within the health care team as a provider of regular, ongoing chronic illness care. I routinely discuss the value of these checkups with patients and their families when describing my perspective and role.

The typology presented here facilitates the development of various preventively oriented psychoeducational or support groups for patients and their families. For instance, groups can be designed to meet the needs of patients dealing with progressive, life-threatening diseases; relapsing disorders; acute-onset, incapacitating illnesses; or the chronic phase of diseases with a stable, constant course. This type of grouping is especially useful when there are not enough families with a particular condition to form a specific illness support group and is particularly applicable in rural settings or for less common illnesses. Thinking about group-oriented services in terms of specific psychosocial types of illness helps overcome such obstacles, while preserving the groups' thematic coherence. Brief psychoeducational "modules," timed for critical phases of particular types of diseases, enable families to digest manageable portions of a long-term coping process. As discussed in Chapter 4, preventively oriented multifamily psychoeducational support groups and workshops for patients and their families provide cost-effective preventive services that can decrease family isolation, increase networking, and identify high-risk families.

PART II

THE FSI MODEL
WORKING WITH COUPLES AND FAMILIES

CHAPTER 4

An Integrated Practice Approach with Couples and Families

The FSI model helps clinicians to understand the quality of fit between the psychosocial demands of a chronic condition over time and critical family processes, highlighting life-cycle issues and belief systems (see Chapters 6–8). This chapter describes the basic principles and clinical guidelines for effective systemic treatment.

LEVELS OF SYSTEMS-BASED INVOLVEMENT WITH FAMILIES

Professionals in varied disciplines and health care settings can adapt the FSI model to suit their context, treatment role, time constraints, and patient population. All providers have a valuable role to play, regardless of how limited it is. Doherty and Baird (1986) articulated a useful five-level framework of systems-based involvement with families.

1. Institution-centered with minimal emphasis on the family.
2. Ongoing medical information and collaboration.
3. Feelings and support.
4. Brief, focused intervention with systemic assessment and consultation.
5. Family therapy.

Each level requires a corresponding knowledge base and therapeutic skills (as detailed in Table 4.1) and considers a clinician's role and responsibilities. Minimally, the FSI model's approach can be mindfully infused into most

TABLE 4.1. Levels of Clinical Involvement with Families

Level 1. Institution-Centered

Interactions with families are institution centered, not family centered. Families are not regarded as an important area of focus, but are dealt with for practical or legal reasons. One-way communication prevails.

Level 2. Information and Collaboration

Knowledge Base: Content information in the professional's specialty.	*Skills:* 1. Communicating information clearly. 2. Eliciting questions and areas of concern. 3. Conducting informative family conferences.
Personal Development: Openness to engage families in collaborative ways.	4. Making pertinent and practical recommendations. 5. Generating mutually agreed-upon action plans. 6. Respecting cultural concerns that families raise. 7. Providing information on community resources.

Level 3. Feelings and Support

Knowledge Base: Family development plus individual and family reactions to stress.	*Skills:* 1. Eliciting expressions of feelings and concerns. 2. Listening with empathy. 3. Normalizing feelings and reactions. 4. Creating an open and supportive climate.
Personal Development: Awareness of one's own feelings in relation to family members and an ability to tolerate family members' feelings without fleeing or trying to fix them.	5. In group settings, protecting a family member from too much self-disclosure. 6. Engaging families in collaborative problem-solving discussion that involves feelings and values as well as rational planning. 7. Tailoring recommendations to the unique needs and concerns of the family. 8. Sensitively exploring cultural issues. 9. Identifying family impairment and psychological dysfunction. 10. Making a referral tailored to the family's unique situation.

Level 4. Brief, Focused Intervention

Knowledge Base: Family systems theory.	*Skills:* 1. Asking a series of questions to elicit a detailed picture of the family dynamics.
Personal Development: Awareness of one's own participation in systems, including one's own family, client family systems, and larger community systems.	2. Developing a hypothesis about the family systems dynamics involved in the problem. 3. Working with the family for a short period of time to change a stuck family interaction pattern. 4. Knowing when to end the intervention effort and either refer or return to level three. 5. Helping the family use its cultural resources to address an issue. 6. Orchestrating a referral by educating the family and the therapist about what to expect. 7. Working closely with therapists and community systems.

(continued)

TABLE 4.1. *(continued)*

Level 5. Family Therapy

The following partial description shows the boundary between Level 4 and Level 5 family therapy.

Knowledge Base: Family systems and patterns whereby distressed families interact with professionals and other community systems. *Personal Development:* Ability to handle intense emotions in families and oneself and to maintain one's balance in the face of strong pressure from family members or other professionals.	*Skills:* 1. Interviewing families or family members who are quite difficult to engage. 2. Working intensively with families during crises. 3. Efficiently generating and testing hypotheses about the family's difficulties and strengths. 4. Working with family impasses and intense conflict. 5. Constructively dealing with a family's ambivalence about change. 6. Working on culturally related stress and conflicts that are impairing the family. 7. Negotiating collaborative relationships with other professionals and systems, even when these groups are at odds with one another.

Note. Adapted from Doherty and Baird (1986).

---

interactions with patients and their families. It provides a way for clinicians to listen with a more refined attunement to what a patient or family member is conveying. For example, a parent may say to a nurse practitioner, "It seems that our son's (Jim) cancer might affect his life in uncertain ways for the rest of his life." This comment includes concerns about the illness course, possible disability, and outcome; living with anticipatory loss (see Chapter 9); about the continued interplay between the illness and Jim's individual development; and about its interaction with the nuclear family's life cycle. Reflecting back to the parent(s) about how the concern was heard on these levels can guide further discussion with the nurse (if time permits), or facilitate referral for a more in-depth mental health consultation. The nurse practitioner may choose to address some of the parents' concerns, such as the illness trajectory and disability (and its psychosocial implications for the patient and family), but defer addressing the impact on individual and family development to a mental health colleague.

Families can easily become overloaded by too many condition-related details and future uncertainties. The FSI model provides a map for each professional to zoom in tactfully on the most immediate and practical concerns, while helping families begin to address longer-term implications.

All providers should be able to conduct a basic preliminary "screening" assessment (level 3) and mental health care clinicians to provide a more thorough consultative evaluation (level 4). It is important that these skill sets be readily available in one's clinical toolbox and be consistent with one's role with families. For many providers, there is a pragmatic dividing line between assessment, psychoeducation, brief supportive consultations, and those situations with significant family dysfunction that call for a referral to more intensive family- or systems-based individual therapy.

BASIC PRINCIPLES OF INTERVENTION

The FSI model is used most effectively in a preventive, normative manner. Ideally *all families facing illness and disability should have from the beginning a psychosocial component of care that includes the key members of the family system and engages them as valued partners and resources.* When all health care team members adopt this approach (at whatever level is appropriate for professionals in their role), then biomedical and mental health care providers, the patient, and the family are powerfully enjoined and avoid unhelpful mind–body divisions. This posture ensures a psychosocial aspect of care from the start and simplifies a referral for more intensive mental health care, if needed, at some future point in the illness course. Every time a psychosocial consultation is included in the initial crisis phase or a provider suggests a "psychosocial checkup" at predictable transitions, it models (1) that it is normative for a chronic condition to affect the family system and its emotional health and (2) that it is possible to be proactive about expected condition-related challenges.

Initial Family-Oriented Consultation

Optimally, all families facing chronic illness or disability would routinely have a family consultation in the initial crisis phase, near the time of onset. As a preventive measure, this accomplishes three vital therapeutic tasks.

1. It includes a systems-oriented behavioral health care consultant as a member of the health care team.
2. It engages the family as a key resource and partner of care.
3. It normalizes the expectation of common psychosocial strains for the entire family in a positive, nonpejorative manner that enables them to utilize psychosocial support effectively, minimizing stigma and shame.

It also reduces feelings of helplessness that can lead to family withdrawal and isolation. Inviting a family early into this kind of collaborative process promotes open and flexible communication among all professionals and family members involved in the caregiving system.

The following assessment and intervention goals should be incorporated into a basic family-centered consultation.

Assessment

- *Elicit family history and information that may be vital to diagnosis and treatment decisions.* This includes a family's multigenerational experience with illness and loss that may hinder or facilitate current coping and adaptation.
- *Understand the cultural, spiritual, and health beliefs that guide the family.* This is essential to fostering culturally sensitive collaborative care and family meaning-making of the illness experience (see Chapter 6).
- *Identify high-risk, multistressed, or dysfunctional patients and families* needing more intensive follow-up care.

Psychoeducation and Intervention

- *Emphasize that all family members are affected* by the strains and challenges of living with a major illness.
- *Address the immediate emotional needs of the patient and family members* such as guilt, shame, and helplessness, and the activation of old family conflicts around illness decision making.
- *Provide information about the illness and treatment* and ways in which family members can be helpful.
- *Provide family psychoeducation regarding a psychosocial understanding of the particular illness over time* in relation to family expectations, offering practical management guidelines. It includes helping the family understand the illness in longitudinal and developmental terms, that is, how different phases of the illness might affect plans and future dreams for the patient, family members, and the family unit.
- *Facilitate communication concerning the illness, its treatment, and caregiving decisions.*
- *Recommend the usefulness of periodic family-centered consultations ("psychosocial checkups")* and brief interventions at nodal points and transitions in the illness course and individual and family development (see Chapter 7).

An initial consultation can be handled in different ways, depending on the service delivery model and resources available. It can be conducted in several meetings over the initial phase of engagement with a clinical service. For instance, in a program implemented with a comprehensive diabetes center at the University of Chicago (see Chapter 18), family-oriented behavioral specialists are located on-site. New patients and their families are given a brochure in the waiting area describing the behavioral component of care. The behavioral specialist sees the patient and family for 10 minutes toward the end of the first medical appointment, explaining his or her role and clinical philosophy, answering basic questions, and scheduling a more thorough one-time family consultation, typically coordinated with the first medical follow-up visit. Recommendations regarding which family members should or can participate are made at this time.

This psychosocial screening consultation does not require a clinician who has advanced family therapy skills. With some basic in-service training in family interviewing skills and a consultation outline, this initial assessment can be completed by a diabetes educator, RN, or medical social worker. Clinicians with advanced individual and family therapy training skills are available for referral of high-risk (e.g., those with treatment-adherence problems), multistressed, or high-dysfunction families.

Understanding and respecting each family's ethnic, cultural, racial, and spiritual background and values are paramount to a successful collaboration. It is important to assess socioeconomic factors, accessibility to care, and service delivery issues that are additional challenges to implementing any psychosocial component of care. Work-shift constraints can make participation in family meetings extremely difficult. An initial inquiry with key family members is vital in clarifying realistic expectations or joint problem-solving strategies. In the context of a diagnosis of a serious health condition, most families welcome an initial consultation.

Who Is in the Caregiving System? What Are the Caregiving Needs?

These are crucial questions best raised in the initial crisis phase, ideally at a first consultation. Key considerations include the extended family, the patient's family of choice (e.g., LGBTQ community), the patient's community (e.g., neighborhood, religious involvement), cultural and gender norms, and geographical proximity. These considerations, in turn, need to be thought about in relation to the specific illness and its psychosocial demands over the long haul and the condition's ongoing interaction with evolving individual and family life-cycle factors. Some disorders, such as a TBI, may involve the need for decades of major caregiving. Others, such as Alzheimer's disease, will necessitate ongoing and gradually increasing caregiving. Yet others, such as type 2 diabetes, may require only a short initial period of intensive family support. Family life-cycle transitions, such as marriage and starting a family, may require a reallocation of caregiving roles for specific family members to fit new demands. An initial consultation can afford an ideal opportunity to explore such current and future caregiving needs.

Family assessment with today's diverse and geographically dispersed family structures must consider the kinship network beyond the immediate household. Clinicians should inquire about members living at a distance or who are estranged, who may potentially provide resources and/or challenges. We can coach shared caregiving roles and strategies. Not infrequently, even limited, pragmatic participation also catalyzes dialogue and repair of old hurts and relationship issues. A family consultation about negotiating shared responsibilities can be very valuable at key illness junctures.

When a serious illness involves major disability or is in the terminal phase, ex-spouses, partners, or nonresidential parents may step up and participate in caregiving. Providers should ask about previous spouses or partners, the nature of their current relationship, and any possible understandings they may have regarding their availability to provide care (including financial support). Stereotypic assumptions that exclude or marginalize a potential resource should be avoided. With remarried couples and stepfamilies, it is important to inquire about the more complex roles, alliances, and strains across generations and households. It may be necessary, for example, to involve an adult stepchild in long-term planning discussions for a parent with a highly disabling illness.

Engaging the Family System

When an initial family-oriented biopsychosocial collaboration occurs, families are less likely to experience feelings of shame or blame when referrals for psychosocial treatment occur later in the chronic or terminal phase. Professionals need to be careful not to unwittingly contribute to these feelings, commonly by making a referral when biomedical treatment has reached its natural limit, treatments have failed, or a condition has progressed. At these junctures, families can easily confuse a physician's frustration at not succeeding, according to his or her own professional standards, with judging them as inadequate and at fault. Sensitivity is needed, especially when a referral is made in the chronic phase, when the course of the condition has worsened, or when an expected cure or improvement has not materialized. If a behavioral consultant was not included initially, families may feel that when a referral is made, it has to mean that they are coping poorly. This situation can easily arise, though, since physicians are often not accustomed to thinking in terms of using a family systems consultant in a preventive fashion.

Communicate Illness Challenges as Normative

During my first contact with the referring clinician and the identified patient and family, whether at illness onset or later in the chronic phase, I convey my philosophy about the primacy of the family or caregiving system. Regardless of the reason for referral, I point out that chronic disorders are challenging for the entire family, and that I am interested in the well-being of all family members. I emphasize that even the strongest families will encounter very challenging periods over the illness course. My primary goal is to join with the whole caregiving system, including the health care team.

Family Consultation as the Foundation for All Behavioral Health Care Modalities

A family-oriented consultation and assessment provide the best foundation for making decisions about the most appropriate kinds of treatment, which may include additional consultations, brief intervention (e.g., 1–3 meetings), or more intensive therapy for individuals, couples, or the whole family. A key goal of my initial consultation is to determine the relative usefulness of each modality. Rather than interpret a request for an individual consultation as resistance to including others, I assume that many referring health care providers and families are unfamiliar with a systems-based treatment model. I use the initial contact with both the referral source and the family unit to inform them about my approach and learn how it fits with their own ideas of getting help. This approach is not intended to convey that I am rigid about meeting only with the entire family. If I do go ahead and meet with one person, I make it clear that part of our agenda will include discussing the pros and cons of including other family members.

Mental Health Care Consultant as a Resource over Time

As much as possible, I want to normalize my joining the family's effort to master their situation. They should see me as a positive and helpful resource, rather than as a source of punishment or shame. At the time of referral, I find that directly inquiring about any feelings of shame to be the best approach. To help counteract such feelings, I routinely tell families that 75% of families who come to our Center have never seen a mental health professional. Emphasizing family strengths and what families have done well in the face of adversity are very helpful. Often, families are surprised when I compliment them during a consultation. They usually have had no way of measuring their skills in coping, resulting in overly harsh judgments about their competence. Rarely do I find that this approach encourages avoidance or denial. When I first meet these families, most of them are overwhelmed, emotionally depleted, and demoralized. Affirming their strengths gives me greater latitude to begin addressing areas of dysfunction.

Several other strategies facilitate the partnering process. Communicating to families that I am flexible is an important one. Where appropriate, I will meet with families according to the demands of the condition. If the affected member is in a recovery phase, I may meet the patient and family in the hospital at the bedside or in their home. This flexibility establishes me as part of the larger health care team and helps dispel myths that mental health professionals form rigid, secretive therapeutic relationships confined to their offices. Privacy is essential, but clinician distancing and secrecy can heighten these families' feelings of stigma and shame.

Collaboration with the Health Care Team: Promoting and Modeling Integrated Care

I almost always directly communicate with the primary health care providers. Frequently a mental health referral comes from a medical social worker. If I limit my contacts to a referring mental health professional, I may reinforce a dysfunctional split between medical and psychosocial care. Many mental health professionals are intimidated by the notion of directly calling the primary physician. The inherent power discrepancy and the lack of medical training can make them uneasy about such an encounter. In this regard, the psychosocial typology provides a useful middle ground for therapists in understanding the essence of an illness in psychosocial terms, thereby facilitating their ability to communicate effectively with a health professional without being medical experts. Calling the physician, going to the hospital, meeting with other health care professionals, and having the family see the consultant involved in such interactions all facilitate a functional joining process and demythologize the behavioral specialist's role. Also, it counteracts the common mind–body split in which parallel biomedical and psychosocial care are disconnected.

Integrated care is optimal (see Chapter 18). Here, the mental health care provider is on-site, and clinical care is partly or fully integrated. In this setting, health and mental health care providers share a biopsychosocial vision with shared expectations for team-based prevention and treatment. Operationally, this includes regular team meetings to discuss complex cases.

Whether conducted on-site or off-site, a meeting that includes the patient, key family members, and health care providers together with the family systems behavioral health care (BHC) specialist is the most effective. For the family, seeing the biomedical and BHC providers together forges a collaborative integrated vision of care. Further, it enables a discussion of the reasons for the referral and the relationship between biomedical and psychosocial treatment objectives. And it clarifies the respective roles of each provider. Such a joint meeting is easiest to arrange if the initial framing event about the BHC provider's role has been established as a collaborative one. This can be accomplished in the referral process, when the behavioral consultant and primary medical provider meet together briefly with the family in order to introduce the former's involvement within a team model (a "warm handoff"). Current technology enables "virtual" inclusion of providers or family members who are unable to be literally in the room. When this is not convenient, the same groundwork can be achieved by the family systems consultant's having early contact with the health care team. This process, which communicates a functional, flexible boundary among providers, needs to be sensitively balanced with family needs for confidentiality about personal issues.

Often health care providers think that mental health care professionals are unapproachable. However, in chronic disorders, ongoing, multiple-system involvement that includes other professionals is inevitable. Because of this fact, strict traditional rules about communication among mental health providers, other health care providers, and family members can become dysfunctional and heighten tendencies toward disengagement. For instance, when family members disagree about the possibility of loss, helping them establish family priorities that are uninformed by medical advice might be destructive and irresponsible. When working with chronic disorders, mental health clinicians need to examine how their rules for therapy may need to be flexibly adapted to facilitate effective collaboration.

These initial partnering strategies serve as a model for families who are learning how to integrate the biomedical and psychosocial aspects of their experience with illness and disability. A number of families have commented that seeing me discuss their situation with their primary physician(s) greatly facilitated such an integrative process. The provider, however, needs to bear in mind the HIPAA rules of privacy and confidentiality, and discuss and negotiate this type of communication with all relevant family members.

TIMING OF CONSULTATIONS

The psychosocial typology and illness time phases, combined with an understanding of individual and family life cycles, offer a coherent framework for timing periodic consultations.

Illness, Individual, and Family Transitions, and Nodal Points

Understanding the natural trajectory of a condition clarifies common transitions and nodal points in the evolution of a disorder (see Chapters 2 and 3). Key psychosocial developmental tasks associated with successful coping and adaptation can be integrated with such a time line. Since most individual and family life-cycle transitions will be affected by a chronic disorder, normative life-cycle tasks will need to be considered in the context of the condition. The interplay of the illness with individual and family development offers a useful way to think about the timing of psychosocial interventions (see Chapter 7). Families can be educated to anticipate nodal points and the psychosocial demands that will have to be faced, and to recognize the warning signs that help is needed. It allows them to request a consultation in a more proactive way.

Psychosocial Checkups

Where feasible, I offer individuals and families the opportunity for psychosocial checkups, usually every 3, 6, or 12 months. This is analogous to a health checkup. Many families like the term and the approach. If behavioral health care is co-located with medical care in a primary or specialty care setting, then these psychosocial checkups can often be piggy-backed with a routine medical appointment. This is time efficient and promotes quality care.

Illness Crises

Sudden disease flare-ups, such as asthma; life-threatening crises, for example, heart attack or hemorrhage; illness progression requiring prompt, intensive medical treatment like a recurrence of cancer; or an especially difficult week with a family member with Alzheimer's disease typically require families to abruptly switch into a crisis mode. Pragmatic juggling of household functions and emotional concerns about the patient's medical status take over. To remain in sync with such families' ongoing reality, therapists need to be adept at shifting from ongoing therapeutic work to supporting families through a health crisis. Mental health providers accustomed to maintaining continuity and therapeutic momentum between sessions can find the inherent power of the illness trajectory a jarring and frustrating reality. It is isomorphic with such families' daily experience. Professional understanding and equanimity are needed to fully empathize with and help such families.

For families with whom I consult on an as-needed basis, my active involvement is useful during medical crises and their aftermath. A medical crisis may be time limited, with recovery expected back to a prior baseline, or it may signal an illness transition with possibly greater permanent disability. With cancer recurrences, for instance, a crisis may represent a transition to a terminal phase. These condition-related issues often benefit from a consultation focused on family emotional and pragmatic processing.

Family Gatherings

Family gatherings afford natural opportunities for psychosocial consultation(s). Because serious illnesses make families more aware of the preciousness of time, holidays, such as Thanksgiving, that were taken for granted may suddenly take on new meaning. The awareness that each family gathering may be the last encounter can be emotionally disabling or empowering. Clinicians can propose consultations to coincide with family get-togethers or coach family members in initiating important conversations or designing meaningful rituals. In one example, a family approached the mother, who was in failing health, with the idea of a family celebration to honor her life. Her reply was, "That's a terrific idea, but let's get together so we can all honor each other as a family."

TREATMENT MODALITIES

A systems-based assessment provides an excellent basis for making appropriate clinical decisions about the relative usefulness of individual, couple, family, multifamily, psychopharmacology, complementary healing (e.g., mindfulness meditation or yoga), or self-help group interventions. I consider a family-oriented assessment the hub of a "psychosocial wheel" from which various individual needs can be addressed in an integrated manner and in relation to their effects on the rest of the system.

Individual and Family Approaches

Questions about how to balance individual needs, especially those of children, with those of the family unit naturally arise. Using a both-and rather than an either-or mindset guides treatment priorities within a systems orientation. Attention to the needs of an individual member can often be accomplished by combining individual and family meetings. Some illness challenges affect everyone and are best addressed in family consultations.

Optimally, the initial consultation should be flexible enough to allow time with the whole family, an adult couple, and individual members. There is no substitute for getting a picture of the entire system. Understanding a family's basic patterns of communication, particularly concerning illness-related issues, is vital. Deciphering patterns of protection—of an affected member, aging parents, or children—is important. Because patterns of protection and secrecy are so common, I routinely allow for separate time with each family member. For couples, certain issues related to shame or guilt (see Chapter 13) may be best addressed separately first. For example, a woman coping with issues of self-esteem and body image after a mastectomy may be more comfortable revealing her concerns in an individual session before she is able to share them with her spouse or other family members. Some conversations, such as intense anger toward a dying, fragile, or cognitively impaired family member, may be more appropriately dealt with in individual meetings.

Any decision to advocate for a more intensive individual intervention has to take into account the long-term consequences for communication patterns within the family. In chronic disorders, especially those involving threatened loss, there is a natural tendency toward protective and secretive communication, particularly with children. Encouraging them to open up in individual sessions may be adaptive in the short run. But if there is no attempt to foster open communication within the family, a child may use this experience of private communication as a model for the future. Eventually, it may lead to an emotional cutoff from the child's nuclear family.

In one case, individual sessions were conducted with a sibling in the initial crisis phase of her brother's diagnosis of cancer. Her parents were at the hospital almost constantly. Although these individual meetings helped at the time, they also resulted in her not discussing concerns directly with her parents. The girl's pattern of holding back out of worry about her ill sibling led to strong resentment against her parents and her brother, who did survive. A family session could have marked the end of the initial crisis phase and affirmed the need for direct communication between the girl and her parents.

There are additional strains in single-parent households. Single parents often do not have another adult at home to validate and support their efforts to cope with the physical and emotional needs of an ill or disabled child. In such families it is especially important to invite extended family or significant friends for consultations since they may represent an essential part of the caregiving network.

Cultural Factors

In sociocentric cultures worldwide, adversity, such as a serious medical condition, is normatively addressed as a family challenge involving the support of the extended kinship network. In the dominant U.S. eurocentric culture and western medical system, individual autonomy is often emphasized. Yet, if a clinician is open to exploring potential resources, illness and caregiving may afford opportunities for families to realize potential strengths in greater and more extended family collaboration and teamwork.

Imbalances in Adaptation

In families facing chronic disorders, the natural rhythm of coping and adaptation is often skewed. This is partly because family members are at different stages of personal development. Also the pace of individual adaptation can vary according to a condition's psychosocial demands and one's caregiving role. When family members understand these imbalances, it enhances communication. Also, it is valuable to normalize adult members being in and out of sync with one another. Different members may need to process parts of their experience according to their own time schedule. Individual sessions can be tailored to a member's personal style and pace of coping and adaptation.

The psychosocial typology and illness time phases of the FSI model can help clinicians understand how these imbalances are manifested. For instance, for a child who suffers a TBI, the difference between what the child needs and what the needs of the rest of the family are is sudden and immediate. Parents may be overwhelmed by caregiving demands at a time when their other children most need support. When a child has a slowly debilitating condition or one with a constant course, such as cystic fibrosis or mild intellectual disability, the discrepancy between the affected child and his or her siblings may become apparent only gradually. This latter situation permits siblings a longer time in which to adjust to inevitable imbalances and losses.

Flexible Use of Individual and Family Meetings

Typically, family treatment with illness and disability requires a clinician to flexibly move back and forth between meeting with different family configurations and having individual sessions. Sometimes meeting with members of each generation separately is useful, for example, with a sibling group when a parent or sibling is ill or disabled. When one parent is seriously ill, the children may form a primary support network so as not to further burden their parents, especially if the well parent is the primary caregiver. In this case, meeting with the siblings separately may uncover a rich network of communication that is hidden when the parents are included. Such sessions can promote bonds of support and caring among siblings and reduce competition and loneliness.

With aging or frail parents (see Chapter 12), it is very useful to convene meetings of the adult siblings. Doing this encourages the development of effective collaborative caregiving strategies and negotiation of specific roles and responsibilities going forward. Such meetings help the process of a generational transition of leadership from the parents to their adult children. These consultations need to be coordinated with conjoint meetings that include both the aging parents and their children.

Family Psychoeducation

Family psychoeducation has been empirically demonstrated to be an essential component of effective treatment with a wide range of chronic mental and physical conditions and stressful life challenges (Anderson, Reiss, & Hogarty, 1986; Lefley, 2009; Lucksted, McFarlane, Downing, Dixon, & Adams, 2012). This approach counters the stigma, blame, and shame families too often experience in traditional treatment settings. It respects families as valued partners and resources in collaboration with health care providers. Family psychoeducation is based on the premise that families need vital information and support in the care of their loved one with challenging mental or physical conditions. This systemic approach provides practical information about the condition, prognosis, medications, and treatment options. Also, it addresses stress reduction, helpful supports, and guidelines for management and problem solving through predictable stressful periods and crises over the condition's course.

Psychoeducational family interventions have been adapted to a variety of formats, including one-time or periodic family consultations, brief time-limited groups, or ongoing multifamily discussion groups. "Modules" can be timed with critical illness phases or transitions, and they can encourage families to accept and digest manageable portions of a long-term coping process. Some examples of modules include postdiagnosis or hospital discharge and community reentry, and the initial crisis, chronic, terminal, or bereavement phases of an illness.

Family psychoeducation can be "packaged" with a regular medical appointment, and with appointments with a nutritionist, a respiratory therapist, for cystic fibrosis, for example, or a diabetes educator for patients with type 1 or 2 diabetes. Multifamily psychoeducation can be delivered as part of a broader educational event with biomedical and psychosocial topics as an integrated whole. In our collaboration with a large diabetes center (see Chapter 18), half-day educational events were provided for adults and children. They included afternoon breakout sessions, where additional family-based psychosocial information and discussion occur in smaller groups on specific topics, such as parenting or adolescent transition to adulthood.

Multifamily and Couple Discussion Groups

Psychoeducational multifamily group (MFG) approaches are helpful for families facing chronic disorders (Asen & Scholz, 2010; Gonzalez & Steinglass, 2002; McFarlane, 2002; Steinglass, Ostroff, & Steinglass, 2011). Considering that a broad range of health care professionals, from nurses to medical social workers, can facilitate MFGs, they have been greatly underutilized.

MFGs are distinct from most illness-specific support groups in that they include both patient and nonpatient family members and attend to the family or couple as a system with the family unit as the focus. By contrast, support groups tend to focus either on supporting the patient or supporting caregivers. Also, multifamily discussion groups are marketed as educational and not psychotherapeutic interventions. This approach greatly facilitates recruitment and participation.

MFGs first became widely used with major mental disorders. They have been used increasingly in health care settings as family-focused psychosocial interventions with a range of chronic conditions, including cancer, diabetes, chronic pain, asthma, and infertility. Most psychoeducational MFGs use a time-limited structure that can vary from a single, one-day workshop to a specified number of meetings, typically four to eight. A modular, time-limited arrangement overcomes concerns about long-term treatments and is palatable to consumers unfamiliar with or wary of psychosocial treatments. It also appeals to insurance payers concerned with cost containment and effectiveness.

Multifamily Group Formats

A four-session format has the advantage of allowing families to absorb information at each meeting and have some intervening time (1–2 weeks) for family discussions before returning for the next meeting. It also tends to foster greater connection and networking among participating families. That said, the 1-day format is generally more cost effective and can serve many more families. The family workshop can be divided, for instance, into four segments covering the same material. Each segment begins with giving the larger group information on a topic (e.g., family communication, individual and family development, living with uncertainty), followed by a small-group discussion with a facilitator for each group. Often, it is easier and more appealing for families to attend a 1-day workshop.

Groups typically consist of four or more patients and their spouses or partners, parents, siblings, and significant kin or friends. The group meetings include a combination of psychoeducational information delivered by the professional facilitators, followed by group discussion. During group dialogue, facilitators promote maximum interaction among the families. Generally, this kind of structured information-giving format is preferred over more unstructured ones in the initial crisis phase. The group context gives families the opportunity to learn from one another and gain support in trying out new adaptive patterns of relating and handling challenges. Family members can relate to the experience of their counterparts in other families, can gain perspective on their own stressful situation, and can feel less guilty, blameworthy, stigmatized, and isolated. Changes in family relationships are less threatening when shared with the mutually supportive network the group provides. Also, the format allows families who are isolated to establish support networks that may extend well beyond the group sessions. This is particularly important in disorders such as HIV or conditions involving disfigurement, in which stigma can foster extreme family isolation. Online support groups can accomplish the same networking goals for families, but they lack the face-to-face advantage and are typically less structured and connected to a clinical service that includes an integrated care component.

At the height of the AIDS epidemic, when our Center first proposed forming a family support group for HIV, the medical team and I were very concerned about families' being reticent to discuss their problems openly. We prepared for this possibility by designing some "warm-up" communication exercises to facilitate the group process. We were completely surprised when, within the first 10 minutes of the group meeting, a gay man and his father, an Irish Catholic police officer, began to discuss issues related to terminal care, and the rest of the group was immediately supportive and shared their own similar concerns. For many of these families, this meeting was their first chance to discuss dealing with AIDS, and making good use of their limited time together was essential.

Sometimes multifamily support groups can empower families in their struggles with other systems. In one instance, a time-limited group was offered through an occupational medicine clinic to families coping with occupationally related respiratory diseases resulting from chemical sensitivity. Many of the cases involved litigation with previous employers concerning who or what was responsible for the condition. These families often felt isolated and rejected. At the last meeting in the psychoeducation series, the group decided to form an information, advocacy, and self-help network for themselves and other similarly affected families throughout the state.

Group Coherence: Using the Psychosocial Type and Time-Phase Framework

Multifamily discussion groups can be organized according to the psychosocial type and illness phase. Bringing together families who are coping with conditions posing similar psychosocial demands promotes a sense of group identity and coherence. I find it very useful to start with a time-limited psychoeducational module in the initial crisis phase followed by an ongoing weekly or monthly multifamily group to address continuing family strains in the chronic or terminal phase. Giving sequential priority to manageable segments of an overall process of coping and adaptation helps prevent feelings of being overwhelmed. For instance, in one oncology service, a multifamily orientation group is formed every few months for families in the initial crisis phase following a recent diagnosis. This consists of a series of four meetings whose purpose is to inform families about salient issues related to caring for a member with cancer, including:

- Understanding themselves as a system
- Learning about key challenges in the initial crisis phase and how to think about cancer in relation to family, couple, and child development
- Developing effective methods of problem solving
- Communicating about emotional issues
- Learning to live with uncertainty and anticipatory loss
- Becoming informed about available community support services
- Knowing when to seek professional help.

The first meeting includes the chief oncologist, who helps families understand the illness, its treatment, and the common psychosocial demands of living with cancer. I have found that participation of a key medical provider in the first meeting is invaluable. It encourages family participation and provides a powerful visible link between the biomedical and behavioral health providers. At the initial meeting, we briefly outline topics that will be addressed as well as solicit suggestions for additional subjects that family members want to have covered. This approach combines a planned agenda with a more loosely structured one adapted to each group's unique interests.

After completing this orientation series, families have a number of options. Some families identify issues they want to address privately in individual, couple, or family sessions. Others may enter an available ongoing MFG or disease-specific individual or family support groups designed to deal with chronic-phase issues. Many support groups are open to everyone—the newly diagnosed and those at the terminal phase. In my experience, it seems preferable to have a time-limited psychoeducational module for those in the initial crisis phase precede entry into an ongoing MFG or general support group. The initial module provides a base of psychosocial knowledge that lessens the discrepancy between illness newcomers and "veterans." This enhances the experience for everyone.

Ongoing MFG Groups

Ongoing multifamily or couple groups are useful alternatives or adjuncts to other types of psychosocial treatment. This is particularly true in dealing with the constant, inevitable biopsychosocial strains involved in progressive, relapsing, and potentially fatal conditions. Ongoing groups can be structured so that families can use the group as needed, including inviting speakers to discuss specific topics. Groups may offer different meetings for specific subsystems, such as couples, siblings, and well partners. In some groups, families themselves have emerged as leaders. Others prefer the continuity of health care professional expertise and facilitation. Both kinds of groups are workable.

Couples' Groups

Groups designed explicitly for couples are uncommon. Yet, there is a tremendous unmet need for them. Support groups for caregivers are primarily geared to provide for the needs of caregivers in that role. They are not intended to address primarily the challenges for couples. In one instance, we developed the Resilient Partners Program for couples facing an MS diagnosis (see Chapter 18 for a description of the collaboration). The program was structured either as four evening meetings on consecutive weeks or 1-day workshops. Many attendees had participated in support groups. Strikingly, although the majority of couples had lived with MS for at least 5 years, very few had met with other couples to focus specifically on the challenges to the partnership or marriage over time. Because of the large number of MS-affected families in the Chicago region (over 8,000), we were able to offer life-cycle-tailored groups for younger couples, who were often involved in child rearing, and for midlife and later-life couples, often coping with greater levels of disability and caregiving demands (e.g., intergenerational caregiving, cognitive impairment).

To conclude, multifamily groups are cost effective; they provide flexible, long-term continuity of care at regular intervals or at nodal stress points; and they offer a valuable adjunct to individual or family-based psychotherapies.

Combined Mental Health Approaches

With the expanding range of therapeutic approaches and the recognition that complex biopsychosocial issues are often not resolved by a single approach, combined modalities have become increasingly common. For chronic psychiatric disorders, such as schizophrenia, or serious physical conditions, research had documented the effectiveness of combining psychotropic interventions with individual, family, and group approaches (Dixon et al., 2001). Likewise, the family-based component of psychosocial care mutually supports treatments such as psychopharmacology, cognitive behavioral therapy (CBT), dialectical behavior therapy (DBT), substance abuse treatment, trauma-focused care, and integrative treatment approaches.

Collaboration among Mental Health Care Providers

Communication and mutual support among mental health providers is as essential as that between health and mental health providers. This minimizes parallel behavioral treatments delivered in separate silos. For example, a family dealing with cancer sees a medical family therapist located in the family's primary care clinic. Concurrently, the patient's spouse sees a clinical psychologist for CBT at the medical center's mental health clinic and attends a caregivers' support group at the cancer center, which is facilitated by a medical social worker. Another member gets antidepressant pharmacotherapy from a psychiatrist. A third member is learning mindfulness-based stress reduction meditation from an integrative medicine practitioner in the community. A fourth member sees a private practitioner in longer-term psychodynamic psychotherapy, which began before the cancer diagnosis. The training and "cultural" distinctions among these mental health providers and the different care delivery settings notwithstanding, often these providers may be insufficiently informed about each other's worthwhile and complementary treatments.

In the context of family-oriented consultation, information about family member use of different mental health professionals or self-help strategies may come to light for the first time. A family therapist can play an essential facilitative role. The norms of optimal collaborative care may require shifting from common private practice rules restricting communication outside a dyadic therapy relationship. Any fundamental differences among mental health providers should be acknowledged. Where possible, mental health providers should seek complementary or sequenced strategies that are mutually supportive. This helps protect families from unnecessary added stress and conflict. With specific patients and families, biomedical providers may need input regarding these various mental health approaches (see Chapter 18).

With a systemic family component of care, other individual-based approaches can be incorporated in tandem or sequentially. Often, the family component can support follow-through with and adherence to other mental health modalities. In my experience, the FSI model facilitates this process. The model can be used flexibly with diverse treatment approaches and modalities, primarily because it provides an overarching framework to guide thinking and is not tied to a particular theoretical perspective or treatment orthodoxy.

CHAPTER 5

Facilitating Family Organizational and Communication Processes

The previous chapters have offered a framework for clinicians to rethink chronic physical conditions in systemic terms according to the pattern of psychosocial demands over the course of an illness. Equipped with this framework, we turn now to the family side of the FSI model. This introductory chapter highlights family organizational and communication processes.

A NORMATIVE PERSPECTIVE

Clinicians need to consider family functioning from the standpoint of the flexibility, stamina, and depth of commitment that coping with a particular disorder will require. The resilience needed by a family dealing with slowly progressive but fatal illnesses, such as muscular dystrophy or Alzheimer's disease, cannot be compared to the resilience needed to cope with the demands of ordinary life.

In a family assessment, clinicians need to be mindful of distinctions between *symptomatic versus dysfunctional behavior*. Most families dealing with disabling or life-threatening conditions can eventually become symptomatic, regardless of how well they initially appear to be functioning. Families commonly exhaust their emotional and material resources under protracted stress. Just as we should not consider the biological decline in an 80-year-old person a failure of the body, so an assessment of normality in families dealing with serious disorders needs to be undertaken in light of the magnitude and duration of the challenge. This is not to imply that symptomatic family functioning does not need attention; rather, we should view the assessment and treatment process through a normative lens that facilitates a collaborative therapeutic relationship that promotes resilience and healing. The process of family consultation and assessment can be a powerful "framing event" that determines whether families create affirming or destructive narratives about living with a serious condition (see Chapter 8 on family belief systems).

FAMILY ORGANIZATION AND COMMUNICATION

Some leading and well-researched systemic models of family functioning incorporate concepts of organization, including adaptability/flexibility, cohesion, hierarchy/power, role functions, and boundary integrity, and communication styles (Lebow & Stroud, 2012). This discussion draws from Walsh's (2016b) conceptualization of family organizational and communication processes outlined in Table 5.1.

In addition to assessing family organizational and communication processes, the psychosocial typology and time-phases framework suggest the areas of family life that will be most heavily taxed by a particular condition. Since all families have areas of relative strength and vulnerability, certain illnesses and time phases may play into a family's strengths, and others, into their vulnerabilities. For instance, some conditions, such as well-controlled hypertension, may necessitate little day-to-day communication; patients take their daily medication, monitor their diet, and keep regular medical appointments. On the other hand, a family coping with a child with cystic fibrosis must communicate with each other on a daily basis about complex, home-based medical procedures and a range of practical and emotional issues.

Family Organizational Patterns

Family functioning requires effective organization to maintain integration as a family unit, to foster the healthy development of its members, and to master challenges over the life cycle. A flexible structure, connectedness, and social and economic resources strengthen family resilience. With the reshaping of contemporary family life, myriad evolving family cultures and structures, such as sole-parent, binuclear divorced, stepfamily, three-generational household, have become normative. With divorce and remarriage and "families of choice" now commonplace, it is important to inquire about and involve individuals who are considered potential key caregivers. Beyond the "household" or legal marriage bond, "family" can include nonresidential parents, ex-spouses or partners, grandparents, aunts or uncles, and children of former marriages.

The Family Constellation

The family constellation includes all members of the current household, the extended family system, and key people, such as close friends and professional caregivers, who function as family insiders.

TABLE 5.1. Key Processes in Family Resilience

Organizational Processes

1. Flexibility
   - Rebound: adaptive change to meet new challenges.
   - Reorganize, restabilize: continuity, dependability, predictability.
   - Strong authoritative leadership: nurture, guide, protect.
   - Varied family forms: cooperative parenting/caregiving teams and household.
   - Couple/coparent relationship: mutual respect; equal partners.
2. Connectedness
   - Mutual support, teamwork, and commitment.
   - Respect individual needs and differences.
   - Seek reconnection and repair grievances.
3. Mobilize Social and Economic Resources
   - Recruit extended kin, social and community supports; models and mentors.
   - Build financial security; navigate stressful work–family challenges.
   - Transactions with larger systems: enlist institutional and structural supports.

Communication Processes

4. Clarity
   - Clear, consistent messages in both words and actions.
   - Clarify ambiguous information; truth seeking.
5. Open Emotional Expression
   - Share painful feelings (e.g., sadness, suffering, anger, fear, disappointment, remorse).
   - Share positive feelings and interactions (e.g., love, appreciation, gratitude, humor, fun, respite).
6. Collaborative Problem Solving
   - Creative brainstorming; resourcefulness.
   - Share decision making; repair conflicts; negotiation, fairness, reciprocity.
   - Focus on goals; take concrete steps; build on success; learn from setbacks.
   - Shift from reactive to proactive stance: prepare for future challenges.

Note. Adapted from Walsh (2016b).

With chronic disorders, it is useful to conceptualize the "health-related family system," which includes both the family system and the system of health care providers or team involved in the ill member's care. With terminal or life-threatening illness, providers become associated with issues of life preservation, anticipated loss, and dependency. With protracted, disabling conditions, it is not uncommon for professionals involved in home health care to become central to family life; they therefore need to be evaluated as part of the day-to-day system. This is most striking in serious disorders that begin in childhood, in which the health-care team then becomes a true "second family."

With disorders, such as HIV, that are stigmatizing or affect groups subject to discrimination, such as the LGBTQ community, caregiving networks emerge that function as a family unit. Clinicians need to inquire about whom the patient considers to be family and be sensitive to possible conflicts that may loom between a family-of-origin and a "chosen" or "emergent" family who may never have met, but who are brought face to face for the first time in a life-threatening crisis.

Family Adaptability: Flexibility and Stability

Family adaptability is one of the chief requisites for well-functioning family systems. Optimal flexibility to adapt to the challenges of chronic disorders depends on an effective balance between change and stability. To function well, a family needs enduring values and traditions and strong leadership with predictable, consistent role functions and patterns of interaction. The family must also adapt to changing circumstances and developmental priorities. Families at dysfunctional extremes tend to be overly rigid and autocratic or chaotically disorganized and leaderless.

In times of an illness crisis or disruptive transitions, a willingness to change must be counterbalanced by efforts to restabilize and reorganize patterns in daily life. In one case, a single mother's cancer diagnosis necessitated repeated hospitalizations for intensive chemotherapy. Rather than experiencing further disruption by moving her kids between households, she and her siblings negotiated their taking turns staying with her children during and immediately after the postchemotherapy-treatment recovery period. This plan enabled her children to maintain familiar "home" surroundings and keep up daily routines and friendships.

Significant losses may require major adaptational shifts in order to ensure the continuity of family life. For instance, in a traditional family, when a husband becomes disabled, family role functions shift as the wife becomes the primary breadwinner. The husband may assume the bulk of homemaking and child-rearing responsibilities. Family adaptability is essential particularly in disorders that are progressive, relapsing, or have acute medical crises.

Family stability is also important to counter disruption and maintain continuity, dependability, and predictability. For instance, childhood illnesses that react quickly to emotional stress, such as asthma and diabetes, may predictably flare up whenever parents' marital disagreements escalate beyond tolerable limits. The child's distress can divert attention from the marital conflict and ease the tension between parents as they focus on the child's current crisis. The destructive, nonadherent behavior of an acting-out adolescent with diabetes may be offset by the angelic behavior of a well sibling, who contributes in a complementary way to the overall family balance. The reciprocal interplay of these behavior patterns may become obvious only when the ill child leaves home and the angelic sibling starts to misbehave in response to interactional cues like those responsible for the diabetic adolescent's behavior. In instances of serious family dysfunction, an individual treatment that succeeds for the adolescent with diabetes (for instance, in terms of improved adherence with treatment) may have little impact on system dysfunction, which may place another sibling, as a substitute, in the symptomatic position. The health care team needs to not focus solely on improving medical status, but also be attuned to these broader family system issues that need attention.

Flexibility is needed to adapt to the changes that serious illnesses may require. Families at the extremes of adaptability will have more problems with certain types of conditions. Because rigid families have particular difficulty adapting to change, their style of functioning may be ill suited to the rapid shifting of roles required by relapsing disorders. Such families may function better with constant-course conditions, such as a permanent injury. Families that are chaotic and disorganized may have more adaptational difficulties with conditions where strict adherence to regimens is required. For instance, successful management of diabetes requires adhering to dietary rules, specific mealtimes, and timely insulin injections and blood sugar monitoring, all of which are a poor fit with disorganized family functioning.

The following sample questions help the family and clinician to understand how a chronic condition has impacted or may impact family organization.

- How has the family had to reorganize itself, or how will it need to do so? At present? Over the course of the condition?
- In what ways have preillness role functions changed for each family member since the diagnosis? Is this different for pragmatic or emotional issues?
- How much disease management responsibility does the affected member assume? How congruent is this with family expectations?
- How do family expectations about the illness fit with recommendations by health care providers?
- Besides the ill member, who has primary caregiving responsibilities for disease management? How was this decided? How does everyone feel about this arrangement? Could other members share responsibilities to alleviate a disproportionate burden on the primary caregiver?
- Overall, given the psychosocial demands of the condition, does the family organization seem realistic? Is there overcompensation, in which the patient has been relegated to a sick, helpless victim role? Is there undercompensation, in which the patient bears too much responsibility given the illness severity?

Family expectations and rules organize interaction and serve to maintain a stable system. Relationship understandings, both explicit and implicit, provide expectations about role-related functions, actions, and consequences that guide family life. Relationship expectations serve as norms within a family. Chapters 13 and 14 describe how couples' relationship expectations and understandings are challenged with illness and disability.

A serious health condition complicates family expectations. In childhood disorders there may need to be rules for the ill child based on the limits and risks imposed by the condition rather than by chronological age. This fosters an imbalance in which, for instance, younger siblings may have more flexible rules than an older ill brother or sister, potentially creating a source of tension and conflict. In relapsing conditions, such as recurrent migraine headaches, a family often needs to establish two sets of expectations—one set for when the affected family member is well and another for when he or she has a flare-up. A clear understanding of when illness norms apply can be challenging, especially in conditions such as pain syndromes in which the transition from one mode to another is often ambiguous.

Connectedness

Connectedness, or cohesion, another central dimension of family organization, has been shown to be a major predictor of how a family copes with illness. Considering that families have diverse cultural values, well-functioning families balance needs for closeness and mutual support with respect for separateness and individual differences. The functional balance of connectedness shifts as families move through the life cycle. For instance, with adolescence, in many cultures the family organization often shifts and places a greater emphasis on the autonomy of its adolescent members. A disabling chronic condition may intensify and prolong these normative transitions. With some conditions, such as intellectual or developmental disabilities, the need for high cohesion may be permanent, challenging family members to redefine normative developmental shifts (see Chapter 7).

For any condition, clinicians need to assess the fit between the psychosocial demands for cohesion and family patterns of closeness. Conditions that require teamwork, such as home-based dialysis for end-stage renal disease, will be especially difficult for a lower-cohesion family that lacks closeness and cooperativeness. Hemodialysis carried out in a hospital with the close surveillance and support of a dialysis team usually fits better with the limitations of a lower-cohesion family.

Clinician attunement to varying cultural norms is crucial to whether the meaning of caregiving and accommodation of life-cycle goals is framed as loyal and honorable or dysfunctional. A highly cohesive family style is normative in many ethnic groups. For instance, in traditional Italian families, a health crisis commonly brings the entire family to the bedside. In one case, involving a father in a coma, a 6-week vigil was an expression of normal family loyalty, not enmeshment. In Latino families, loyalty and meeting the caregiving expectations of an ill or disabled family member might normatively necessitate a young adult to subordinate his or her life plans to the needs of the family of origin (Falicov, 2013). Unlike the dominant U.S. culture's emphasis on independence and self-reliance, most cultures highlight family and community commitments and interdependence over individual priorities (Walsh, 2016b).

Boundaries

Family boundaries are important structural requisites that need to be clear and consistent, yet sufficiently permeable and flexible to respond to stressors such as major illness. Although family organizational styles vary enormously with cultural norms, dysfunctional family patterns tend to be characterized by extremes of fusion–enmeshment or disengagement. A *fused–enmeshed* family pattern limits or sacrifices individual differences to maintain a cohesive sense of unity. Members are expected to think and feel alike: differences are regarded as threats to family life (Bowen, 1993). A *disengaged* family pattern of too little connectedness reinforces individual differences, separateness, and distance at the expense of family relatedness, which at the extreme results in fragmenting the family unit and isolating individual members, who must fend for themselves.

Extremes of closeness or distance are clearly risk factors for successful family coping and adaptation. Families may be overprotective and inhibit the development of autonomy with regard to self-care and pursuing realistic life goals. This pattern is an issue for chronically ill children and adolescents as they strive for normative independence. Also, as discussed in Chapter 3, the transition from the crisis to the chronic phase is a particularly vulnerable period. The normative need for high cohesion in a health crisis can mask enmeshed family patterns, which become more apparent as a family enters the chronic phase, in which autonomy within the constraint of the disorder is a central goal. Such families maintain rigid boundaries around the family unit and tend to be wary of outsiders. Conditions that necessitate outside professional help, especially in the home, may be problematic for them. They perceive health care provider involvement as a threat to family well-being. In such cases nonadherence needs to be understood within that context.

Generational boundaries help maintain the culturally defined hierarchical aspect of family organization. Within cultural norms, leadership and authority need to be clear; distinguishing among grandparent, parent, and child role functions, rights, and obligations. An effective parental/marital relationship with shared leadership is vital, particularly with respect to chronic disorders of childhood (see Chapter 11). It helps prevent dysfunctional split role functions in which one partner becomes overly responsible as a reaction to the distancing and less-responsible behavior of the other. There may also be a vicious cycle in which one parent becomes increasingly authoritarian as the other becomes more and more lenient.

Most family systems models consider generational boundaries to be blurred when a parent uses a child as a parental surrogate. However, if the illness or disability involves a parent, it may be functional and even necessary for older children to assist parents with certain responsibilities, such as caregiving, household maintenance, childcare, and financial support. This is particularly common in single-parent or large families (see Chapter 12). Optimally, children are assisting the adults, who maintain authority, and the added functions are shared with other family members as much as possible. However, burdening a child with extensive, continual surrogate role responsibilities can sacrifice his or her individual developmental needs. Understanding cultural norms is crucial in managing conditions with high caregiving demands.

Triangulation

The dysfunctional process of *triangulation* refers to the pattern of two family members, for example, the parents, drawing in or scapegoating a third person to deflect rising tension. Typically, triangles breach generational boundaries. In one version, a couple may avoid conflict by rallying together in mutual concern about a symptomatic ill child. For instance, if the child is exhibiting behavior problems associated with an illness, such as refusing medication, the parents may unite to focus on, or sometimes blame, the child. In another version, a triangulated child may assume the role of go-between for parents, thereby balancing loyalties and regulating tension and intimacy. In a high-conflict marriage or divorce, one parent may draw a child into a coalition against the other parent.

Chronic conditions greatly increase the risks of triangulation, particularly when unresolved, conflictual family issues already exist. An illness can serve to shift the balance of power. Imagine a woman caught between loyalty to her husband and to a close-knit family of origin, both of which expect and compete for her attention. An illness in any member of this triangle will alter family dynamics. If either the husband or one of her aging parents becomes ill, that person can legitimately expect more of her time and energy. If she becomes ill, the family of origin and the husband may vie for primary caregiving rights. Another typical cross-generational pattern occurs when, due to gendered role expectations, a mother becomes preoccupied with caring for an ill child and her husband feels shut out or distances himself.

A common triangle presented by divorced families is one in which the parents have not emotionally separated, and the conflict is played out through their children. The intense emotions and caregiving needs generated by a life-threatening illness in one of their children can force warring ex-spouses and remarried families together in an implosive way. Sometimes, however, such a crisis can provide an opportunity to lay aside or resolve old difficulties.

An illness can function as the third leg of a triangle in a dysfunctional couple's processes. The ill partner can use an illness or disability as a means of secondary gain and to wield power in a struggle for control of a relationship, secondary gain here referring to any rights and privileges associated with the "sick role." In disorders with ambiguous or invisible symptoms, such as pain syndromes, the potential for manipulation is much greater since it is difficult for family members to gauge the severity of the patient's complaint.

In some cases *the hospital, the health care team, or one provider can become the third leg of a dysfunctional triangle.* When dysfunctional family processes are apparent, clinicians should watch for evidence of splitting: Competing family factions may unite against or ally with a provider or an entire health care institution. This pattern needs to be distinguished from normal situations of despair, such as during the terminal phase of an illness, when families sometimes express their grief and suffering by angrily blaming the health care system or specific providers for not being able to cure or save the patient.

Social and Economic Resources

Family–community networks can be vital lifelines for family functioning and support in times of crisis. Well-functioning families are characterized by a clear sense of the family unit, with permeable boundaries connecting the family to the community. Many facing serious illness easily become isolated and need social networks for support and connectedness to the community. A chronically ill child with a significant disability is at risk of being isolated from his or her peers and community activities. Clinicians need to familiarize themselves with typical social networks, such as schools, religious institutions, and workplaces, in which families are involved. It is valuable to explore with families the possible impact of a member's illness on relationships with those networks, as well as the supports they may provide. For instance, gross misunderstandings about HIV transmission have severely affected the ability of affected children to attend and function normally within many schools. In situations where families are not supportive, friendship networks can become valued "families of choice," as in the LGBTQ communities (Green, 2012).

Illness-based organizations, such as the National MS Society, the Juvenile Diabetes Research Foundation, and the Alzheimer's Association, can provide enormous benefits to patients and their families. A broad range of disease-specific consumer-based organizations typically provide vital biomedical treatment updates; cutting-edge research; and psychosocial support information, networking, and advocacy. These benefits can be accessed through web-based resources and more locally through state and regional chapters, which typically conduct educational events and support groups. They facilitate networking, and for many families they are a vital illness-related community that promotes resilience.

Most specialty care systems, such as cancer or heart disease centers, host a range of support groups that assist and network affected patients and their families. As valuable as these consumer and health care systems resources are, psychosocial programs that are geared to the family or couple system remain relatively scarce. Support services for patients or caregivers, while very useful, typically lack a systems foundation. Multiple family discussion groups offer an excellent vehicle for timely family-oriented psychoeducation and for networking with families that have similar conditions (see Chapter 4).

For patients and families coping with disabilities, having access to services that would allow for independent living is often inadequate or lacking. At the same time, families are often unaware of available resources through religious affiliations, illness-specific organizations with local chapters (the National MS Society, the Caregiver Action Network), and neighborhood/community formal and informal supports.

Communication Processes

Effective communication is essential for family mastery of illness and disability. Clinicians need to attend to both the content (facts, opinions, and feelings) and the relationship (defining, affirming, and challenging the nature of the bond) aspects of communication. The statement "Take your medicine" is an order with the expectation of adherence. It implies a hierarchy of status or authority, as between a parent and child. All verbal and nonverbal behaviors (e.g., spitting out a pill), including silence, convey interpersonal messages— "I won't obey you!" In families facing major, long-term health conditions, communication cannot regularly be left unclear or unresolved without resulting in unhealthy consequences. At the same time, a clinician needs to be mindful that cultural norms vary enormously in terms of sharing medical information and emotional expression. In some cultures, health care providers apprise family members, but not the patient, of a diagnosis and prognosis. In some, expressing one's suffering or distress to family members is considered culturally inappropriate. In others, it is synonymous with being connected and responsive. Several useful basic questions include the following:

- In your cultural or ethnic traditions, how do families communicate about an illness? Among family members? Or with health care providers?
- What are your expectations of providers or other family members for effective communication?

Collaboration among the patient, the family, and health care providers is addressed in Chapter 18.

Clear and Consistent Communication

Clarity is essential. In a family evaluation, clinicians assess family members' norms and ability to communicate openly about both pragmatic and emotional issues. Cultural norms vary considerably regarding the directness and degree of expression of opinions and feelings (McGoldrick, Giordano, &

Garcia-Preto, 2005). Here are some questions that I find useful in determining the effect an illness is having on family communication patterns:

- How has the condition affected family members' ability to talk directly and openly with one another?
- Is the illness or disability discussed openly? By whom? With whom?
- Is anyone protected in, or excluded from, these discussions (e.g., the ill member; children; or aged, frail, or seemingly vulnerable family members)?
- Are certain topics off-limits? For everyone? For children? Why (for example, due to cultural norms or fear)?

Emotional Expression

A climate of mutual trust encourages the open expression of a range of feelings and empathic responses, with respect for differences. Troubled families, in contrast, tend to perpetuate mistrust, with repeated blaming and scapegoating. High emotional reactivity can fuel destructive cycles of conflict and escalate to violence. The cascading effects of criticism, stonewalling, contempt, and mutual withdrawal contribute to despair and divorce (Driver, Tabares, Shapiro, & Gottman, 2012). Noteworthy patterns include (1) toxic or sensitive subjects, such as the possibility of death, in which communication falters; (2) the constraints of gender-based socialization; for instance, often men are good at practical tasks related to illness caregiving, but guarded in sharing emotions or revealing vulnerability; (3) specific relationships in which communication is extensive and intimate and others in which it is blocked or distant; for instance, anger may be expressed, but not love.

Communication about emotional issues is generally more difficult, particularly with disorders that involve threatened loss. In this situation, I ask specifically about the effect a condition is having on the overall family emotional climate and on members' willingness to communicate about specific emotional issues. Some illustrative questions include:

- How has the family mood been affected by the disorder? Has it become more or less optimistic, warm, affectionate, and playful or angry, sad, depressed, and helpless?
- Which relationships have become closer or more distant? How?
- What feelings seem easiest and most difficult for the family to express?
- Living with chronic conditions can be very frustrating at times. To whom do you express this frustration?
- Do family members refrain from expressing these kinds of feelings to the affected member? If so, how do they feel about being protected in this way?

As part of an initial consultation, I often find it helpful to meet separately with particular family members to assess any constraints to open communication that commonly occur with regard to sensitive topics, such as threatened loss and feelings of shame. Here are some questions I often ask at these initial meetings:

- Are there issues related to the illness that you think about to yourself, but do not discuss openly? What issues? Why do you keep them to yourself?
- Under what circumstances, for example, when a child is older or when the patient becomes terminally ill, would you discuss these private thoughts?
- With whom would you feel most and least comfortable talking about these issues (e.g. the ill member, a friend, a minister)? Why?

Achieving success and confidence in discussing these topics provides a foundation for addressing more sensitive ones.

Collaborative Problem Solving

Collaborative problem solving is essential for successfully coping with chronic conditions. Well-functioning families are characterized not by an absence of issues, but by their joint problem-solving abilities. Families can have difficulties solving pragmatic issues (e.g., reorganizing household responsibilities after a mother's heart attack) and the more emotional aspects of illness, such as sharing the grief and fear associated with a diagnosis of cancer. They can falter at various steps in the problem-solving process (Ryan, Epstein, Keitner, Miller, & Bishop, 2005): identifying the issue, communicating with appropriate people about it, brainstorming possible solutions, deciding on an alternative, taking the initiative, following through, and evaluating the effectiveness of the process.

Resilient families build on small successes and view mistakes as learning experiences. In the context of illness and disability, families become more resourceful as they learn to anticipate, prepare for, and avert future challenges. Creative brainstorming increases the possibilities for overcoming illness adversities. Proactive planning is vital. Families can benefit by shifting away from a crisis-reactive mode in preparation for anticipated illness challenges, as well as by considering alternatives for disease-related uncertainties (see Chapter 7 on life-cycle planning).

A systemic assessment emphasizes the process the whole family used in resolving issues and how successful the group was, viewing individual effectiveness within the context of such matters as the family's division of labor, power structure, and available resources. Observing joint problem-solving processes and inquiring about how crucial decisions are arrived at constitute important information about shared power and communication.

Regarding ongoing health issues, it is useful to ask families what kinds of important decisions are significantly affected by their family member's condition. Are there particular types of challenges they have difficulty trying to solve? For instance, one family with an aging parent with advanced dementia knew the grandmother needed to go to a nursing home and had gathered all the background information necessary to make a sound decision. They discussed the pragmatic aspects of the issue very effectively, but the decision to carry out the plan was so emotionally wrenching that they got stuck at that point in their efforts.

CONCLUSION

No single family style is inherently optimal (Walsh, 2012). Assessment of family functionality should emphasize the fit of a family's organizational and communication style with the functional requirements of an enduring chronic condition within developmental and social contexts.

CHAPTER 6

Understanding Multigenerational Experiences

A family's current behavior and therefore its response to illness cannot be adequately comprehended apart from its history (Bowen, 1993; Byng-Hall, 2004; McGoldrick et al., 2016; Walsh & McGoldrick, 2004). A multigenerational inquiry helps to clarify areas of strength and vulnerability. It also identifies high-risk families, burdened by past unresolved issues and dysfunctional patterns, who will require mental health care to absorb the challenges of a serious condition. A basic genogram and time line are useful means of tracking key events and transitions (McGoldrick, Gerson, & Petry, 2008). Such inquiry helps explain the family's current style of coping, adaptation, and meaning-making.

A chronic-illness-oriented family genogram focuses on how the current and previous generations organized and adapted over time to illnesses and unexpected crises. A central goal is bringing to light areas of consensus and "learned differences" (Penn, 1983) that are sources of cohesion, resilience, and potential conflict. Patterns of coping, replications, changes in relationships (e.g., shifting alliances and triangular patterns or complete cutoffs), and a sense of competence are noted. These patterns are transmitted across generations as sources of family pride, myths, negative expectations, and belief systems (Seaburn, Lorenz, & Kaplan, 1992). Also, it is useful to note other forms of loss, such as divorce or migration; crisis situations, such as a job loss; and protracted adversity, including poverty, racism, war, and political oppression. Positive family-of-origin experiences with illness, loss, and adversity can provide transferable sources of resilience and effective coping skills to draw on in adapting to the current situation (Walsh, 2016b).

DIFFERENT DISCIPLINES AND SETTINGS

Clinicians frequently raise questions about the amount of multigenerational information that is useful, particularly given the significant time constraints of most health and mental health providers. Whether to solicit such information and how much to gather are two separate issues. In my experience, it is almost always important to conduct a basic inquiry when someone has a chronic condition. How much information is needed depends on the clinical context and time limitations. A brief screening interview by a primary care physician, nurse, or medical social worker is different from a psychiatric consultation or psychotherapy evaluation. Here I present a comprehensive approach, with the understanding that posing only a limited number of key questions may be feasible in a crisis situation or given typical time constraints. When psychosocial care is regular or intermittent, I generally gather multigenerational information over a number of consultations or toward the beginning of treatment.

In one family practice center, the genogram was placed on the first page of the patient's chart. Routinely, the primary care physician initiated the genogram at the first appointment. As new family information was gathered or emerged, any health care provider could add or modify the genogram information. This method engaged the entire health care team. Its placement at the front of the chart emphasized its importance for excellent comprehensive care.

In this chapter, I give a brief introduction to a basic family genogram and then discuss a family health genogram through case illustrations of common multigenerational patterns and issues in health care. For a more comprehensive overview of genograms, the reader is referred to McGoldrick et al.'s (2008) excellent book *Genograms: Assessment and Intervention*.

USES OF THE FAMILY GENOGRAM

A family genogram is a very useful means of graphically presenting a family tree and showing key multigenerational patterns. A tool whose use can be learned by a broad spectrum of health care professionals, it facilitates "joining" with and getting to know families. It provides a context for other parts of a thorough systemic evaluation and enhances a clinician's ability to see the interplay of important family system events and ways of functioning. It furthers continuity and comprehensiveness of care by offering a versatile, succinct, clinical summary that can be used to quickly familiarize consultants or other providers of intermittent care with a particular case.

As McGoldrick et al. (2008) point out, "The genogram helps both the clinician and the family to see the 'larger picture'—that is, to view problems in their current and historical context. Structural, relational, and functional information about a family can be viewed on a genogram both horizontally across the family context and vertically through the generations" (p. 5). Helping a family or couple view its current situation in relation to multigenerational patterns is a valuable learning experience and furthers rapport between clinicians and families. Often, a family finds this process of sharing its history an easier first step than discussing current emotionally charged issues. Gathering multigenerational information leads the clinician to ask factual questions, which often reduces family members' anxiety. The structured genogram format helps families regain a feeling of control, an important therapeutic first step, and promotes constructive solving of condition-related challenges.

The genogram helps assess the relationship of immediate family members to one another as well as to the broader network of extended family, friends, and community supports, and to their cultural milieu. Highlighting the significance of ethnic and racial diversity, Watts-Jones (1997) describes the importance of including in genograms nonbiological "kin," who have or currently play a significant role in the patient's or family's life. Placing present issues in the context of multigenerational family patterns enables clinicians and the family to move back and forth between current and past patterns of organization, communication, and beliefs that helped or hindered families in meeting earlier adversity. It provides a means of addressing family concerns by beginning to reframe, detoxify, and normalize emotionally charged information.

Three steps are useful in creating a genogram: (1) mapping the family structure; (2) recording information about the family, including its cultural and spiritual background; and (3) describing family relationships. Excellent software programs, such as Genogram Analytics (*www.genogramanalytics.com*) and GenoPro (*www.genopro.com*) are tailored to health care contexts and family health data collection.

THE BASIC FAMILY GENOGRAM

The basic family structural map is a pictorial representation of nuclear and extended family members and significant nonfamily persons or organizations, usually encompassing three generations. Figure 6.1 shows some of the common relationship and illness symbols used later in this chapter.

Family Information and Relationships

The family structural map is fleshed out by adding information about demographics, family functioning, and critical family events. Demographic data include the ages, dates of birth, dates and causes of death, occupations, levels of education, religious affiliations, ethnic backgrounds, and geographic locations of different branches of the family.

Functional information covers medical, emotional, and behavioral patterns of key family members. Recurrent patterns, such as repeated illnesses,

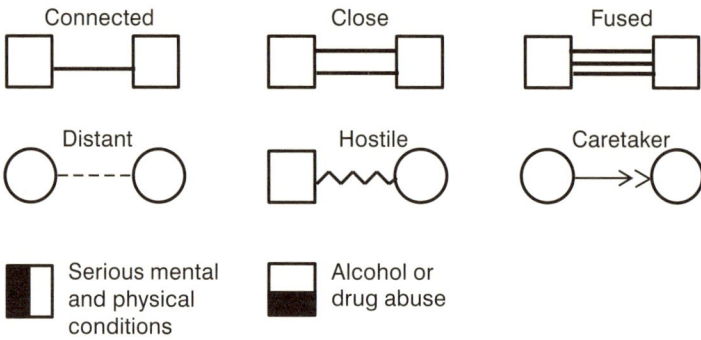

FIGURE 6.1. Genogram relationship and illness symbols.

are noted; these point to an increased biological risk of particular diseases. Less obviously, a wife's excessive anxiety about and overprotection of her husband following a mild heart attack becomes more understandable when it is learned that her father died of a massive coronary when he was the same age as her husband. Research shows that the impact of an illness is much greater when it involves a close emotional figure or one who is the primary source of financial support.

Mapping family interaction patterns helps identify healthy and problematic relationships that have to be taken into account when a family needs to establish a caregiving system. Historical examples of resilience might include strengthening family bonds, healing prior relationship hurts, and meaning-making that allowed living well in the face of adversity. Problematic patterns include substance abuse, rigidly defined gender roles, unresolved losses, and estranged survivors' relationships when a family member dies. Mutually supportive bonds, as well as particularly conflictual, distant, or ruptured relationships in the nuclear and extended family, are especially noteworthy. Dysfunctional triangles may be revealed. In cases of divorce and remarriage, relationships with biological parents, stepparents, and step- and half-siblings should be noted. Finally, the impact on relationships and family functioning of unexpected and untimely life-cycle events, such as a childhood-onset illness or divorce, is important. Descriptions of relationships and people's attributes are highly subjective; nevertheless, hearing different versions of a key family story is valuable. Understanding key family members' perspectives fosters effective collaboration.

Cultural and Spiritual Background

Developing a genogram offers a wonderful opportunity to gather vital information about a family's ethnocultural and spiritual background and beliefs.

Family traditions and beliefs are powerful factors in health behavior, especially when an illness strikes (see Chapter 8). A fundamental question to ask is what ethnic groups, religious traditions, national and racial groups, and communities do you consider yourself part of.

TIME LINE

In conjunction with a genogram, a *time line* is a very useful format for recording the dates and chronological sequence of critical family events, such as a major illness, important shifts in relationships, transitions (e.g., divorce, remarriage, job changes), migrations, losses, and successes. A time line highlights periods of great stress or change, any accumulation of multiple stressors, and meaningful anniversaries. It can also highlight the concurrence of such events with illness onset or exacerbation. For example, a child's illness flare-up may occur at the time of his noncustodial father's remarriage, especially if the father's contact and support have been erratic.

THE FAMILY HEALTH GENOGRAM

With illness or disability, a multigenerational assessment involves the same information gathering process involved in a basic family genogram, but the assessment focuses on a family's past experiences with illness, loss, crises, and adversity. It is valuable to know how each adult's family of origin organized itself as a system in response to these situations, in both current and previous generations, and how systemic patterns evolved over time. This information helps anticipate areas of conflict and consensus. Both untapped sources of resilience and unresolved multigenerational issues related to illness and loss, triggered by a current chronic condition, may suddenly reemerge.

PSYCHOSOCIAL TYPOLOGY AND TIME PHASES

The psychosocial typology and time-phases framework can be a focus for a multigenerational assessment. Tracking family members' illness experiences gives the clinician a sense of a family's breadth of experience and of its history with a particular kind of illness or a specific disease. Clinicians can use their time most effectively by attending to the most relevant experiences with illness and adversity—those with psychosocial type and time-phase characteristics similar to the current condition. How did a family organize itself to cope with a specific condition, and how did the resulting system evolve in relation to the practical and emotional demands required over time?

At the most basic level, the clinician can evaluate each adult's degree of exposure to illness and disability and his or her general beliefs about coping and coping skills. This evaluation will reveal whether the family was flexible in organizing itself to meet varying issues or tried to impose a rigid, monolithic model for adapting, regardless of the demands of different conditions. Did the family show a particular skill or vulnerability in relation to phases of an illness? Although a particular family may have handled crises and losses effectively, it may have been unable to deal successfully with a long-term condition requiring pacing and endurance. Such a family might feel vulnerable in a future encounter with a protracted illness, such as Parkinson's disease.

What has the family learned from past experiences? One family, despite its psychosocial difficulties with their father's heart condition, learned improved coping skills from that experience and adjusted accordingly when their mother developed a similar illness. Another family may be unable to learn from experience and repeat dysfunctional patterns across generations; confronted with threatened loss and death, this family may repeatedly reenact patterns of denial, inadequate preparation, and avoidance of mourning and bereavement.

One can direct historical inquiry more effectively if it is based on the anticipated psychosocial demands of the current condition. Consider a family that faces an acute-onset, unpredictable, somewhat disabling, and possibly fatal condition, such as the aftermath of a heart attack. Besides a general inquiry about the family's previous experience, one could ask specifically about illnesses or situations that involved acute or rapid change, uncertainty, disability, and living with the threat of loss and death. Asking about earlier encounters with heart disease would naturally offer the closest approximation, but encounters with similar psychosocial types of illness, such as strokes or certain cancers, would also be useful. Experiences with a disabling injury might provide insights about a family's ability to adapt to acute change and disability.

This inquiry tells us whether a family has certain standard ways of coping with any illness and whether there are vital differences in its style and success in adaptation to different types of conditions. For instance, asking about different illness types may reveal that a family dealt successfully with non-life-threatening illnesses but reeled under the weight of a mother's metastatic breast cancer. Such families might be well equipped to deal with less-severe conditions, but be particularly vulnerable if another life-threatening illness were to occur. Another family may have experienced only nonfatal illnesses and be uninformed about how to cope with the uncertainties particular to life-threatening conditions. Both families face challenges in coping with probable loss and death, but for different reasons: the former because it has been sensitized by a negative legacy, the latter because of lack of experience with a possibly fatal condition. Cognizance of these facts will draw attention to areas of strength and vulnerability in a family facing cancer or any life-threatening illness.

This information can help guide clinicians in choosing the appropriate interventions. For a high-risk family burdened by negative experiences and legacies, a brief intervention focused on relevant multigenerational patterns can help prevent a dysfunctional reenactment. Simply drawing attention to parallel situations makes covert linkages overt. Such focused intervention early on can help families to make better use of psychoeducational or ongoing support groups. Families that lack exposure to chronic conditions typically welcome early psychoeducational approaches.

Tracking a family's coping capabilities in the crisis, chronic, and terminal phases of previous chronic illnesses highlights legacies of strength and phase-specific difficulties in adaptation. One man grew up with a father who was partially disabled with heart disease and witnessed his parents' successful renegotiation of traditional gender-defined roles when his mother went to work, while his father assumed household responsibilities. This man, now with heart disease himself, has a positive legacy about gender roles from his family of origin that facilitated a flexible response to his own illness. Some families are able to express their emotions in a crisis, but may feel constrained in a later phase. One family that had a member with chronic kidney failure functioned very well with the practicalities of home dialysis. However, in the terminal phase, their limitations in expressing their emotions left a legacy of unresolved grief. In this case, tracking attuned to time phases helps clinicians to see both family strengths and vulnerabilities, and counteracts the tendency to emphasize the difficult periods and label the family as dysfunctional. A history of even partial success can be harnessed and amplified to help with the current illness situation.

LIFE-CYCLE COINCIDENCES ACROSS GENERATIONS

Coincidental dates on which life-threatening events occurred across generations is often significant. The common statement "All the men in my family died of heart attacks by the age of 55" is a multigenerational statement of biological vulnerability that signifies a legacy and expectation of untimely death. In one instance, mental and somatic symptoms began as a son approached the age at which his father had died of a sudden, unexpected heart attack in early midlife. This man distanced himself from his wife and family, believing he would spare them the pain he had suffered when his own beloved father died. In a similar case, a man vulnerable to stomach ulcers began to eat indiscriminately and drink alcohol excessively, despite medical warnings, when he reached the age of 43, precipitating a crisis requiring surgery. His failure to comply with treatment created a life-threatening situation. It was only after his recovery and upon his 44th birthday that he remarked that his own father had died tragically at age 43, and that he had felt an overpowering conflict about surviving past that age.

Knowledge of such age-related multigenerational patterns can alert a clinician to the risks of unexplained medical symptoms, such as pain, and somatization, adherence issues, blatantly self-destructive behaviors, and realistic fears that may emerge at the time of an illness diagnosis or at a particular life-cycle phase of the patient or a family member (see Chapter 7). It is not uncommon for the onset of a family member's symptoms, particularly somatic complaints, to coincide with the diagnosis of a serious disorder or death of another member. A similar pattern is sometimes seen in pain syndromes in which a medical workup is inconclusive. Uncovering a temporal relationship between the onset of symptoms and a concurrent or previous traumatic family crisis facilitates a clearer biopsychosocial treatment strategy that helps prevent or interrupt such a multigenerational family pattern.

FAMILY PROCESSES

Clinicians can get a picture of multigenerational family processes related to major health conditions in an adult's family of origin.

Structural and Practical Issues

Organizational patterns that were used to cope with past conditions suggest the preferred system a family will fall back on in a health crisis. This includes family hierarchy, designated roles, and boundaries within the family and between family members and their community and health care team. Some questions to consider exploring to elicit family organizational strengths and vulnerabilities include:

- Did these organizational shifts represent a sharp change for the family? This question provides information about the family's ability to adapt its usual organization to the increased and distinct demands of chronic conditions.
- Were these family structures appropriate and functional for the particular situation?
- Did the family "illness organization" persist dysfunctionally beyond the situation? This question clarifies whether a family became frozen in time at a particular illness phase or never completely recovered. Did this happen through inertia, a lack of understanding, or an inability to let go or move on?
- What particular role did each adult and their parents play in these situations?
- What did their experience mean to them and what did they learn?

Affective Issues

Clinicians can also learn how a family managed affective issues by asking questions, such as the following:

- Did communication about an illness stick to just pragmatic issues, or was there an ability to share emotions? Were certain emotions, such as anger, sadness, grief, fear, and love, avoided?
- Were there gender-related patterns in which men displayed anger, but not grief, and the opposite was true for women?
- Were there particular patterns for adults compared with children, for example, a generational barrier that allowed parents, but not children, to communicate feelings?
- Were these patterns cultural, based on fear of losing control, a previous catastrophic experience, or other factors? Secrecy, as distinct from communicating age-appropriate information, is often dysfunctional with chronic conditions.

Past Experience with Health Care Professionals

It is valuable to know the family's history and pattern of relationships with physicians and other health care providers (see Chapter 18). Some questions to consider are the following:

- Did the family tend to delegate one family member (often the wife or mother) to communicate with the health care provider(s)?
- Did the family make its own wishes known, or did it modify a usual style of assertiveness to one of deference to accommodate a physician who wanted to be completely in charge without being questioned?
- What norms existed about sharing feelings with one's physician?
- Did family members hide their feelings from any of the health care providers? If so, why?
- Did the physician relate to the family in an unemotional, technical, businesslike way to which the family responded in kind?
- Did a warm relationship with a family doctor make it difficult to deal with the segmented, more hierarchical relationships that are common in large, impersonal hospitals or that are dictated by a disease requiring a number of specialists?

Personal Roles

It is useful to know what the practical and emotional responsibilities of individual family members were. What did they learn from those experiences that influences how they think about the current illness? What would they want to do similarly or differently? Are there aspects of the current situation that they feel confident, insecure, or terrified about? Did members emerge from relevant experiences with a strong sense of competence, failure, or fear?

When they were children, were parents given too much responsibility or shielded from involvement in family affairs? In one case involving a family with three generations of hemophilia transmitted through the mother, the father, as a child, had been shielded from the knowledge that his older brother, who died in adolescence, had developed a fatal kind of kidney disease. He had not been allowed to attend his brother's funeral. That trauma gave rise to a strong commitment to openness about disease-related issues with his two sons, who had hemophilia, and with his daughters, who were genetic carriers.

GENERAL EXPERIENCES WITH CRISIS AND ADVERSITY

Often families do not understand how their experiences with other forms of adversity can be applied resourcefully to a major health condition. Clinician inquiry enables families to link the two experiences and tap into resources and stories of resilience that they may not have considered. For instance, one family's experience with a flood that destroyed its home generated important insights about how the members pulled together in a crisis, juggled strong emotions simultaneously with huge logistical problems, and made use of resources outside the family. This past experience gives the clinician some idea of how the same family might manage illnesses with an acute-onset, moderate-to-severe sudden incapacitation, or rapid relapse. Managing such conditions require quick and efficient family mobilization of crisis skills.

Similarly, a family's protracted struggle with poverty, for example, may give vital clues to its hardiness when confronted with a persistent condition such as a TBI or developmental impairment in a child with autism or cerebral palsy—conditions that require endurance, perseverance, and skill in dealing with prejudice. A family history of effective coping with ongoing major stressors is a good predictor of family adjustment to these types of illness.

Individuals can vary tremendously in terms of their experience with illness, despite evidence of resilience with other adversity. A mother may have endured the complexities of divorce and abandonment by her father, yet never dealt with a serious illness. A clinician can help her draw appropriately on her earlier experiences and coping skills so that she can apply them to her current situation of caring for a husband whose cancer is fatal. The strengths she acquired as a child can assist her in dealing with her own children as they confront their father's death. Awareness of traumatic experiences that were beyond her control as a youth are important in facing an illness whose outcome may be beyond personal control, but a clinician can also help her differentiate the present situation from the past and guide her in making pragmatic choices today about how to cope with her children's distress.

CASE EXAMPLES

Inexperience

A family consultation highlights the importance of gathering a family history to uncover dormant areas of inexperience.

Joe, his wife, Pat, both of Scottish ancestry, and their three teenage children presented for a family evaluation 10 months after Joe's diagnosis of moderate-to-severe asthma. Joe, age 44, had been successfully employed for many years as a spray painter. Apparently, exposure to a new chemical in the paint triggered the onset of asthmatic attacks, which necessitated hospitalization and job disability. Initially, his physician had told him that once he ceased spray painting, his condition might disappear, improve somewhat, or progress to include other triggers in his daily environment. The physician was noncommittal concerning the possible chronicity of the asthma and how severe it might become. Although somewhat improved, Joe continued to have persistent, moderate respiratory symptoms.

Joe had a history of alcoholism that had been in complete remission for 20 years. There was no family history of other emotional difficulties.

During the 8 months after his initial diagnosis, Joe's condition did not improve, and he developed symptoms of asthma at home in response to other environmental triggers. His continued breathing difficulties contributed to a depression, uncharacteristic angry outbursts, alcohol abuse, and family discord. This finally led to hospitalization for alcohol detoxification and treatment for depression.

During the initial assessment, I inquired about the family's previous experience in coping with chronic disease and learned that this was the nuclear family's first such encounter. In their families of origin, they had limited relevant experience. Pat's father had died 7 years earlier of a sudden and unexpected heart attack. Joe's brother had died in an accidental drowning. Neither had any history of experience with disease as an ongoing process. Illness for both had meant either death or recovery. Joe had assumed that improvement meant cure. The physician and family system were not attuned to the hidden risks for this family going through the transition from the crisis to the chronic phase of his asthma—the juncture at which the permanency of the disease needed to be addressed. The history of alcoholism presented another risk factor that compounded this couple's difficulty in coping with a chronic illness in which the prognosis was uncertain.

Retrospectively, it is evident that this crisis could have been prevented if a provider took the uncertain prognosis into account in conjunction with the family histories during a physical and psychosocial checkup roughly 6 months after Joe's diagnosis. At that point, enough time would have elapsed for the physician to offer a revised prognosis, one that involved the likelihood of chronicity, and family members probably would have had sufficient time to deal with their disappointment and make the transition to acceptance of a chronic condition before a downward emotional spiral could lead to a family crisis.

This case highlights the importance of gathering multigenerational information from the entire family. Sometimes one member's lack of, or negative, experience can be counterbalanced by another member's successful experience in coping with a similar type of illness or adversity. One member can guide another and provide within-family psychoeducation.

In terms of the FSI model, this family lacked experience with a relapsing, intermittently disabling chronic illness. This vulnerability, combined with the history of alcoholism, made them susceptible to the stress inherent in the transition from the crisis to the chronic phase, particularly in terms of the developmental task of accepting the condition's permanency.

Illness Type, Time Phase, and Unresolved Loss

The following case example illustrates the difficulties in coping with a current illness that were fueled by unresolved issues related to a particular disease type or phase in one's family of origin.

Mary, her husband, Bill, and their 8-year old son, Jim, were a Catholic, Italian–Irish working-class family. They presented for treatment 4 months after Mary had been injured in a life-threatening head-on auto collision. The teenage driver of the other vehicle was at fault. Mary had sustained a serious concussion. Initially, the medical team was concerned that she might have suffered a cerebral hemorrhage. Ultimately, it was determined that this had not occurred. Mary's physicians assured her that there was no bleeding and that she could expect a full recovery. Nevertheless, over this time, Mary became increasingly depressed and, despite strong reassurance, continued to believe she had a life-threatening condition and would die from a brain hemorrhage.

During the initial consultation, she revealed that she was experiencing vivid dreams of meeting her deceased father. Her father, with whom she had been extremely close, had died of a cerebral hemorrhage after a 4-year history of a progressive, debilitating brain tumor. Toward the terminal phase, his illness had been marked by progressive and uncontrolled epileptic seizures. Mary was 14 at the time, and was the "baby" in the family, her two siblings being more than 10 years her senior. The family had shielded her from his illness, culminating in her mother deciding to not have Mary attend either her father's wake or the funeral. This event cemented her position as a child in need of protection, a dynamic that carried over into her marriage. Despite her hurt and anger and lack of acceptance of her father's death, she had avoided dealing with her feelings with her mother for over 20 years.

Additional family history revealed that her uncle had died from a work-related head injury. Further, her maternal grandfather had died of a stroke when Mary's mother was 7 years old. Her mother had had to endure a wake with an open casket for 3 days at home. This traumatic experience was a major factor in her mother's attempt to protect Mary from the same kind of memory.

Mary's own life-threatening head injury triggered a catastrophic reaction and a dramatic resurfacing of unresolved traumatic losses involving similar types

Understanding Multigenerational Experiences 101

of illness and injury. In particular, her father's, uncle's, and grandfather's deaths from head injuries and central nervous system disorders had sensitized her to this type of problem. The fact that she had witnessed the slow, agonizing, and terrifying downhill course of her father only heightened her catastrophic fears.

Her mother's protection of Mary is largely clarified by the genogram in Figure 6.2 and sessions in which she was involved. Her mother had felt traumatized by the open casket in the living room at the time of her own father's death. As a result, she vowed that she would never let her own children experience the same kind of trauma. As is common in multigenerational patterns, the mother's attempt to spare her own daughter the trauma she endured had the opposite effect when her own daughter had to deal with death. This pattern unfortunately created a new problem of unresolved loss that surfaced in the context of Mary's head injury.

The recurring pattern of treating Mary as the child to be protected was solidified at the time of her father's death. One important expression of this pattern was that Mary's mother always communicated important sensitive information through Mary's husband. Over the years of their marriage, he had colluded in treating Mary protectively, which served as a source of power for him in their marital relationship. Mary, for her part, had never discussed her feelings about not being permitted to attend her father's funeral because she felt her mother had had a hard enough life without reviving old hurts.

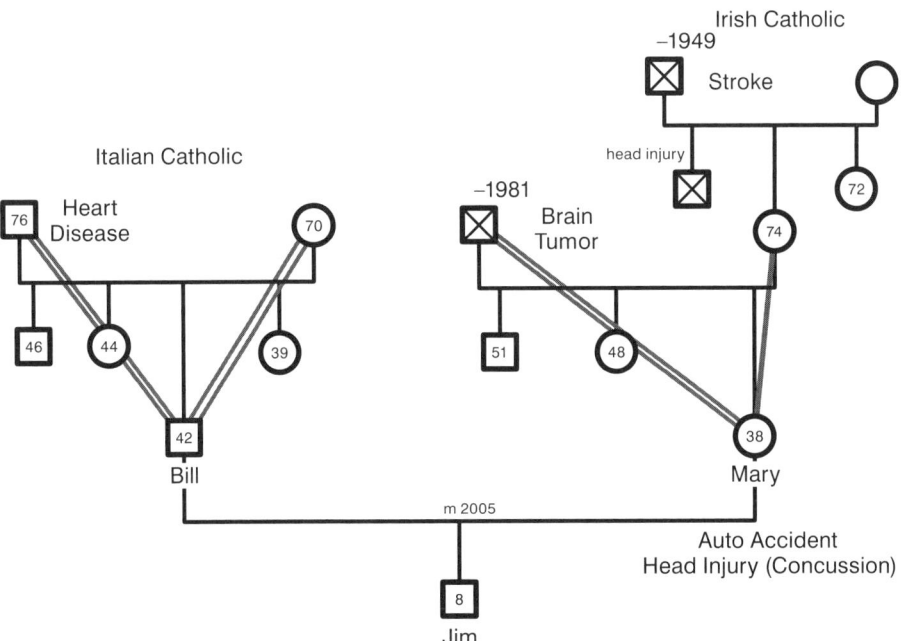

FIGURE 6.2. Multigenerational legacies based on illness type, time phase, and unresolved loss.

A clinician might wonder whether Mary was vulnerable to any physical problem or major stressor. In fact, a kidney complication that developed during her first pregnancy had precluded her from having more children and, naturally, affected the couple's family planning. At that time the couple grieved; but Mary did not develop the sort of disabling, catastrophic reaction that had occurred in the present situation, in which the prognosis was favorable. As happens in many cases, an unresolved loss or catastrophic fear can remain encapsulated and walled off until rekindled by a crisis—in this instance medical—whose characteristics closely resemble the original experience. In Mary's situation, the initially life-threatening involvement of the central nervous system was a sufficient stimulus.

The family therapy focused on a series of tasks and rituals that involved Mary's family of origin. Her husband, Bill, participated in most sessions and, on occasion, her 8-year-old son did as well. For several reasons it was particularly important to include Bill. First, interventions focused on changing her pattern of interaction with her mother would likely alter the customary pattern of interaction and hierarchy in the marriage, which closely paralleled that with her mother. Second, Bill had aging parents with heart disease and preferred to minimize the risks of losing them. Bill could have undermined Mary's efforts to address issues of threatened loss and death in her own family, because of his fears regarding his own aging parents. Conjoint sessions provided an opportunity for both Mary and Bill to address these issues together.

Because Mary had enormous difficulty expressing anger, she was coached to write a letter to the teenager who had been responsible for the accident. Although she did not mail the letter (owing to pending litigation), writing and sharing it with her husband were very helpful to her.

Next, Mary initiated a series of conversations with her mother about her feelings of having been excluded from her father's funeral and about the pattern of mutual protection between mother and daughter in the past. A more open relationship between mother and daughter facilitated the next stage of treatment, which involved Mary's saying good-bye to her father. Her first attempts to write a good-bye letter seemed as if she were writing to someone still alive, trying to enable him to catch up on the last 24 years. Over a 3-month period, Mary did compose a real farewell letter to her father, experiencing the grief that she had bypassed for so long. Bill needed reassurance because he initially interpreted her grief as regression, while also activating concerns about the looming loss of his own parents.

The final phase of treatment involved a graveside ritual in which Mary, with her family of origin and nuclear family present, read her good-bye letter to her father. This ritual brought closure, for all the family members, to unfinished family issues related to her father's death.

The choice of treatment was critical in this case. At first, Mary was extremely depressed. Many clinicians might have chosen to treat her immediately with antidepressants. Although I considered that option, I found that focusing on the connection between her reaction to her head injury and her unresolved issues related to loss reduced her level of depression and panic sufficiently to obviate the need for pharmacological intervention. Making these connections gave her a better sense of control. Validation of her unfinished story by me as a health care provider and by her husband as her best friend laid a foundation to reenter, rework, and finish the story.

Replication of System Patterns

An evaluation of the system that existed and evolved around a previous illness includes assessment of the pattern of relationships within that system. In many families, relationship patterns are adaptive, flexible, and cohesively balanced. In other families, these relationships can be dysfunctionally skewed, rigid, enmeshed, disengaged, and triangulated. Particular coalitions that emerge in the context of a chronic illness can be isomorphs of those that existed in each adult's family of origin. The following case is a good example.

Matt and Ann had been married for 9 years when their 6-year-old son, Jeff, developed type 1 diabetes. Soon thereafter, Ann became very protective of her son and made frequent calls to their pediatrician expressing persistent concerns about Jeff's condition. This occurred despite Jeff's doing well medically and emotionally and frequent reassurances from the physician. At the same time, the previously close marital relationship became more distant, characterized by Ann arguing with her husband, and Matt distancing himself from his wife and son.

Ann had grown up with a tyrannical, alcoholic father. She had witnessed intense conflict between her parents. During her childhood and adolescence, she had tried to rescue her unhappy mother. To counterbalance her victimized mother, she tried to tend to her mother's needs and cheer her up. She talked frequently to her family physician about the situation at home. However, she felt that she had failed at helping her mother since she continued for many years to be stuck and depressed.

Matt grew up in a family in which his father developed disabling heart disease when Matt was 5. His mother devoted a great deal of time to taking care of his father. Not to further burden his parents, he reared himself, remaining distanced from the primary caregiving relationship between his parents. He supported his mother's caregiving efforts by mostly taking care of his own needs, and he stoically viewed this strategy as successful. (See Figure 6.3.)

With their son's illness, Ann, burdened by feelings of guilt at being a failed rescuer, had a second chance to "do it right" and assuage her guilt. Her son's diabetes gave her this opportunity, and it is a culturally sanctioned, normative role for a parent, particularly a mother, to be the protector of an ill child. These factors—her unresolved family-of-origin issues and the culturally sanctioned roles—promoted the overprotectiveness that developed with her son. Moreover, since she had derived support from the family physician concerning her situation as she was growing up, she actively sought and expected support from her son's pediatrician.

Ann unconsciously pushed her husband away, because in her family of origin she had viewed rescuing her mother within the context of battling her father. She fully transposed the pattern of relationships by rescuing her son while keeping her husband at a distance.

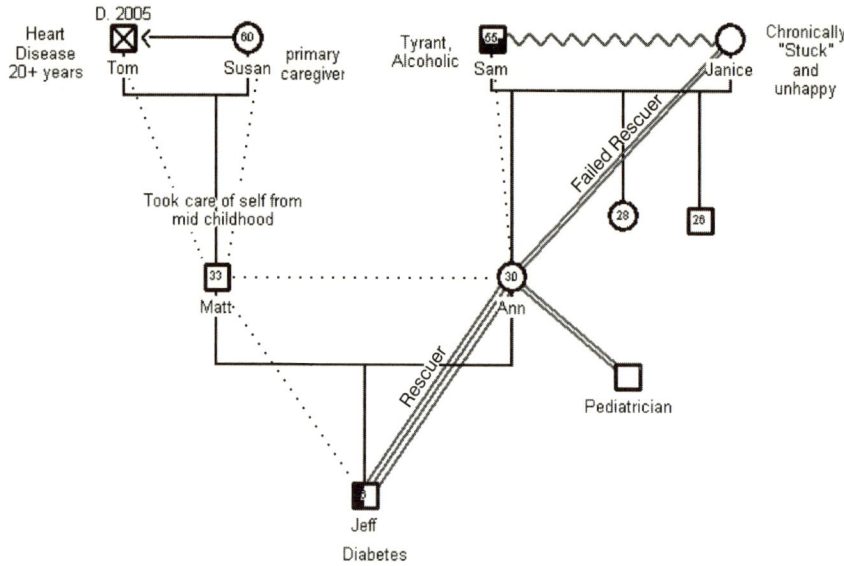

FIGURE 6.3. Multigenerational replication of patterns of involvement with illness.

In this situation, Matt, though outwardly objecting to the coalition between his wife and son, honored their relationship, as if it would make up for the one he had forfeited with his own mother. Further, despite his unmet needs as a child, he believed that the structure, and his role in it, had worked. Hence, he distanced himself to allow the paradigm to flourish, that of the caregiving relationship he saw between his parents and now between his wife and son.

Both Matt and Ann replicated their particular positions in triangles from their families of origin. In a complementary way, Ann was a rescuer in a coalition, and Matt was in the distant position in the triangle they created with their son. The roles of each person in this triangle fit traditional cultural norms. The mother was appropriately concerned and attending to her ill child. The father was in a more distant, instrumental provider position. For this reason, it can be more difficult for a clinician to ferret out a traditional pattern from the beginnings of a dysfunctional reenactment of family-of-origin patterns.

Early assessment of multigenerational patterns such as these helps distinguish normative from problematic responses. Additionally, it helps identify the source and degree of commitment to gender-defined caregiving roles. Particularly in crisis situations, such as illness onset, couples may fall back on traditional divisions of labor, particularly if they have worked well in previous situations of illness or crisis. The climate of fear and uncertainty itself is a powerful stimulus for seeking the familiar, time-tested methods of coping. Or, as this case highlights, a sense of failure around a gender-based role can act as a powerful push toward reenactment in the current situation. In this case, Ann felt she let her mother down in relation to her father's alcoholism. Psychoeducational guidelines can help her to distinguish what forms and degree of responsiveness are appropriate from those that are excessive and unhelpful. Also, tasks that can be done by the husband and couple jointly would be useful to increase a more balanced, shared involvement in coping with the burdens of a chronically ill child and would counteract the peripheral position of the father.

In this case, an early referral by the pediatrician was essential in preventing entrenchment of a dysfunctional relationship pattern. At this early stage, the parents were able to reflect upon the situation, recognize the connection to family-of-origin issues, and disengage from a destructive path. A brief intervention of three sessions was sufficient. If these kinds of problems are not detected early, they typically progress over a period of years to highly enmeshed, intractable systems. The likelihood of morbidity is high and may be expressed in a poor medical course and adherence issues, a possible divorce, or child and adolescent behavioral problems that end up in the hospital's emergency department.

Reenactment of previous systemic illness patterns can occur as an unconscious, automatic process (Byng-Hall, 2004). Moreover, the dysfunctional complementarity can emerge specifically within the context of a chronic disease. When asked, couples frequently reveal a tacit, unspoken understanding that if an illness occurs they will reorganize to reenact unfinished business from their families of origin. Typically, the roles chosen represent a repetition or a reactive opposite of the roles played by them or the same-sex parent in their family of origin. This process resembles the expression of a genetic template that is activated only under particular biological conditions. It highlights the need for a clinician to distinguish between what constitutes a functional family process with and without illness or disability. For families that present in this manner, placing primary therapeutic emphasis on the resolution of family-of-origin issues may be the best approach to prevent or rectify an unhealthy pattern.

Multiple Chronic Disorders

Many families facing chronic conditions have had functional multigenerational patterns of adaptation, but an assessment reveals multiple, stressful, chronic conditions in the immediate or extended family—a prescription for potential caregiving overload. Couples in later life are a prime example. A typical scenario might involve a couple in the child-rearing phase who have two sets of aging parents. It is vital to inquire about the health of all living parents. A situation in which one of the wife's parents has a progressive disease might be compounded by the failing health of the husband's sole surviving parent. Chapter 12 discusses clinical issues for families with aging parents.

Any family may falter in the face of multiple disease and nondisease stressors that converge in a relatively short time. For progressively disabling conditions or the occurrence of illnesses in several family members, a pragmatic approach that expands the use of resources outside the family is the most productive. It is useful to know both multigenerational patterns and the cultural norms for a family's inclusion of extended family, friends, community-based support groups, and professional caregiving services (e.g., home health aides, visiting nurses, and/or mental health professionals). Families with flexible rules for inclusion of others have an advantage.

Multigenerational Dysfunctional Family Patterns

Distinct from families that have dormant, encapsulated "time bombs" are those in which illnesses become embedded within a web of pervasive and long-standing dysfunctional patterns. In this situation, clinicians should avoid collusion with a family's resistance to addressing preexisting issues by focusing excessively on the disease itself. If clinicians collude, they become involved in a detouring triangle with the family and the patient, analogous to the dysfunctional triangles formed by parents deflecting unresolved marital issues by overly focusing on an ill child (Minuchin, Rosman, & Baker, 1978).

Some families express difficulties psychosomatically. It is valuable to identify multigenerational patterns in which stressors are easily translated into somatic reactions or in which family communication is problematic or blocked and is transacted through bodily symptoms (Griffith & Griffith, 1994). This dysfunctional psychosomatic pattern needs to be distinguished from the more normative clustering of illnesses commonly found during periods of major family or personal stress. Persistent patterns that tend toward more immediate somatic reactions differ from the physical letdowns that can occur in the exhaustion phase of an illness or in the aftermath of any major stressor.

Families with multigenerational psychosomatic patterns have distinct safety valve mechanisms. Somatic expression can signal impending system overload and modulate what are perceived as dangerous situations and transactions. These families can resemble some of those that are coping with chronic mental disorders. When a chronic physical disorder exists, the risks of serious recurrences may be higher because the pathway of somatic reactivity now includes a physically vulnerable member, such as one with severe asthma.

In the traditional sense of "psychosomatic," this kind of severe family dysfunction predisposes a family to a higher level of baseline reactivity. When an illness enters its system, the reactivity can get expressed somatically through poor treatment adherence and medical course. Multigenerational assessment of the origins and severity of the dysfunction and a potential resistance to change can inform a clinical approach, but initial interventions may need to be more focused on current nuclear family processes than on multigenerational patterns.

In one case, Joe, a 40-year-old man with a history of chronic depression and repeated hospitalizations, was admitted to a psychiatric day treatment program. He had always lived with his parents and received disability income. He had a longstanding somatic preoccupation with his lips and mouth, considering them deformed. This symptom metaphorically and literally kept his lips sealed about important family matters. His father suffered from a chronic heart condition.

Joe initially responded extremely well to the treatment program and became more forthcoming. Within a week, his father developed a life-threatening exacerbation of his heart condition. The admitting clinician was not aware of a multigenerational pattern. The history later revealed that on at least two other occasions, one in Joe's nuclear family and one in his extended family, open communication had been followed by serious physical crises. Over the years, Joe's mental condition had acted as a thermostat that regulated all communication perceived as dangerous. Whenever change began, their basic mechanism to deal with an unacceptable risk, through physical and mental symptoms, could be used by a vulnerable member, in this case the father.

Had this history been known at the outset, a different therapeutic strategy sensitive to this family's somatic reactivity would have been chosen. It might have included a family assessment in the home at the time of Joe's admission to the day program. The assessment would have included his disabled father, who could not participate at the program site. Also, a more thorough tracking of the possible functions that Joe's symptoms served for the family and of the risks to the entire system that change might bring would have facilitated a more strategic intervention. An emphasis on small changes might have allowed family concerns to emerge in a less dramatic fashion.

This kind of more serious family dysfunction needs to be distinguished from common presenting situations in which communication is avoided because of an exaggerated fear of killing a vulnerable member or causing a medical crisis by upsetting someone. An awareness of the real medical vulnerabilities and probabilities associated with different disorders is crucial. Clinicians need to be mindful that avoidance of family meetings can collude with the family's own fear of the destructive impact of open dialogue. The key for providers is how to intervene most effectively, and they may need to actively interrupt dysfunctional interactions and guide families to communicate within safe limits so that important and needed discussions will take place.

CHAPTER 7

Addressing Life-Cycle Issues with Chronic Conditions

The dimension of time becomes paramount when a condition is chronic. The family as a whole and each member face the formidable challenge of focusing on the present while looking toward the future. They must master the practical and emotional tasks of the immediate situation, while charting a complex and uncertain course forward. Families and clinicians need an effective way to utilize the dimension of time for comprehending both the present and future. This understanding can shape decisions on the timing and types of consultations or interventions. Placing the unfolding of chronic conditions in a developmental framework facilitates this endeavor. To do this effectively requires understanding the intertwining of three evolving threads: illness, individual members, and family development.

The psychosocial typology and time phases of illness framework furthers an understanding of the illness thread. The ongoing interaction of individual and family development should always be considered. The particular impact of a chronic disorder on the development of each family member will depend on their ages at diagnosis, their core commitments, their future plans, and the timing in the family life cycle. With a serious health condition, the phase in the family life cycle significantly shapes—and is shaped by—each member's developmental stage. For instance, the relational imbalances that often develop between spouses require both an individual and a family developmental perspective (see Chapter 14).

As noted previously, individuals are living longer with serious health conditions. Adults in their seventies and beyond increasingly lead productive and satisfying lives. Children and younger adults with serious, life-threatening disorders, who in the past would have died early, now may live for decades, even into old age. For instance, formerly, children with cystic fibrosis rarely survived to adulthood. Now most of those affected reach young adulthood, albeit with long-term challenges. Medical advances have swelled both the number and proportion of families managing chronic conditions for many years.

Chronic diseases can severely disrupt the usual sense of continuity and the rhythm of the life cycle. Illnesses and losses that occur earlier in the life course tend to be developmentally the most disruptive. The timing of an unexpected illness event shapes both the form of adaptation and subsequent developmental pathways. It's useful to link individual and family developmental perspectives through the core concepts discussed next: life-cycle phases, life structure, and the evolving psychosocial demands of a chronic illness.

CORE LIFE-CYCLE CONCEPTS

The Life Cycle

A life-cycle framework encompasses major life phases and transitions. These include expected events, such as birth, childhood and adolescence, marriage or partnership, child rearing, later life, and death, and less predictable events, such as divorce, migration, and untimely illness.

Older life-cycle models assumed a universal progression of sequential life stages, with individual, family, or illness judged by normative standards. Contemporary life-span research and contextual postmodern perspectives have eschewed a single model of "healthy" development in light of the growing diversity and fluidity of individual and relational patterns over the life course (Elder & Shanahan, 2006; Walsh, 2012). Divorce, remarriage, repartnering, stepparenting configurations, and periods of single living are increasingly common. Many lives evolve into more complex, expanding relational networks over time, within and across households. Some individuals begin a family at midlife; some people with adolescent or grown children remarry and start a second family; others have no children. Yet, most envision a life course that includes a committed relationship, procreation, and child rearing. Most plan their lives in relation to these hopes and dreams, which can be interrupted and altered by serious illness.

Family life-cycle models have tended to divide family development into stages demarcated by nodal events, such as marriage or the birth of a first child. McGoldrick et al. (2016) describe the following family life-cycle stages: (1) emerging young adults, (2) couple formation: the joining of families, (3) families with young children, (4) families with adolescents, (5) launching children and moving on in midlife, (6) families in late middle age, and (7) families nearing the end of life. While not all individuals experience this sequential progression, predictable emotional processes and life challenges and tasks are associated with each life-cycle stage. Beginnings and endings, such as birth, illness, aging, and death, while varying in timing and specificity, remain part of our human condition.

Life-cycle issues also must be considered in relation to the major influences of ethnocultural, socioeconomic, gender, religious, and racial variations, and access to community resources and health care. The dominant European American ideal of the two-parent nuclear family, guided by the values of individualism and autonomy, has been touted as the hallmark of healthy development. Viewed from a diverse multicultural perspective, this narrow ideology is at odds with the values of collectivistic, extended family systems favoring interdependence and mutual help throughout life (Falicov, 2013). For example, many white middle class families experience elder caregiving as a burden that interferes with individual strivings. Groups guided by family-centered loyalty traditions, such as Latinos, Asians, or African Americans, may view elder care more as an expected and honored family life phase.

Life Structure

A second core concept is life structure, which refers to the elements of individual and family life at a particular point in the life cycle (Levinson, 1986). Examples of such elements include work, love relationships, child rearing, religious and spiritual resources, community involvements, leisure, and caregiving. Although life structure was originally studied in the individual, the general concept can be usefully applied to the family as a unit. It encompasses reciprocal relationships with various significant others in the broader ecosystem (e.g., the community, various institutions, and the larger culture). Life structure evolves over the life cycle, with the relative importance of different components (e.g., love relationships vs. occupation) changing over time.

What illness, individual, and family development have in common is the notion of phases, each with its own priorities. For instance, the major tasks of emerging adulthood are to redefine one's relationship to the family of origin and to begin establishing an early-adult life structure. A basic goal in later adulthood is gaining a sense of integrity about the life one has lived in light of approaching mortality.

Levinson (1986), in his model of individual adult development, describes how life structures can alternate between periods of transition and periods of building or maintaining stability. In a transition period one weighs different possibilities for personal and family life, eventually deciding on and drawing up blueprints for the next phase, and then living them out in the ensuing building/maintaining period. The actual timing and possibilities may be affected by assets or barriers related to culture, race, class, gender, and sexual orientation.

Transition periods are sometimes quite fluid. Previous individual, family, and illness life structures are reappraised in light of new developmental challenges that may involve major changes rather than minor alterations. As I will illustrate later, alternating transition and structure-maintaining phases are particularly relevant to chronic disorders.

Major events, such as a disability, can color the nature of a developmental period and, in turn, be colored by their timing in individual development. A combat-related TBI in a young adult returning from military service could profoundly affect that person's abilities and options for meaningful adult relationships and a career. If the young adult is single, he or she might return to the family of origin for economic support and caregiving. If he or she is married, the injury could significantly affect the young couple in myriad ways, including plans for having children.

Family Life-Cycle Phases: Child Rearing and Non-Child Rearing

The typical family life cycle oscillates between developmental phases that require intense bonding and an inside-the-family focus, as in early child rearing, and phases during which the external family boundary is loosened, often emphasizing increased personal identity and autonomy (Combrinck-Graham, 1985), which are characteristic of families with emerging young adults. This suggests a fit between family developmental tasks and the relative need for family members to direct their energies inside the family and work together to accomplish those tasks.

Unifying Concepts

To summarize, the following concepts provide a foundation for understanding the experience of chronic disorders and the fit among the phases of illness, individual, and family development. Each phase in these three kinds of development poses priorities and challenges that progress more or less in sync.

1. Transition phases and life-structure building or maintaining phases alternate in both individual and family development.
2. Child rearing and non-child-rearing phases in the family life cycle require relatively greater or lesser degrees of family teamwork.
3. There are typically periods of higher and lower psychosocial demands over a chronic condition's course.

The FSI model uses these overarching concepts in concert with specific life-cycle events as a way of directing our attention to the interaction of individual, family, and illness development.

INTEGRATING INDIVIDUAL, FAMILY, AND ILLNESS DEVELOPMENT IN CLINICAL PRACTICE

In clinical assessment, basic questions include:

- What is the relationship among the practical and the emotional demands of an illness, the family and individual life structures, and the developmental challenges at this particular point in time?
- How will this change as the illness unfolds in relation to the family life cycle and the developmental passages of each member?

The nature of the fit between life cycle and illness will influence the kinds of challenges faced.

Serious health conditions tend to push individual and family developmental processes toward transition and an increased need for cohesion and teamwork. This tendency varies tremendously according to the specific type and phase of a condition. In family developmental models, periods of increased cohesion can begin when a new child is born, which propels the family into a prolonged period of socialization of children. Analogous to the addition of a new family member, illness onset sets in motion an inside-the-family focused process of socialization to illness. Illness symptoms, a loss of functioning, the demands of shifting or acquiring new illness-related roles, and fears of further disability and/or death all motivate a family to work together.

Non-Child-Rearing Phases

If an illness onset coincides with non-child-rearing phases, it may conflict with individual and family developmental priorities and may derail a family's natural momentum. For example, the inherently great demands of a new illness for cohesion and caregiving may collide with other salient demands in the post-launching period in the family life cycle. For an affected early adult, this may require a heightened dependency and return to the family of origin for caregiving. The greater autonomy and separate developmental pathways of parents and young adult are affected if separate interests and priorities must be relinquished or put on hold, as in the following case.

Alan, age 25, was a passenger in a serious automobile accident 5 years earlier, while away at college. He suffered a severe TBI and was hospitalized for almost a year, undergoing more than 15 operations, followed by rehabilitation. Subsequently, he returned home to live with his mother, Mrs. S., a widow for 10 years. His older brother, who was married, had a blossoming career, and lived at a distance.

At the time of referral, Alan had tried unsuccessfully to return to school, but found the workload beyond his capacity. He had been at home for 2 years, helping around the house, with no plans for the future. Unable to drive, his mother had to take him to appointments or to visit family or friends.

Mrs. S., in her early 50s, had a full-time job and a romantic relationship of 6 years. After the accident, she was forced to table tentative plans to move forward and live with her partner. Moreover, she looked after her own mother and her father, both close to 80, who still lived independently in a nearby apartment. Her father had had a minor stroke a year before Alan's accident.

This case is typical of families that I have worked with at this life-cycle phase. Alan's head injury halted his early adult career plans and the family's developmental course, particularly his own and that of his mother. Mrs. S., a widow in the post-child-rearing phase, became the sole caregiver for her young adult son, on top of caring for her elderly parents, both of which affected plans to move forward in her evolving couple relationship. They adaptively constructed a more cohesive family structure to cope with the ongoing demands of Alan's TBI, which was now in the chronic phase, and living with long-term disability.

The goal of treatment was to try to resume, to the extent possible, their more natural developmental trajectory within the real constraints of Alan's permanent disability. This meant that the family needed to consider making the following changes.

1. Alan had to redefine his career goals more modestly by entering vocational rehabilitation.
2. Alan had to gradually attempt some independent activities, such as exploring other modes of transportation and initiating social contacts.
3. Mrs. S. had to focus more on her own needs and ask Alan to do more chores at home, spend more time with her partner, and explore assisted living and caregiving options for her aging parents.

Two years later, Alan has his license and a job, drives himself to work, and has been considering the possibility of getting his own apartment. Mrs. S. regularly spends weekends with her partner and is again making future plans to live together. Her parents have moved into a retirement community that provides meals and other social support services.

Sometimes, when people are diverted from personal developmental goals, they need to go back to the point at which they were sidetracked and attempt to resume their original developmental path, even if it may be unrealistic. Clinicians need to help other family members understand that failing to achieve their original goal may be a necessary step in the grieving and loss process. Alan's disability precluded returning to college, but he needed to try it before he could more fully accept his limitations and move on. This developmental need for closure has to be balanced against the possible physical risks involved in challenging limits or in situations of destructive denial. For example, a young man who had a massive heart attack and was at a high risk for a life-threatening recurrence had to give up rejoining his training class to become a police officer.

Family processes, as well as disease severity, influence whether the family's reversion to a child-rearing-like structure is a temporary detour or a long-term reversal. The more severe the condition, the more difficulty a family will have in resuming its previous developmental course. In the case of Alan, even with a successful intervention, the permanence of his brain damage imposed some real limits on eliminating an ongoing support system. This need will continue to impose an inward pull on the future life-cycle phases of all involved family members.

Child-Rearing Phase

When disease onset coincides with the child-rearing phase in family development, it can prolong this period. At worst, the family can become enmeshed and stuck. When the inward pull of the illness and the phase of the life cycle coincide, there is a risk that they will amplify one another. In families that functioned marginally before an illness began, this timing can trigger a runaway process increasing family dysfunction. An illness may reinforce preexisting enmeshed patterns by providing a focal point for other family problems (Minuchin et al., 1978). This is particularly common with childhood-onset conditions, such as asthma and type 1 diabetes. For instance, in a family with intense marital conflict, a chronically ill child can become triangulated with the parents to deflect marital distress. Serious exacerbations of the child's illness, such as asthma attacks, can become physiologically intertwined with family dysfunction. The threat or occurrence of a serious medical crisis serves to moderate conflict that might escalate beyond control.

In other families, difficulties surface dramatically in adolescence, when the developmental push for greater autonomy conflicts strongly with the longstanding need for a highly cohesive system during the period of raising a child who is chronically ill. Clinicians need to be attentive to a family's propensity for quietly absorbing an illness when it is organized in an inwardly focused, highly cohesive manner, as when rearing small children. Over time, this initially adaptive pattern can rigidify, impeding the natural evolution to a more-autonomous, less cohesion-demanding phase that facilitates adolescent development.

Alternatively, with chronic disorders, there is a risk of labeling the family as *enmeshed* if the clinician disregards the normative lengthening of developmental phases for the child and family. Often, families coping with a chronically ill child are tentative about giving him or her more autonomy, not because of the dysfunction, but because they seek to protect the child or they anticipate further loss. With major health conditions, previous norms concerning family organization may need greater flexibility. Blurred generational boundaries can be overdiagnosed as family dysfunction. The real demands on older children and adolescents to assume more adult functions, in the interest of family well-being, should be distinguished from rigid, pathological descriptions of "parentified" children.

When a parent develops a chronic condition during the child-rearing phases of development, the family's ability to stay on course is severely taxed. For more serious debilitating conditions, the impact of the illness is like the addition of a new member, one with special needs that will compete with those of the other children for potentially scarce family resources. With psychosocially milder health problems, an efficient reallocation of roles may keep family development on course, as a recent case of a family with young children illustrates.

Sally and her husband, Tom, were seen 4 months after Sally's diagnosis of chronic fatigue syndrome, which made it difficult to manage the demands of raising their two young children, ages 2 and 4. Tom worked long hours in a small construction business with his father and brothers. Sally became increasingly upset with his unavailability to share housework and childcare burdens that left her exhausted. Tom felt she did not appreciate his job demands and loyalty to the family business, while she resented his rigidity and prioritizing of family-of-origin commitments ahead of her needs. Marital strain soon escalated into serious conflict.

For Sally and Tom, sufficient resources were available within the marital system to accommodate her condition and ongoing parenting tasks. Yet, their concept of marriage lacked the necessary role flexibility to master the challenge. The concurrence of Sally's condition with the child-rearing demands in this highly cohesive phase of the family life cycle overloaded the system. The conflict between Tom's loyalty to his family of origin and his nuclear family heightened tensions further. Intervention in this case focused on having the couple rebalance their roles, particularly that of Tom, who rigidly thought of himself only in terms of being the family provider, a view that had become stronger after the children were born.

If a health condition affecting a parent is severely debilitating, it may cause a major loss of parental functioning. In two-parent families, the couple needs to flexibly alter parenting and job roles; in single-parent families, extended kin, especially grandmothers, are commonly called upon to step in. In acute-onset illnesses, when family resources are often inadequate to meet the combined demands of working, child rearing, and caregiving, parents commonly turn to their children and extended kin to share responsibilities. Children can gain competencies and a positive sense of involvement in team efforts, but the arrangement can become maladaptive if they are overburdened, or their own needs are neglected. It can also cause a developmental setback for grandparents, who may be called upon to resume childcare, and can overstress those who have their own health problems. These forms of family adaptation are appropriate if structural realignments are flexible, shared, and sensitive to competing age-related developmental needs. Strong extended kin networks facilitate family adaptation. We need to be careful not to pathologize structural changes that may be necessary and encourage families to forge creative coping strategies.

Psychosocial Typology

The need for cohesiveness varies enormously with different illness types and phases. The tendency for a condition to draw a family inward increases with the level of disability or risk of progression and death. Progressive diseases inherently require greater cohesion than constant-course conditions. The ongoing addition of new demands keeps a family's energy focused inward, often impeding the development of other family members. After an initial period of adaptation, a constant-course disorder (without severe disability) permits a family to get back on track developmentally. The following case of a couple at midlife illustrates how the inward focus exerted by a progressive illness can increase the risk of reversing or freezing family development.

Lemont, a 54-year-old African American, had become increasingly depressed as a result of severe and progressive complications of adult-onset type 2 diabetes over the past 5 years, including a leg amputation and renal failure that had recently required instituting home dialysis four times a week. For 20 years, he had had an uncomplicated, constant course, allowing him to lead a full, active life. He was an excellent athlete and engaged in several recreational group sports. Lemont and his wife, Shirley, had a stable marriage in which both maintained many independent interests. Short- and long-term family planning had never focused on his illness. This optimistic attitude was reinforced by the fact that two relatives in Shirley's family of origin had diabetes without complications. Their only child, a son age 26, had uneventfully left home after high school and recently married. In short, the family had moved smoothly through the postlaunching phases of the life cycle.

Lemont's disease transformation to a progressive phase, coupled with the disabling and life-shortening nature of his complications, had reversed the normal postlaunching process for all family members. His advancing illness required Shirley to take a second job and give up her involvements with their church. Their son and his wife moved back home to help his mother take care of his father and the house. Lemont, unable to work and deprived of his athletic social network, was isolated at home and spent his days watching television. He felt that he was a burden to everyone, was blocked in his own midlife development and from making future plans with his wife, and foresaw a future filled only with suffering.

The goal of family treatment centered on reversing some of the system's overreaction to achieve a more realistic balance. For Lemont this meant coming to terms with his losses and his fears of suffering and death and identifying the capabilities and possibilities still available to him. This involved reworking his life structure to accommodate his actual limitations, while maximizing his chances of remaining independent. For instance, although he could no longer participate on the playing field, he could remain involved in sports through coaching. For Shirley and their son, this meant developing realistic expectations that reestablished him as an active family member with a share of family responsibilities. This helped the mother and son to become autonomous again in key areas within an illness–family system that could be more flexible about handling future life-cycle transitions.

The on-call nature of preparedness required by many relapsing illnesses keeps the family partly focused inward despite asymptomatic periods, and potentially hinders the natural flow between phases of development. In such situations, families can be helped to understand the need for ongoing higher cohesion; for developing strategies in which caregiving-related tasks are distributed equitably among family members; and for exploring various extended family, community, and health care provider resources.

When Illness Time Phases Are In or Out of Sync

One can think about illness time phases as transitioning from an initial crisis phase, requiring intensified cohesion, to a chronic phase, often demanding relatively less cohesion. A terminal phase, if it occurs, forces most families back into being more inwardly focused and highly cohesive. In other words, the "illness life structure" that a family develops to accommodate each illness phase is influenced by the need for cohesion dictated by that time phase. The initial crisis phase, because of its high psychosocial demands and its analogy to childhood (here as a period of socialization to illness), promotes a tendency toward higher cohesion. The primary task of the chronic phase is that of maximizing autonomy and living well within the constraints of the illness. The terminal phase, in which increasing psychosocial demands accompany physical decline, is like the later life phase: both foster an inward focus for the family because of increased caregiving.

These natural trends toward higher or lower cohesion in different stages of family development may or may not be in sync with the phases of illness. Consider a family in which illness onset has coincided with a relatively autonomous phase of its development, such as a family with young adult children in which the father has had a heart attack. In addition to the sheer level of demands placed on this family initially, the inward pull of the initial crisis phase conflicts with the family's being at an outwardly directed, more independent phase, and would become a source of family stress. One expression of added complexity might involve a young adult son or daughter having to postpone life plans and return home for an indeterminate period to assist in caring for the father. This scenario contrasts sharply with that of a family that has middle- and high-school-age children still at home and in an earlier, more inwardly and cohesion-focused child-rearing developmental phase.

The transition of the father's heart problems to the chronic phase may permit the family to resume its original developmental trajectory to some extent. At that point, if the father's recovery from his heart attack is progressing well and he can return to work, the children can pursue their early adulthood plans.

Overlapping Transition Periods

All transitions inherently involve beginnings and endings. A diagnosis may force the family into a transition in which one of the family's main tasks is to accommodate the possibilities of further loss and untimely death. When illness onset coincides with a transition in the individual or family life cycle, issues related to previous, current, and anticipated losses tend to be magnified. Transition periods are often characterized by upheaval, a rethinking of prior commitments, and an openness to change. Such times often hold a greater risk for the illness to become either embedded or ignored in planning for the next life phase. During a transition period, the process of thinking through future commitments can bring to the forefront family norms regarding loyalty through sacrifice and caregiving. Normative feelings of indecision about one's future can be diverted to an excessive focus on a family member's physical problems. Sometimes, this can be a major precursor of family dysfunction.

By adopting a longitudinal developmental perspective, a clinician can stay attuned to future transitions, particularly overlaps in those of illness, individual, and family development. Offering prevention-oriented family consultations at major transitions is extremely useful. The following example highlights this point.

In one second-generation Latino family, the father, a factory worker and primary financial provider, had a mild heart attack. He also suffered from emphysema. At first, his level of impairment was mild and stabilized, allowing him to continue part-time work. Because their children were all teenagers, his wife was able to undertake part-time work to help maintain financial stability. The oldest son, age 15, seemed relatively unaffected. Two years later, the father experienced a second, more serious heart attack and became totally disabled. His son, now 17, had dreams of going away to college. The specter of financial hardship and the perceived need for a "man in the family" created a serious dilemma for the son and the family. Moreover, the parents had worked hard to move out of the housing projects to ensure that their children could get a good education and have a better future.

In this case, there is a fundamental clash between developmental issues of launching a child and the prolonged demands of a progressive, chronic disability on the family. Simultaneous transition periods were at odds: (1) the illness transition to a more incapacitating and progressive course; (2) the adolescent son's transition to emerging adulthood, along with individuation, leaving home, and his desire to pursue a college degree; and (3) the family developmental transition from a "living-with-teenagers" to a "launching-young-adults" phase. It also illustrates the significance of the type of illness. An illness that was relapsing or not as life threatening, progressive, and disabling might have interfered less with this young man's emerging adulthood. If his father had an intermittently incapacitating condition, such as a disc disease, the son might have moved out, but would have tailored his college choices to remain nearby and thus be available during acute flare-ups. Culturally, in this Latino family a strong emphasis on loyalty to family needs would normatively take priority over individual goals, especially with a major illness or disability.

Illness Onset in a Life Structure-Maintaining Period

Illness onset that coincides with a life-structure building or maintaining phase presents a different challenge. The life-structure maintaining phase is characterized by living out one's choices made during the preceding transition. Relative to transition periods, family members try to protect their own and the family unit's current life structure. Mildly disabling and nonfatal conditions may require some life-structure revision but not a radical one. A severe condition can require a more complete family transition at a time of inertia when the family seeks to preserve a stable phase.

For instance, in the previous example, when the father's heart disease progression coincided with the oldest son's developmental transition period, he might have felt very threatened about losing his status as a single young adult to that of a caregiver, altering his life structure. The nature of the strain in developmental terms would be quite different if his father's disease progression occurred when this young man was 26, had already left home, finished college, secured a first job, and possibly gotten married and started a family. He would have made some developmental choices and been in the process of living them out. His life structure would be highly cohesive and inwardly focused on his newly formed family. Fully accommodating to his family-of-origin needs could require a monumental shift of his developmental priorities, creating a potential crisis between being loyal to his family of origin and his new nuclear family. To navigate this kind of crisis successfully, the son might have needed to transform his previously stable life structure back to a prolonged transitional state. The shift would have happened out of phase with the flow of his individual and nuclear family's development, and would almost invariably have placed a greater strain on his marriage. One complex way to resolve this dilemma of divided loyalties might be the merging of the two households. This approach can sometimes alleviate the strain of travel between two different families, thereby allowing for consolidation of meal planning and other household obligations, and the young couple's movement back and forth between caregiving and child rearing.

For some family members, giving up the creation of a new life structure that is already in progress can be more devastating than making changes in a more transitional period, when future plans may be more preliminary and less firmly formulated or clearly determined. An analogy would be the difference between a couple's discovering that they do not have enough money to build a house versus being forced to move out of a house they have already built.

CASE ILLUSTRATION

Thus far this discussion has considered separately the interplay of a chronic disorder with higher and lower cohesion, transition periods, and stable, structure-maintaining phases of family and individual life cycles. In reality, there is a dynamic interplay between the illness and the development of the family and individual members over time. I have been fortunate to have close friends who have been willing to share with me their individual and collective stories.

Jim and Nancy are married and have one daughter, Janet. Jim has MS. He first developed symptoms as a college freshman, at the age of 17. The first 3 years of his illness were particularly severe, marked by a number of flare-ups and rapid progression. His major disabilities included a loss of coordination and muscle strength, difficulty walking, and impaired eyesight. His last major flare-up requiring hospitalization occurred at age 24. Since that time, his condition has progressed very slowly.

During the initial period of Jim's illness, between the ages of 17 and 21, he was undergoing his early adult transition. For him, this was a time to develop an initial plan for an independent adult life outside his family of origin. For men in particular, this typically means starting a career. Before his illness, Jim had entered college with ambitions to become a lawyer and had an active social life. His diagnosis and its initially rapidly progressive and life-shortening trajectory became superimposed on this developmental phase. Jim felt he might die an early death, as happens with approximately 10% of MS patients. Based on this ominous prognosis, he decided to pursue a career that offered more immediate personal gratification and would benefit others. He volunteered his time to help advocate for local and regional environmental preservation. Jim adaptively revised his early adulthood and life structure to accommodate more immediately achievable goals.

Typically, emerging adulthood is a time of exploring and developing a capacity for intimacy, mutuality, and often, long-term relationships. The onset

Addressing Life-Cycle Issues with Chronic Conditions

of a chronic condition can severely affect this developmental process. Jim described how the uncertainties about his prognosis, his insecurity because of his new disability, and his relative lack of experience with intimacy all interacted to block his pursuit of close relationships. In essence, learning how to manage his illness and intimate relationships simultaneously in the context of threatened loss was too much to handle. After several disappointing experiences, Jim realized that he needed to learn how to cope with his condition before he could resume exploring intimate relationships. This was an adaptive way to create and prepare himself for a wider range of achievable options in the next phase of his life.

During this vulnerable initial period, he might have found a partner who needed to fill a caregiving role. Often, a young adult, like Jim, who felt overwhelmed and insecure, might find a partner who is drawn to become a caregiver because of unresolved issues in his or her family of origin. One example might be a young adult who as a child assumed the role of a parent or rescuer in a family dealing with a chronic disorder such as alcoholism. Any relationship that begins when one partner is in an initial crisis phase is vulnerable to dysfunction. This risk is much greater if the couple is also at a stage in their personal development when both are beginning to learn about intimate relationships.

Through his early and mid-20s, the initially rapid progression of Jim's illness ceased and stabilized into a more typical, slowly progressing pattern with no major flare-ups. This change in prognosis, coupled with Jim's gradually learning how to live with his disability in its more chronic phase, altered his perspective on time. He could realistically entertain longer-range career and relationship possibilities. Moreover, he had achieved a level of confidence in coping with his condition that enabled him to resume thinking about developmental goals more fully, and with less need to compromise.

As a result of this changed perspective, during his transition into his 30s, Jim began a long-term relationship with his future spouse, Nancy. They married when Jim was 31. To Nancy, who was trying to understand his illness, Jim's "willingness to be open, direct, and supportive with regard to my questions and anxieties was absolutely fundamental." Nancy stated, "My ability to set limits on what I would do, to express my own needs and have him accept them as legitimate, was essential to our being able to forge a mutual relationship."

Nancy had grown up as the oldest sibling of an alcoholic mother. During her 20s, she had sought professional help to work out unresolved issues from her family of origin that interfered with relationships. This therapy allowed her to approach a relationship, even with someone with a chronic illness, more assertively. For both Jim and Nancy, their coming together partially reflected the overcoming of obstacles to intimacy they had faced in their 20s.

During the early phase of their relationship and marriage, Nancy undertook additional education to advance her career and then established herself in her first job. During this time Jim continued his volunteer work and supported Nancy during her career transition. Although dealing with the disability required time and energy, their relationship was organized to maximize individual goals outside the home.

Three years into their marriage, Jim and Nancy had settled into a comfortable relationship. Jim's illness had progressed very slowly, with no new major complications and at a rate to which they could easily adapt. Nancy was established in her new career and had turned 37. New life-cycle dilemmas surfaced because of competing biological clocks. Nancy was approaching midlife. Her fertility clock, like the one for Jim's progressive illness, was ticking. Initially they had agreed to defer a decision about whether to have a child. To accommodate Jim's need to stay in familiar surroundings, with an elaborate support network to which he was well adapted, Nancy had rejected opportunities for career advancement in a large city and settled for a less interesting and prestigious position. As she entered her midlife transition, she was reevaluating her choices. She decided that she wanted either to have a child or to move so that she could advance her career more ambitiously. She felt too compromised if she had to give up both having a child and advancing her career, seeing it as unhealthy for her personally and for the relationship. Her ability to maintain a sense of legitimacy about her own needs, given Jim's limitations, was healthy.

At the time, Jim had been medically stable for 10 years. His disease was progressing slowly, particularly with regard to his eyesight and his mobility. He had abandoned his original career ambitions in his early 20s because of the threat of an early death, and he did so again at 30 so that he could pursue a relationship. He had made active choices while fully recognizing his physical limitations and the risk of a flare-up if he became overstressed. He felt pressure to go back to school to increase his career options while he still had the physical stamina and the ability to read. But he wondered, "Should I even consider these choices, because . . . I don't want to blow it?"

As a couple, Jim and Nancy were at a crossroads. Jim's illness dictated a limit on their reserves as a couple. Could Jim handle school? Could they manage an infant? If they chose not to have a child, how would they define the future of their relationship and each person's goals? Decisions that were appropriately deferred must now, under the time pressure of life-cycle demands, be addressed. Both Jim and Nancy had parents who died in the past year, which had heightened their sense of life's fragility and the impetus to actively shape their lives and have a child. The ongoing, likely progressive illness trajectory weighed on all other developmental choices and forced decision making into more of an either-or framework than would be the case for couples less burdened by adversity.

Consistent with their "can do" philosophy, this couple chose a modified both-and approach. Jim entered graduate school on a part-time basis, in order to feel his way and leave enough slack to overcome any hurdles without overreaching his physical limits. Also, they decided to try and have a child. Nancy quickly became pregnant; and a year after their decision, Jim was attending school and they had a baby.

Jim and Nancy were least prepared for the transition from a lower-stress family system of two relatively autonomous adults to the considerable demands of an inwardly focused, cohesive family unit with an infant. During prenatal visits, the physician minimized the special needs they might have. As Nancy said, "I too desperately wanted to preserve the glossy picture of raising a child together, so I didn't question things," but "Jim's limits that normally don't come into play got accentuated." For instance, their baby, Janet, had a period of colic during the first few months. The pediatrician told Nancy that their baby was not getting enough food and suggested that timely and efficient bottle-feeding was needed. Jim could feed Janet but, because of his coordination difficulties, he was slow. The pediatrician's definition of the problem created a dilemma: Jim's disability would prevent "efficient" feeding and exacerbate the colic. Jim argued with Nancy, "I can do it fine, my own way." Nancy was torn between her need to be a good mother and her wish to protect her husband from disappointment. Jim felt inadequate, and their glossy picture of mutual infant care was tarnished. They needed time to socialize themselves to the added complexities of parenthood within the context of a chronic illness that they had mastered in the previous phase of the life cycle. This part of their story highlights the need for clinicians to be mindful of life-cycle transitions that may require helping a family to redefine mastery in terms of new developmental tasks.

From this experience Jim learned to anticipate the complexities related to his daughter's future development. For instance, he realized that, given his visual impairment, it would be difficult to read bedtime stories to Janet. Instead, he began a ritual of making up bedtime stories that sidestepped his disability, while preserving special time with his daughter before sleep.

For Nancy and Jim, having a child inevitably heightened their relationship difficulties. Because of the limits imposed by Jim's illness, Nancy had to bear the bulk of homemaking and childcare responsibilities on top of her job. It was crucial for the well-being of their relationship that they maintain a balance so that Nancy did not have to assume responsibility for all aspects of family life, which could cause resentment. Although Jim was limited in his physical capabilities, he could handle any of the family's emotional needs. But to keep that balance required open, direct communication and a willingness to challenge gender-role stereotypes (see Chapters 8 and 13 for further discussion).

Twenty-Year Follow-Up

Janet is now a young adult, who completed college several years ago, has an excellent job, and recently got married to George. Jim's MS has slowly progressed over the intervening years. He now uses a walker at home and a wheelchair outside their apartment. Signs of some mild cognitive impairment, particularly with memory, have slowly developed in recent years. Janet has a close relationship with both parents and is open and understanding about Jim's condition. Personally, their commitment to living with the challenges of MS resiliently without it defining their family's or Jim's identity has had a positive impact on Janet's development and the health of Jim and Nancy's marriage. The strain on Nancy as the primary parent and caregiver in terms of meeting her husband's physical needs and being the financial provider for the family has been a formidable, ongoing challenge. Continuing open, sensitive, and direct communication has been essential to their success.

Thinking forward developmentally, Jim, Nancy, and Janet had discussed potential future caregiving needs and expectations for Janet. Jim and Nancy expressed their strong wishes for Janet to have a full life and have set limits on caregiving expectations for her. Janet voiced her own desire to live close by, so as to be available to her parents and also to make grandparenting more accessible to them. In turn, as Janet and George's relationship developed, they proactively discussed her commitment to live near her parents and be available to assist, while establishing reasonable limits to protect their nuclear family, which includes having children. All four agreed to review these decisions periodically in the context of the evolution of Jim's MS and any planned or unanticipated individual or family developmental transitions.

GENERAL CLINICAL DISCUSSION

At the time of diagnosis, it is important to know the life-cycle phases of each family member, not just the ill one. Chronic disease in one family member can profoundly affect the developmental goals of another. For instance, an infant's disability can be a serious roadblock to parents' preconceived ideas about competent child rearing, or a life-threatening illness in a young married adult can interfere with the well spouse's readiness to become a parent. The ability of each member to adapt, and the rate at which he or she does so, is related to each one's own developmental phase and role in the family. Successful long-term adaptation is maximized when family members are attuned to one another's developmental processes, while being flexible about pursuing alternative means to satisfy developmental needs. *An overarching goal is to handle the developmental demands of the illness, while preserving family members' own and the family's development as a system over time.*

Some characteristic patterns of strain that emerge over time in unanticipated illnesses include the following:

- Because diseases have an inward pull on most families, they can be more disruptive to families during non-child-rearing phases.
- The transition period generated by the onset of a serious illness is

particularly untimely if it coincides with a life-structure maintaining phase in individual or family development.
- If the particular illness is progressive, relapsing, increasingly incapacitating, or life threatening, its evolution will be punctuated by numerous transitions. A family may need to alter its life structure more frequently to accommodate the new and increasing demands of the disease. This level of demand and uncertainty keeps the illness in the forefront of a family's consciousness, impinging on its developmental strivings.
- The transition from the crisis to the chronic phase is often the juncture at which the intensity of the family's socialization to living with chronic disease lessens. This transition offers an opportunity for the family to chart a new normal developmental course or reestablish an old one.

Many health care providers believe that conditions that occur in the child-rearing period can be most devastating because of their potential impact on a family's financial and other responsibilities. Again, the actual impact will depend on the psychosocial type of illness. Families will adapt best with flexibly defined roles concerning who should be the primary financial provider and caregiver of children.

The process by which life-cycle decisions are reached is particularly important. A clinical objective might be to help a family become more flexibly cohesive and share responsibilities in such a way that, although everyone's life is somewhat affected, no one person is disproportionately or radically compromised. This value placed on sharing the burden more widely can help protect the individual developmental goals of core nuclear family members.

The degree to which individual and family developmental priorities are preserved or altered is an excellent barometer of family processes. It is useful to know whose plans are the most and least affected. Did factors, such as gendered role expectations, influence the process? How does each family member feel about the impact on his or her developmental plans? By posing these sorts of questions, a clinician can learn a great deal about general family functioning.

Are sacrifices warranted? Often, families overreact in the initial crisis phase, such as with a heart attack that begins in a dramatic or life-endangering manner. A family that initially thinks a condition is severe may prematurely cancel plans that could be preserved through postponement or creative alterations. When family members change their life plans prematurely, an amplifying cascade effect follows that can tragically alter the whole life course of an individual or an entire family. This is particularly true for conditions in which the uncertainties about the prognosis, which may continue indefinitely, can solidify an initial crisis-phase caregiving arrangement that eventually becomes unnecessary.

Early in the illness experience, families may find it particularly difficult to appraise the need for temporary detours or permanent changes in life-cycle plans. Once developmental plans are derailed, the inherent inertia of chronic conditions makes it more difficult to find one's original path. This underscores the importance of timely prevention-oriented psychoeducation and consultation for families.

A clinical orientation that is sensitive to the future means asking family members when and under what conditions they contemplate resuming plans put on hold or addressing future developmental tasks. This approach enables a clinician to anticipate key developmental junctures. Questions, such as the following, are useful.

- What individual, family, or illness transitions will be coming up in the next year? In the next 5 years?
- Are family members aware of major developmental issues that will become salient at that time for themselves? For other members? For the entire family?
- What are family expectations for the next phases of the illness?

These questions encourage a family to think in developmental terms. They help a family to focus on key issues and provide a new frame of reference for more effective problem solving. These questions can also be aimed at a particular nodal event rather than at a general long-term plan. For instance, one might ask the following questions of a family with teenagers, in which the father has heart disease.

- In 2 years, when Joe is 18 and finishing high school, what issues will he, other family members, or the whole family, need to consider? Whose life might be most affected at that time?
- How will those issues be affected by Dad's heart disease?
- How will those issues be affected if Dad's heart disease worsens and he has another heart attack?
- Given Dad's illness, are there certain expectations about how Joe should plan for the next phase of his life?

These questions help reveal how much life-cycle planning will be needed depending on the status of Dad's condition. Finding out about expectations is critical because it provides a window into loyalty issues, ethnic or cultural understandings, and other beliefs that will become guideposts for decision making during the upcoming transition.

In ambiguous illness situations, such as a cancer in remission, it is useful to ask, "If Mom were cured tomorrow, what would each person or the whole family do differently in terms of planning for the future?" This question elicits the degree to which life-cycle plans have been affected. It helps a clinician

Addressing Life-Cycle Issues with Chronic Conditions 127

and the family understand the extent to which a disorder currently governs and is expected to control family life in the future. Issues suggesting that an illness has assumed too much influence over family planning may emerge. The discussion can invite follow-up questions, such as "If you were to view Bill's diabetes and potential complications as less powerful in your relationship, how would that affect your marriage now and your plans together for the future?"

When normative life-cycle tasks must truly be abandoned, anticipating this possibility can further adaptation. Consider young couples in which one member has a disabling condition, such as MS, that may worsen. Suppose they are beginning to discuss having children. By thinking ahead, a clinician may ask, "Given your interest in having children, and given your disability and the uncertainties of MS, if you decided that not having children of your own was an option, are there alternative ways you could satisfy your interest in becoming parents?" "What would need to change in order to accept this alternative as good enough?" When childbearing or child rearing is precluded, individuals and couples need to be guided in finding other ways to express developmental generative needs and to dispel feelings that they are inherently deficient if they do not have a child.

A forward-thinking clinical philosophy that uses a developmental perspective as a way of gaining a positive sense of control and opportunity is vital for families dealing with chronic disorders. Often beneath a surface optimism concerning the present lies an undercurrent of unacknowledged dread of the future. Much of this negative thinking is associated with anticipatory loss, which will be discussed in Chapter 9. A life-cycle framework offers families a way to think about different dimensions of their life (e.g., work, relationships and family, and recreation) now and in the future and the relative priority of each one. It also facilitates thinking about how each domain might be affected, positively or negatively, by illness or disability.

CHAPTER 8

Tapping the Power of Family Belief Systems

When illness strikes, families strive to create meaning for the illness experience that promotes competence and mastery. Because serious illness is often experienced as a betrayal of our fundamental trust in our bodies and belief in our invulnerability (Kleinman, 1988), it can be a formidable challenge to make meaning with an empowering narrative. Family health beliefs can help us grapple with the existential dilemmas of our fear of death and our tendency to deny our own mortality. Beliefs provide coherence to family life, facilitating a continuity between the past, present, and future. They offer an approach to new and ambiguous situations, such as a serious illness, and serve as cognitive maps guiding decisions and actions (Antonovsky, 1998; Hansson & Cederblad, 2004; Reiss, 1981). Our appreciative inquiry into family beliefs is a powerful foundation for collaborating with patients and families. Wright and Bell (2009, p. 10) wisely write: "It is beliefs about the clinical problem or illness that serve as the greatest source of individual and family suffering . . . beliefs also lie at the heart of healing."

This chapter describes how shared belief systems related to health and illness profoundly shape family adaptation to major health conditions. I address the key elements and the forces that shape these beliefs over time. Using the psychosocial typology and illness phases, I highlight ways to assess and sensitively help families modify their beliefs, emphasizing ones that optimize coping and adaptation.

OVERVIEW

Our beliefs are represented and continually revised in the narratives we construct together to help make meaning of our world and our place in it

(Freedman & Combs, 1996; Hoffman, 1990; White & Epston, 1990). Core beliefs predominate when major life challenges, such as serious health conditions, arise. Collaborative health care emphasizes the cocreation of narratives about health conditions that incorporate the belief systems of patients, families, and health care providers.

THE EXPERIENCE OF ILLNESS: LEVELS OF MEANING AND INFLUENCE

Arthur Kleinman (1988) conceived three health levels of meaning—*disease, illness,* and *sickness.* I've expanded these levels to an ecosystemic, family-oriented perspective that includes the *biomedical level, the human experience level,* and *macrosystem level of meaning.* A biopsychosocial understanding requires an appreciation of the ongoing mutual influences among these levels of meaning over the illness course.

The *biomedical level* refers to a purely biological description or understanding of a patient's condition. Health professionals function mostly at this level, consistent with how they have been traditionally trained. From this perspective, when they ask, "Tell me about your pain," they want to know where it is, when it occurs, how intense it is, what treatment has already been tried, and what other physical symptoms are associated with it. These questions are intended to discover a physical explanation for the pain.

Patients and their families live primarily in the realm of the *human experience of illness,* at the level of symptoms and suffering. This refers to "how the sick person and the members of the family or wider social network perceive, live with, and respond to symptoms and disability" (Kleinman, 1988, p. 3). The experience of illness involves the synthesis of biological phenomena with personal, family, and cultural meanings.

At a third *macrosystemic* (larger system) *level,* health meanings are derived from larger cultural, macrosocial, economic, political, or institutional forces that are often beyond a patient's and family's control. For example, some health conditions are strongly influenced by poverty, racism, and technological oppression (e.g., flawed environmental policies), or are viewed pejoratively as due to an "immoral" lifestyle. The policies and ideology of our health care delivery system, which limits universal quality care for everyone, actually causes health care disparities. Diseases, such as lead poisoning, cancer, asthma, and HIV, which are more common in inner cities, need to be viewed through this larger societal lens. Affected patients and their families internalize the messages about their conditions that they receive from the dominant cultural milieu. This process can profoundly influence their illness experience.

In the traditional biomedical model, the health care provider decodes and reduces descriptions of the human experience of illness to biological diseases that can be treated. In turn, a diagnosis can alter a family's prior understandings or beliefs. Over time, a recursive process evolves, characterized by new biological or treatment information, the personal or family experience of living with illness, and revised meanings. Throughout, the family lives in the world of its personal experience of the condition, yet it is also influenced by societal and medical perspectives. Belief systems can be conceptualized as mediators between biological conditions and the family's personal experience, as diagrammed in Figure 8.1.

Clinicians need to carefully navigate the biomedical, human experience, and macrosystem levels of meanings. Years ago, when I began to interview families about their experience with illness and disability, I realized that for many of them, it was the first time anyone had taken an interest in the totality of their illness experience. I asked about their core family beliefs and their experience with a particular condition or health concern—from their own viewpoint. Repeatedly, families expressed feelings of being misunderstood by health care providers. What this generally meant was that no one (particularly their physicians) had inquired about their core personal beliefs or the meanings they attached to their family member's condition.

Chapter 18 addresses the fit of beliefs between health care providers and families. The essential point here is that the process of inquiry about belief systems and meanings is integral to establishing a mutual, viable relationship, regardless of the consensus between professionals and families. Taking into account the perspectives of the patient and family acknowledges the importance of beliefs. This extra effort protects against a disconnection that too often results when a professional operates solely in the world of disease and the family in one of personal experience (Frank, 1998).

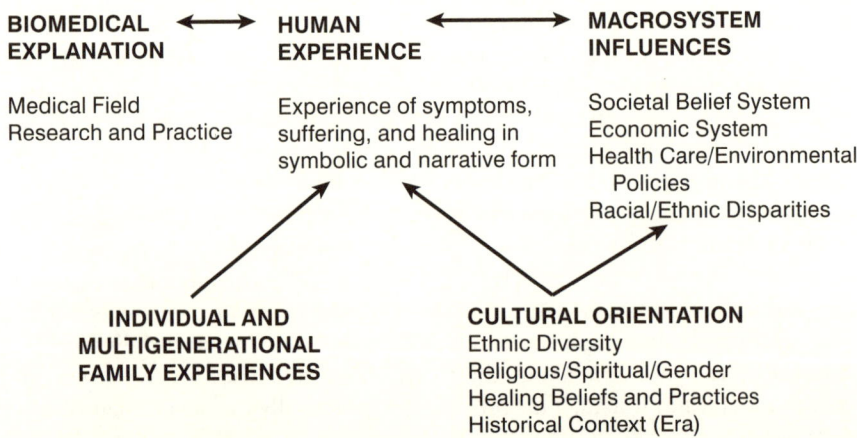

FIGURE 8.1. Levels of meaning: Illness and healing.

Families may disengage if they feel unacknowledged or misunderstood when a health professional fails to consider their beliefs or their particular experience of a health issue. Often a negative outcome of this process is labeled as noncompliance by the patient or family. In fact, a clinician's disregard of these other levels of meaning interferes with a necessary joining process. Mindfulness to belief systems enables the clinician, patient, and family to work flexibly together to address the biomedical, human experience, and macrosystem levels of meaning.

To summarize, belief systems are a tremendous force in illness. When disregarded, they can damage relationships and block healing. When approached sensitively, they empower all relationships and provide a foundation for biological, psychosocial, and spiritual healing.

ASSESSMENT OF HEALTH BELIEFS

As part of early consultation(s), particularly in the initial crisis phase, it is useful to inquire about the key beliefs that shape families' meaning-making and coping strategies. First get a sense of the *core beliefs* that contribute to a family's overall identity (Walsh, 2016b) beyond the health challenge. Core beliefs provide a foundation on which health beliefs are constructed. It helps to gain an appreciation of the family beliefs evoked by bearing the strains of a chronic disorder and the meanings associated with the particular condition. I pay attention to the family's health beliefs about the following:

- Normative illness experience
- Ethnic, cultural, and spiritual influences
- Gender-related expected roles and behavior
- Mastery, control, and acceptance
- The cause(s) of an illness
- Factors that can influence the course and outcome
- Sense of hope or optimism, or pessimism
- Particular symptoms (e.g., chronic pain), types of illnesses (e.g., life-threatening), or specific diseases (e.g., HIV/AIDS) by a family, ethnic group, religion, or the wider culture
- Family rituals
- Fit of health beliefs among family members as well as between the family and the health care system and the wider culture (also see Chapter 18)
- Integrative healing practices

I will discuss each of these areas, highlighting assessment or inquiry about a family's beliefs, connecting with a patient and his or her family by validating their beliefs, and techniques to facilitate helpful beliefs and modify unhelpful ones. Rather than making a sharp distinction between assessment and intervention, I consider the process of assessment itself as an intervention.

Normative Illness Experience

Family beliefs about what is normative or abnormal can influence their adaptation to chronic disorders (Rolland, 2012; Walsh, 2012). When family values normalize the psychosocial challenges of an illness without stigma, it encourages families to seek outside help and maintain a positive identity. When families view seeking help as weak and shameful, it can undercut their resilience and foster suffering. Essentially, difficulties are to be expected with chronic disorders, and professionals and outside resources are often needed.

Two useful questions for families are: (1) "How do you think other families would *typically* deal with a situation similar to yours?" and (2) "How do you think families *ideally* cope with your situation?" The first question explores family members' sense of the range of experiences and common coping strategies. Are they making comparisons to situations with similar psychosocial demands, or are they making unrealistic ones? A family in the initial phase of a member's TBI might inappropriately compare its coping ability and strategies with those of a family facing a seizure disorder or with age peers who are healthy.

The second question invites a family to share its beliefs about what is most healthy or optimal. Does a family compare itself with superstars featured in the media in a similar situation, or does it have a more realistic view of typical coping that includes the anticipated challenges and struggles with emotional highs and lows? Sadly, families facing illness and disability often have a romanticized view of healthy adaptation that is unrealistic and leaves them feeling inadequate.

In one situation, a courageous young woman with metastatic cancer was filmed for a documentary about coping with life-threatening illness. The film captured her positive approach extremely well, but left out the problematic times. During her low physical or emotional periods, she would decline, and family or friends would protect her from the film crew. Thus, the film did not record the poignant, normative, low points at which she and her loved ones expressed frustrations and demoralization and thoughts about giving up the fight. The portrayal of her remarkable experience was sanitized and incomplete. She and her family were rightfully concerned that other patients and their families who viewed this film could develop unrealistic expectations for their own journey with illness.

Families that value high achievement or perfectionism are prone to apply unachievable standards in a situation of illness. Untimely conditions that occur early in the life cycle come with additional pressures to keep up with socially expected developmental milestones of age peers. Life goals may take longer to achieve or need revision. Sustaining hope requires having a flexible belief about what is normative and healthy.

A young couple's ability to define what is expected or typical can be impeded both by a lack of exposure to similarly afflicted peers and by ambiguities in social interactions. For instance, distancing by friends can be interpreted as, "You're not normal," when it may be due to their emotional difficulty in facing their own vulnerability. Because most families lack an illness-relevant comparison group, multifamily discussion groups and support networks can meet their need for a valuable normalizing context.

Unlike families tested by adversity, those who have been more fortunate in life and spared the "slings and arrows of outrageous fortune" may have unrealistic expectations shaken by unexpected illness and disability. They may have greater difficulty in coping when faced with the inevitable challenges.

Normalizing Mind–Body Interaction

Through advances in the neurosciences, traditional psychosomatic notions of mind–body influence have become outdated. Mental health theories and research that were pathology-oriented tended to emphasize character traits or emotional states that could adversely affect the body. Significant advances in understanding the importance of positive attitudes in coping and healings stress the interconnection of mind and body (Bolier et al., 2013; Carr, 2013; Cousins, 2001; Csikszentmihalyi, 2014; Levine, 1987; Siegel & Sander, 2009). Practices, such as mindfulness meditation (Kabat-Zinn, 2003; Khoury et al., 2013) and yoga and guided imagery, and a range of spiritual resources (Koenig, 2012; Walsh, 2009) can significantly affect coping and adaptation, and in some cases, influence an illness course. As clinicians, we need to become aware of our own belief biases, which are often fostered in professional training that is skewed toward pathology, disease, or dysfunction (see Chapter 17).

It is helpful to ascertain how families think about biopsychosocial–spiritual influences and body physiology. They may attach importance to emotional states and have spiritual beliefs that maintain physical health and promote or interfere with physical healing. They may believe in the role of willpower—or a higher power—in illness control and healing (see later in this chapter).

Almost all health conditions are affected in both negative and positive ways by psychological, relational, and life-circumstance factors. This is good news. Rather than viewing psychosomatic interactions in traditional pejorative ways that blame individuals or families for their physical problems, practitioners can enhance successful coping and adaptation when we normalize a mind–body interaction. We might say to a family dealing with asthma, "Families notice that asthma is affected by stressful times; many worry that this will be interpreted as a sign of emotional problems. I want you to know that asthma normally worsens during the inevitable strains that arise in family life. It is important to keep me informed about major family stresses so that I can decide with you whether adjusting Susan's medication might be helpful or find better ways to reduce stress." This promotes a positive attitude toward the potential role of psychosocial factors to influence the disease course and the patient's quality of life, yet without blaming the patient. Rather than considering psychosomatic interactions a shameful liability, a family can approach such an interaction as an opportunity to make a difference by decreasing stress and increasing its sense of control.

Ethnocultural and Spiritual Influences in Illness and Health

Ethnocultural and spiritual beliefs in the context of dominant societal norms can strongly influence family values, concerns about health and illness, and family pathways in healing (Falicov, 2013; Kirmayer et al., 2014; McGoldrick et al., 2005; Rolland, 2006b). Practitioners need to be mindful of the diversity of belief systems of ethnic and religious groups in their community and of how they are expressed in different behavioral patterns. Simultaneously, we need to avoid cultural stereotyping and recognize and respect the unique perspectives of each patient and family. Cultural norms and religious expectations vary as to:

- The appropriate "sick role" for the patient.
- The kind and degree of open communication about the condition and its prognosis.
- Who should be included in the illness caregiving system (e.g., extended family, friends, health professionals).
- Gender-based expectations for caregiving and for the primary caregiver role.
- What treatment or healing approaches (e.g., Western medical practices, faith healing practitioners, Eastern or indigenous traditional beliefs about causes and curative practices) can be helpful.
- The proper rituals (e.g., hospital bedside vigils, healing-related, last rites, funerals or memorial tributes, and burial or cremation), at different illness phases.
- Within-family diversity (e.g., parents' German and Mexican cultural differences in handling a son's diabetes).

As practitioners we need to hold a broad view of spirituality as a dimension of human experience and expand our systemic orientation to embrace a holistic biopsychosocial and spiritual view (Walsh, 2009). Spirituality involves overarching and deeply personal faith beliefs and practices, both within and outside formal religious structures. Spiritual resources may include prayer, meditation, or sacred rituals; belief in a higher power; a faith community; and/or involvement in nature, the creative arts, or social activism.

Suffering invites us into the spiritual domain (Wright, 2009, 2017). Clinicians need to explore how spiritual beliefs may contribute to suffering, such as the belief that a loved one's cancer was caused by sinful living. More often, spiritual beliefs are a wellspring for resilience, offering the meaning, support, comfort, and strength needed to endure illness-related challenges. Mounting neurobiological evidence reveals that strong faith and contemplative practices can promote health and healing; reduce stress; and strengthen neurological, immune, and cardiovascular systems (Khoury et al., 2013; Koenig, 2012). Couple and family studies find that shared spiritual beliefs and practices strengthen relationships and the ability to transcend troubled times (Marks, 2006; Walsh, 2009).

I routinely explore how patient and family members' core ethnocultural and spiritual beliefs influence illness, healing, and well-being. Some guidelines for inquiry include:

- Exploring the importance and role of spiritual beliefs and practices (religious or nonreligious) in individual, couple, and family life.
- Exploring beliefs about psychological, social, cultural, and spiritual influences in illness and health, suffering, and healing.
- Exploring how the dominant culture affects the health care and relationships experienced between minority groups and providers.
- Encouraging members to draw on cultural and spiritual resources for resilience suited to their belief systems and preferences (Walsh, 2009, 2016b).

Clinicians' understanding in these areas can facilitate collaboration and sensitive tailoring of biopsychosocial and spiritual healing strategies. We can identify areas of strength and vulnerability and explore ways of including a family's cultural and spiritual beliefs and practices in biomedical treatments.

We need to be mindful of the tremendous diversity among cultures and within families. With immigrant families, clinicians need to inquire respectfully about indigenous beliefs and healing practices that differ from Western medical approaches. For example, in traditional Latino culture, espiritismo, or the belief in benevolent and malevolent spirits, is essential to the cause and cure of an illness (Falicov, 2009). In many traditions, group prayer or sacred rituals focused on the well-being of the ill person are believed to gather curative energy fields (Kirmayer, 2004).

Practitioners may need to address problematic spiritual differences within families. Profound religious beliefs regarding end-of-life decisions can tear families apart. In some cases, the more religious family members may try to impose their healing practices on a patient who does not share their beliefs and is upset by their unwanted intrusion. One woman, declining rapidly in later stages of ALS, was profoundly distressed by the concerted effort of her devoutly Christian siblings to perform a miracle ritual upon her.

Collaborating with chaplaincy services and pastoral professionals or the family's faith community can foster a cohesive biopsychosocial–spiritual approach. Practitioners must also be sensitive to family members who are not religious. Exploration of secular humanist values and existential concerns about life's meaning and purpose can be important conversations, especially with terminal illness and end-of-life care.

Clinicians need to be mindful of cultural and religious or spiritual differences between themselves, the patient, and family members to forge a collaborative alliance through a long-term illness (Seaburn et al., 1996). Flexibility is needed in addressing core religious beliefs that proscribe certain standard forms of medical care (e.g., receiving blood transfusions for Jehovah's Witnesses), accepting that patients retain final responsibility for decisions about their bodies.

Gender-Based Beliefs: Influences on Patient and Caregiver Roles

Although most contemporary couples and families strive toward flexible and equitable gender role relations (Knudsen-Martin, 2012), it is important to recognize the influence of culturally based gender norms for patient status and caregiving roles. Across cultures, women have been expected to provide the bulk of caregiving and attend to the emotional and practical needs of the patient and family (Qualls & Zarit, 2009). Men have been socialized to take charge of financial and instrumental problem-solving responsibilities. Masculine (macho) stereotypes tend to idealize rugged individuals, who are "in control," and minimize weakness, vulnerability, and dependency needs. This can constrain their emotional involvement and support.

Gender-based issues can peak at important transitions in coping with severe disability or terminal illness, such as the decision for the patient to receive home-based care versus long-term hospitalization or to be transferred to an extended care facility. Because the primary caregiver role is typically assigned to the wife, mother, or daughter, she is apt to bear most burdens. She also may subordinate her feelings or needs and assume caregiving responsibilities without complaint when critical decisions with health care providers are made. Clinicians should be cautious when families present this kind of united front, and sensitively raise an awareness of gender-based caregiving norms and of the potential overwhelming demands of home-based care. It's crucial to explore a family's expectations about caregiving roles. We can encourage flexibility and a shift from defining one female member as the caregiver to that of a collaborative caregiving team that includes male and female siblings and adult children. This intervention helps avert the risk of disproportionate caregiver overload, resentment, and deteriorating family relationships. (See the further discussion of gender in Chapter 6 on multigenerational themes and in Chapter 14 on couples.)

Beliefs about Mastery and Control in Facing Illness

It is useful to explore how a family defines and values mastery and control in general and particularly in situations of illness (Thompson & Kyle, 2000). When mastery is seen as having control over negative forces, illness is sometimes viewed as a clash with our bodies. The dominant American ethos and Western medical training promote mastery *over* illness. A more flexible view of mastery involves *doing* what is possible.

Other cultural belief systems, such as Asian and indigenous traditions, and the core principles of integrative medicine (see "Integrative Medicine and Healing Practices") emphasize striving for harmony with nature rather than control over it. They view health and illness as natural aspects of the human condition, with disorders often arising or worsening when the person has not attended adequately to self-care, personal relationships, or the larger environment. We can help families master the illness-related psychosocial challenges, not just the biological disease.

Beliefs about Control

Early studies related mastery to the concept of health locus of control (Lefcourt, 1982), referring to a belief about one's influence over the course and outcome of an illness. To what extent do family health beliefs emphasize internal control, "powerful" others, or chance and destiny? Individuals who have a high internal locus-of-control orientation believe that they can significantly influence the course and outcome of a situation. They believe individuals are directly responsible for their health and have the power to recover from illness (Wallston, 2004). Those with an external orientation minimize personal control or agency, believing that others exert major influence over their bodies and illness course, such as physicians, "powerful" family members, God, vengeful persons or spirits, or societal forces. Yet others view illness in terms of chance and may hold that illness occurrence and recovery are mostly a matter of luck or misfortune, passively accepting what happens to them.

These three orientations are best seen as tendencies in families, rather than as fixed and absolute convictions. A family may adhere to a different belief about control when dealing with biological illness as distinct from other life challenges. Also, the balance between these orientations may shift, depending on the type or phase of a health problem and the issues surrounding it. Therefore, it is valuable to understand: (1) a family's core values, (2) beliefs about control of a serious illness, and (3) the specific disease. If a family views all facets of life, including health conditions, as a matter of fate and beyond their personal control, psychosocial interventions may be best tailored to that belief. However, a family normally guided by a belief in personal agency might shift to a reliance on medical experts or hope for a miracle if they feel helpless in the face of a serious condition, such as metastasizing cancer. Shifts in a particular situation may reflect societal values, a family's ethnic background, or a powerful multigenerational experience with serious illness. We might explore how a family's core beliefs are shaken by the specific disease in order to foster a positive sense of personal agency that fits the circumstances they are dealing with.

Regardless of the actual severity or prognosis in a particular case, a serious condition such as cancer may be equated with "death" or "no control" based on medical statistics, cultural myths, or prior family history. Forms of heart disease with a similar life expectancy as cancer may be seen as more manageable through lifestyle modifications, because of health care information gleaned through the media. In one family traditionally guided by a strong belief in personal agency, the powerful family patriarch died at midlife from a rapidly progressive and painful form of cancer. As a result, the family developed an encapsulated exception to their usual beliefs about control that was specific for cancer, and they generalized it to other life-threatening conditions. Other families may have enabling stories about a relative or friend who, despite having cancer and a shortened lifespan, lived a "full" life centered on effectively prioritizing the quality of relationships and goals. Clinicians can highlight such positive narratives to help counteract cultural beliefs that define success exclusively as control over biological events.

A family's beliefs about mastery and control can affect treatment adherence and its participation in a member's treatment and healing process. When families view disease outcome as a matter of chance or beyond their control, they tend to establish marginal relationships with health professionals. When poor minority families receive inadequate care or lack access to care, it fosters a fatalistic attitude and lack of engagement with health care providers, who may not be trusted to help. Because any therapeutic relationship depends on a shared belief system about what is therapeutic, it is essential to establish a workable accommodation of fundamental beliefs among the patient, family, and health care team.

Time-Phase Considerations

The goodness of fit between family beliefs about mastery and the need for provider and technological care can vary with the illness phase. For some disorders, the initial crisis phase involves protracted care outside the family's direct control, such as in the recovery period after a stroke, which may begin in an intensive-care unit and entail extended care at a rehabilitation facility. Dealing with this phase may be stressful for families that prefer to tackle their own problems without outside involvement or control. To forge a workable alliance, clinicians should involve families in some aspect of care from the beginning, no matter how great the technological component of care is. Research finds that family members, and especially children, adjust better when they can be usefully involved in some way. The patient's return home, often part of the transition to the chronic phase, allows members to reassert their competence and leadership more fully.

In contrast, a family that is more comfortable with intense involvement and control by health care providers might have more difficulty when their ill family member returns home from a rehabilitation hospital and they lose their locus of competency, the professional caregiving system. It can be useful to inquire about and address concerns in advance of discharge, including rehearsing caregiving scenarios. Sometimes, when deemed "medically necessary," having a longer period of home-based health care provider assistance can help a family shift their strong dependence on the health care team into greater self-directed proficiency. Care guides and home health aides are valuable resources.

When a total takeover by professionals is necessary, in an ICU, for example, a clinician can empathize with the family's need to relinquish physical control temporarily and can inquire about and encourage family rituals or prayer, a meaningful sharing of music and readings, and time with companion animals. Such activities can brighten spirits, complement medical interventions, and allow expression of a family's basic beliefs about mastery.

Family Beliefs about the Causes of Illness and Disability

When a significant health problem arises, most of us wonder "Why me (or us)?" and "Why now?" (Franks & Roesch, 2006; Roesch & Weiner, 2001). Taking into account the limits of current medical knowledge and the tremendous uncertainties about the relative importance of myriad factors, individuals and families cannot help attributing an illness to many varied causes. It is important to clarify each family member's perspective. Framing inquiry in a curious, open manner, clinicians should invite collaborative dialogue and avoid blaming or judgmental implications. For instance, "All of us come up with reasons for how or why something happens, but we may not get an opportunity to share it. I am interested in what influences each of you thinks might have *contributed to* Fred's heart attack." Such questions help foster a meaning-making process and suggest the possibility that multiple factors may be involved. A family's responses reflect their fund of medical information, their core beliefs, and their past experiences with illness.

Various explanations may include biological, religious, or societal factors or individual or family dysfunction. It is useful to distinguish between beliefs about external factors often beyond the patient's control (e.g., lack of access to adequate health care) and those that blame individual members or the whole family. Clinicians should be cautious not to join in scapegoating a member or unfairly blame families stressed by misfortune. At the same time, they can acknowledge contributing factors, such as substance abuse in liver damage, smoking in lung cancer or emphysema, or obesity in type 2 diabetes. Beliefs about the cause of illness might include punishment for earlier misdeeds (e.g., an affair, an ancestor's transgressions); blaming a particular family member (e.g., "Your nagging gave me a heart attack"); a sense of injustice (e.g., "Why am I being punished? I have been a good person"); genetics (e.g., cancer runs in one side of the family); negligence by the patient (e.g., careless driving) or by parents (e.g., sudden infant death syndrome [SIDS]); religious beliefs (e.g., God's punishment for sinful living); or simply bad luck. Inquiry about culturally based beliefs or syndromes is valuable. For instance, Latino families may believe that nervios, an increased susceptibility to stress and symptoms of nervousness, has caused a cancer.

Optimal family narratives respect the limits of scientific knowledge, affirm basic competence, and promote the flexible use of multiple biological and psychosocial–spiritual healing approaches. In contrast, causal attributions that invoke blame, shame, or guilt are particularly important to uncover, as they can derail family coping and adaptation. In such cases, a referral for more intensive family therapy is generally indicated. With a potentially fatal illness, a blamed family member may be held accountable if the patient dies (e.g., "You neglected his care!"). Decisions about treatment can become confounded and filled with tension. As the following case illustrates, every transition to a further progression of an illness can escalate the cycle of blame, shame, or guilt.

Case Example: A Parent with a Terminally Ill Child

Lucy and Tom, a couple in their early thirties, have one child, Susan, age 4, who is terminally ill with leukemia. Following the diagnosis 2 years earlier, the initial treatments were moderately successful; but over the past 6 months, her condition has worsened. The pediatric oncologist has offered the parents the choice between an experimental treatment with a low probability of success or halting treatment; he supports either choice.

Tom's position is "Let's stop; enough is enough." Lucy, on the other hand, feels "We must continue; we can't let her die." The couple cannot reach an agreement, and the physician is immobilized. He requests a consultation for the couple.

I first inquire about each parent's understanding of the options and find out that both comprehend the choices, but have reached strongly opposing positions. When I ask, "How do you each try to explain or make sense of how your daughter got leukemia?" critical stories emerge. Tom basically sees it as bad luck. Lucy, however, has a very different belief. During her pregnancy with Susan, Lucy's father had a heart attack and died several months later from a second episode. Lucy experienced this as a time of great stress and grief, which she feels adversely affected the intrauterine life of Susan. After Susan's birth, by normal delivery, Lucy was still mourning the loss of her father, and feels that the stressful situation affected the quality of her bonding with Susan. She believes that led to a hidden infant depression. Further, Lucy had read of research linking depression with lowering of the effectiveness of the immune system, which could, in turn, decrease normal surveillance and clearing of cancer cells from the body. She believes this combination of factors caused her child's cancer, and that if she had been a more competent mother, this never would have happened.

Lucy said she had never told this story to anyone, including her husband, because no one had ever asked and she was very ashamed. She had hoped for a cure so that the whole issue could be resolved. She cannot accept stopping treatment because, to her, it means feeling that Susan's death will be her fault. Tom was stunned to learn that his wife harbored such a belief.

This case highlights a number of clinical issues. First, Lucy's beliefs about causing her daughter's illness emerged in full force in the terminal phase of the disease, although she had had these thoughts from the beginning. Frequently, destructive beliefs about what caused a condition can remain hidden, here fueling her secret suffering and self-blame, which only surfaced with compassionate inquiry at a clinical crossroads.

Second, the individual pieces of the story are stitched together from real-world data and beliefs: there are accepted theories about major stressors, such as grief, affecting intrauterine development and about inadequate attachment as a cause of childhood depression. Research findings in psychoneuroimmunology show links among depression, immune system compromise, and decreased surveillance of stray cancer cells—as well as a relationship between bereavement and altered physiology. As a whole, Lucy's story goes well beyond its parts and the research evidence. The oncologist and I encouraged her to reconsider her blame-laden assumptions, taking into account the current limits of research and fact that the baby was fine at birth and developed normally throughout infancy.

This case highlights the social construction of beliefs. The most striking, of course, is the gendered belief system of mother blaming in European American culture and in the mental health field. Early maternal attachment was widely viewed as essential for positive child development, and deficiencies in maternal bonding were assumed to be prime determinants of any subsequent development problems. It was important to normalize her preoccupation with her father's death and to expand the parental frame to include the father's important role in early childhood attachments. I questioned her assumptions about maternal bonding deficiencies and contextualized societal expectations of mothers by asking her, "Who might think that about you?" Tom assured her that he did not hold those beliefs or blame her in any way. He thought she overestimated the extent of her physical or psychological absence. He reminded her of his involvement with Susan and strongly affirmed her competence as a mother and spouse.

Brief couple therapy, lasting four sessions, broadened the discussion of Lucy's beliefs about Susan's condition. The oncologist, invited to the second session, added his own second thoughts about whether a different treatment strategy might have been more successful. This process, including the physician's viewpoint, enabled the couple to gain a more coherent and helpful shared narrative regarding the cause and course of their daughter's condition, while strengthening their mutual support and facilitating expressions of grief about their impending loss.

A preventive approach seeks to identify toxic beliefs early and avert unnecessary suffering. Often, feelings of guilt or shame—including worry about judgments by extended family or others—constrain individuals from openly disclosing their beliefs and feelings. This is one reason I usually allow some time during an initial consultation to meet with family members separately (see Chapter 4). Early intervention is particularly critical when family members blame themselves and other family members concur, as these beliefs often remain hidden and can heighten the risks of conflict, estrangement, or destructive behavior. In one case, a husband's belief that his drinking caused his wife's heart attack and death fueled increasingly self-destructive drinking. An out-of-control spiral led to his being fired from his job and, finally, caused a near-fatal auto accident while he was intoxicated.

It is crucial to ask children about their causal beliefs, as in the following case.

Case Example: A Child's Beliefs

Sam, a 6-year-old boy, required a life-saving lower leg amputation for a bone cancer. His 5-year-old brother, Richard, when asked if he had any ideas about what might have caused Sam's condition, said, "I gave my brother cancer when I kicked him during a soccer game. We were on different teams and I was really getting mad at him." Richard secretly believed that his anger (normative sibling rivalry) had gone through his leg to Sam's leg, causing the cancer. Strong parental reassurance and the physician's age-sensitive explanation to both brothers averted what could have fueled guilt-related psychosocial difficulties.

In my clinical experience, families with the strongest, sometimes extreme, core beliefs about personal responsibility and control and those with the most conflictual relational patterns are more likely to attribute the cause of a medical condition to themselves or blame each other. Acknowledging the vicissitudes of life as a causal factor reduces blame, shame, and guilt. In highly dysfunctional families with unresolved conflicts and intense blaming, attributions of what or who is responsible for an illness can escalate into scapegoating and long-term family power struggles or cutoffs.

To make sense of suffering and the unknowable, family members frequently blame themselves in some way or some members fight over assignment of blame in order to deflect unbearable pain. This tendency can be eased through a more empathic interaction that acknowledges the pain of what has happened and can't be changed and promotes the patient and family's active agency on the path ahead. Questions that can open doors to the future move from why something happened toward what can be done about it (Kushner, 1981).

Beliefs about Agency and an Illness's Future Course

Just as it is important to ascertain family members' beliefs or attributions about what caused a condition, it is also important to find out their beliefs about what can influence its future course. In what active ways can family members support patient and family well-being? Abundant research on a "sense of coherence" finds that positive adaptation is facilitated by believing that our adverse situation is comprehensible, posing challenges that are meaningful and manageable to tackle with available resources (Antonovsky, 1998; Reiss, 1981).

Belief-System Flexibility

Because illnesses vary enormously in their responsiveness to psychosocial factors, both families and providers need to distinguish between beliefs about their overall participation, or active agency, in long-term disease management and beliefs about their ability to control the biological progression and outcome. Clinicians can encourage a family's flexible participation in the overall illness and treatment process, independent of whether a disease is stable, improving, or terminal. Proactive attempts to influence a biological course can make a difference, such as when parents stop serving sweet desserts so as not to tempt an adolescent with diabetes. Or, family life might be adjusted to help maintain the health of a member with cancer in remission by adjusting members' roles, communication patterns, diets, type of exercise, and the balance between work and recreation.

Flexibility on the part of the family and the health care team is a key variable in optimal functioning. Rather than linking mastery in a rigid way with survival or recovery, families can define mastery in a more "holistic" sense. Involvement and participation in the overall process can be the main criteria defining success. Psychosocial–spiritual healing may influence the course or outcome, but a positive disease outcome is not necessary for a family to feel successful. This flexible view of mastery permits the quality of relations within the family or between the family and medical providers to become a central criterion of success. The health provider's competence is valued from both a technical and a caregiving perspective, and not solely from a biological one.

Families with flexible belief systems are more likely to experience the death of a loved one with a sense of equanimity rather than as a profound failure ("We did what we could, but..."). Optimally, when an ill family member loses remission, and a family enters the terminal phase, participation as an expression of mastery is transformed from influencing the outcome to easing suffering and supporting palliative care (see Chapter 10).

Clinicians need to be mindful that families with the strongest and most rigid beliefs about personal responsibility and control may function well during earlier stages of an illness but become vulnerable if the condition progresses beyond their control. An attitude that conveys, "We understand the risks, and we are going to try our best to beat this thing" fosters resilience, whereas, "We *must* beat this thing or we've failed" fuels a sense of defeat. If disability or death becomes equated with a failure of will, effort, or competence, this attitude can have a profound, negative impact on a patient's and family's sense of well-being.

Marlene, a successful African American professional in her early forties, was referred because of a recurrence of breast cancer. At the initial consultation, I asked how I could be of help. Her immediate response was, "I need help because *I gave myself a recurrence* of breast cancer." Marlene had grown up in dire poverty. Her enormous willpower was instrumental in overcoming the odds against her throughout her life. This was the first time she had "failed," attributing this to her insufficient will. When I contacted the oncologist, she told me that Marlene had been informed that her cancer had over a 90% recurrence rate and a poor prognosis. The cancer and its prognosis were hard enough, but her inflexible beliefs about responsibility and control led to intense self-blame and suffering. Our work focused on a revised, more adaptable belief about mastery and competence in relation to her cancer, while honoring her overall life narrative.

Clinicians need to think longitudinally about the viability of strongly held beliefs over the entire course of an illness. As this case illustrates, the need for a flexible belief system becomes most evident at major nodal points in illness, individual, or family development. At these times families' mastery of new challenges may require modifying time-honored beliefs. What is adaptive at one point may not be helpful later. Treatment early on that explores the underpinnings of rigidly held beliefs can increase flexibility and thus avert a belief system crisis later, as when a cancer recurs or recovery from a stroke plateaus. The following questions can open a dialogue with a family. "You seem very committed to your beliefs about beating this illness. Do any of you foresee any conceivable problems with this?" or "What would it mean for you to redefine your beliefs about success with regard to your (or your family member's) condition in a more flexible way?"

Working with Hope and Optimism

Abundant research supports the psychological and physiological value of hope (Cheavans, Michael, & Snyder, 2005). Hope is a future-oriented belief that is essential for mastering the challenges of illness. Clinicians should avoid either/or thinking about the value of hope and optimism versus direct confrontation and acceptance of painful realities. Often both are needed, and what is hoped for or accepted may well change over the illness course. Weingarten (2010) describes *reasonable hope*, which includes fluctuations of doubt and despair as part of hope's complexities. The healthy use of minimization or a selective focus on the positive and the ability to find moments of humor in a threatening situation should be distinguished from the concept of denial, which can clearly interfere with effective health behaviors.

Epidemiological research finds that with "positive illusions," information, such as a poor prognosis, has been accurately heard (Taylor, Kemeny, Reed, Bower, & Gruenwald, 2000). Other studies found that cancer patients with positive outcome biases didn't necessarily live longer, but they enjoyed a more positive quality of life and were glad they made the effort to do their best (e.g., following the treatment regimen, changing diet, getting more exercise, and reducing stress). One needs to make an informed decision or choice to believe in the possibility of overcoming poor odds, such as a high recurrence rate for cancer. It fuels active agency to take steps that could increase the odds of success without any guarantee.

Having hope and minimization can reduce family terror related to anticipated loss in the initial crisis phase, particularly if there is an extended period of uncertainty, as in treating life-threatening cancer. Hope can enable family members to adjust to living with arduous conditions involving continual long-term caregiving that is required for a serious head injury or for Parkinson's disease (Forgeard & Seligman, 2012; Hurt et al., 2014; Rasmussen, Scheier, & Greenhouse, 2009); it helps them through an inevitable period of trial and error in learning how to best cope with an ongoing condition. Assisting families in prioritizing immediate challenges can significantly reduce its sense of overload and increase its sense of competency. This is analogous to a couple's developing a comfortable style of parenting. If we knew all the trials and tribulations of parenthood beforehand, many of us might never have children, or we might develop very rigid, constricted, protective child-rearing methods devoid of creative spontaneity. Family adaptation to chronic conditions involves a similar socialization process. As families approach the chronic phase, their initial optimism without much illness-related experience develops into familiarity tinged with positive illusions.

A clinician needs to assess when family members have heard the essential information about a risky treatment, discussed the risks of loss frankly, decided to try it and then adopted a positive outlook toward a favorable outcome. This is different from avoiding an acknowledgment or a discussion of risks (denial) and deciding blindly for or against a risky procedure. Clinicians who are confronting a family with a painful medical reality need as well to respect a family's core optimism. Failure to join the family at this underlying level can impede its ability to confront immediate issues.

Families that are generally optimistic about their ability to master adversity emphasize their overall quality of life and attributes of family identity that transcend biology and the challenges of illness. When a family lacks a sense of competence, hope can flourish or vanish as an illness takes its course. Consultations or more intensive treatment should aim to help build family competencies with illness challenges and to identify important values and aspects of family life, in order to put an illness into perspective where hope for successful treatment is balanced with optimism about the quality of family relationships or making the most of precious time.

Time-Phase Considerations

Direct communication about threatened loss is important at any significant transition in the illness, family, or individual members' development. Clinicians should not regard broaching this topic as dashing family hopes. In fact, when such subjects are avoided, dread is often heightened, leading to more pervasive and dysfunctional denial and restricted patterns of family communication. Timely, frank communication preserves a family's ability to sustain functional hope while addressing new developmental issues.

Illness Narratives and Metaphors

Beliefs about the cause of a condition, which was discussed earlier, are one facet of the overall meaning that families construct concerning a physical condition. Clinicians need to appreciate the fuller narrative, which melds a number of themes, including meanings attached to the disease label itself, beliefs promoted by the health care providers and system, timely cultural metaphors, and personal and family meanings.

Illness Narratives

As Kleinman (1988) points out, "The personal narrative does not merely reflect the illness experience, but rather it contributes to the experience of symptoms and suffering" (p. 49). The story that family members develop about an illness experience is a synthesis of their core family beliefs and their attempt to restore order out of chaos and fear. A simple, direct inquiry, "Tell me about your illness and what it has meant for you and your loved ones," often suffices to elicit this story.

A central clinical goal is to draw out family members' narratives so they can share them with one another. In this process, different perspectives can be explored and clarified, leading to an acceptance of varied positions or consensus building. Empowering life themes can be gleaned from accounts of courage, overcoming adversity, or repairing injustice. Clinicians can affirm each member's meaning-making efforts to facilitate the joining process needed in a collaborative therapeutic process. This ought to be done in an empathic, respectful manner, without blame, and with an emphasis on family strengths and aspirations.

Diagnosis and Labeling

The labeling language used to communicate a diagnosis conveys a revealing message about the locus and extensiveness of pathology. Do family members and professionals refer to diabetes in a family as "Joe has diabetes," "Joe is a diabetic," or even "Joe's diabetic family"? The way all the parties involved communicate about a condition strongly influences the meanings and beliefs that shape enduring narratives. These narratives, in turn, shape the identity of the affected person and of the family system. "Joe is a diabetic" implies that a physical disorder has become the whole person. This is more common in conditions, such as diabetes, that affect the whole body physiologically or in others that are highly visible ("an amputee"). Conditions that have a high level of uncertainty about their cause, control, or cure or have associated stigma lend themselves to more extensive labels (Sontag, 1978).

When families refer to the ill member or themselves in all-encompassing terms (for example, "our alcoholic family"), the entire family is pathologized. Clinicians need to be mindful of their own way of speaking about an illness or disability and encourage families to refer to a chronic condition in more circumscribed terms in order to facilitate healthy adaptation.

Some labels have ambiguous or multiple meanings that make it more difficult for families to demarcate the health condition. Couples dealing with fertility problems can come to view their whole relationship as barren. If they refer to themselves as infertile—or if providers do so—it constrains their ability to absorb a probable significant loss and to continue defining their relationship in hopeful terms despite their difficulties.

Some conditions are associated with embarrassment and shame, particularly those with visible characteristics and public reactions. Examples include psoriasis, Tourette's syndrome (which includes uncontrolled tics, guttural sounds, and cursing), musculoskeletal disorders (e.g., MS, Parkinson's disease, or muscular dystrophy), seizure disorders, and physical deformities. Other conditions can foster shame because of the stigma attached to cognitive impairment. These include intellectual disabilities; TBI; and major mental disorders such as schizophrenia, Alzheimer's disease and other forms of dementia, and substance-abuse-related organic brain syndromes. Some conditions, such as inflammatory bowel diseases, can have hidden shame-laden features (e.g., a colostomy) or entail risk of public embarrassment. Mastectomy for breast cancer can be particularly problematic because of the cultural association of breasts with a woman's beauty and desirability, as well as with the maternal qualities associated with breast-feeding. Conditions that disfigure the face or produce facial signs of emotional and physical pain become outward, public signs of suffering and the changed identity of the afflicted person. The following case is illustrative.

> Bill, a 30-year-old gay man with HIV/AIDS, had kept his diagnosis secret for 3 years, except from his widowed mother. He had carefully concealed his sexual orientation and social life throughout his adulthood. Loyal to his mother, he continued to live in his hometown, a small, conservative community where he felt that his status and livelihood as a bank teller depended on concealing his lifestyle and diagnosis. He received his medical care in a nearby city, telling neighbors and friends that he suffered from a chronic respiratory condition that fatigued him. A crisis arose when Bill developed Kaposi's sarcomas (large purplish lesions characteristic of advanced AIDS). When they spread from his legs and chest to his face, Bill could no longer hide his condition and his mother could not manage his care without outside help.
> In the terminal phase, Bill chose to disclose his "real" life to his extended family and friends for the first time. He had always relied heavily on his handsome appearance in social situations. Genuine support in his period of physical decline and facial disfigurement forced Bill to reevaluate his belief that his appearance was the primary reason that other people valued him.

When diagnoses involve stigma, clinicians need to address dysfunctional family processes that contribute to or reinforce a health problem, such as denial of a member's problematic alcohol abuse. This is distinct from the common tendency in families to avoid the shame-laden labeling of a member or the whole family as "alcoholic." When clinicians confront presumed family denial, it is important to acknowledge their sense of shame. If left unappreciated, it may heighten their experience of shame and increase their failure to address crucial issues.

Metaphors

Metaphors that become attached to biological conditions are critical organizers of families' illness narratives and behavior. Kleinman (1988) maintains that "To understand how symptoms and illnesses have meaning we must first understand normative conceptions of the body in relation to the self and world. These integral aspects of local social systems inform how we feel, how we perceive mundane bodily processes, and how we interpret those feelings and processes" (p. 13). Normative conceptions of the body guide our attributions about illnesses and the narratives families construct about them. For instance, North American culture places enormous value on physical appearance, including qualities such as an unblemished skin and a youthful and sexually desirable body. Illnesses or phases of a disorder that are visible tend, in our culture, to create a nodal point of meaning and a crisis in self-esteem.

Symptoms like pain or fatigue, however, are invisible and poorly understood and can evoke an aura of mystery. These symptoms can ebb and flow and be highly responsive to context, such as emotional states or stressful family interactions. Words, like pain, have multiple meanings that can be used to describe both a biological phenomenon and a social quality. Statements such as "I am in pain," "You are a pain," or "You are making my pain worse" can be interpreted literally or metaphorically. Thus, words such as *pain* or *fatigue* have flexible meanings and an ambiguity that promotes use of metaphors. Clinicians can help patients and families to address this kind of ambiguity and use more direct and clear communication.

Families coping with chronic disorders often become hyperaware of bodily functions and symptoms. Over time, their language tends to incorporate medical terms to describe a range of physical states and feelings. Physical and emotional fatigue or depletion can easily become interchangeable in conversation. This next case illustrates the evolution of an illness metaphor.

Jane, a 20-year-old, single, African American woman with lifelong sickle-cell disease lives with her mother and sister. She has been admitted to the hospital with recurrent frequent bouts of pain (a symptom of her disease) and depression. She requires narcotic medication for her pain. In the past 2 years, she has visited the emergency room with increasing frequency, nearly weekly in recent months. She does not adhere to home medical regimens and routine follow-up visits. Recently, she entered a community college program and is feeling overwhelmed. Her primary physician and emergency-room staff doubt that she experiences pain. Jane tells a psychiatric consultant that her main problem is that "No one believes my pain, so why bother?"

Three years earlier, at age 17, Jane was psychiatrically hospitalized following a suicide attempt. At that time she confided that she had been sexually molested by her father since age 13, but had never revealed it to anyone. Hospital notes state that her father denied the allegations and refused family meetings and that the rest of the family went along with the father's story. Jane was discharged to individual outpatient treatment, which she soon discontinued. Three months later, the father left the family without explanation, and the sexual abuse was never mentioned again. Also, 6 months after Jane's discharge, at age 18, she was transferred from the pediatric service at one hospital to the adult service of an affiliated hospital.

In this case, Jane's experience of pain and feelings of loss are central themes in which "disbelief of pain" has become the metaphor describing the totality of her experience. Her feelings about family disbelief and denial of her claims of sexual abuse and the subsequent loss of her father are now being reactivated in losing the pediatric health professionals and hospital home to which she was very attached for many years. This loss, like the loss of her father, has not been adequately addressed. Her family has not heeded her emotional or physical pain. She felt disregarded by the psychiatric service when the sexual abuse charges were dropped after her father and family denied them. Now, her new doctors question her complaint of physical pain as indicative of manipulation and malingering. Another factor may be gender bias, whereby female patients' experiences of pain too often are not acknowledged as "real" by health care providers, in some cases leading to an inappropriate psychiatric diagnosis.

In life-cycle terms, Jane is in her emerging adult transition, a normative period for setting up an independent life. Faced with a life-threatening illness and disability, issues related to threatened loss cloud her future vision. Emotional pain, in the form of anxieties and self-doubt about achieving the typical goals of early adulthood, is being felt most acutely, as Jane takes on the stressful challenges of college, further strained by her physical limitations and related fatigue.

Effective intervention with Jane required affirmation of her pain and losses by the therapist, the family, and the health care professionals. Ambiguities related to her father's leaving and disbelief of her story of abuse needed clarification. Additionally, exploration of the issues of threatened loss as a young adult with sickle-cell disease was needed to transform what had become her unheeded communication about pain (see Chapter 9).

Larger-System Illness Metaphors

Sontag (1978) has described how certain life-threatening conditions that are poorly understood in terms of cause and treatment, such as HIV and cancer, can tap into larger societal issues of the era and evoke powerful, multilevel metaphors. At any point in history, certain concerns come to the forefront of society. For instance, in the late twentieth century, cancer had become the illness associated with fears about death beyond our control and, metaphorically, with certain problems of modern civilization, such as the rapid technological expansion of society and polluted, stressful, urban environments. Also, cancer predisposition was purportedly linked to familial or personal characteristics, such as repressed feelings or helpless, defeated attitudes.

Clinicians can ask families about the influence of cultural, religious, or societally stigmatizing meanings attached to their illness and how these interpretations have affected them. Some families withdraw, becoming isolated from social support. Others become energized and often become involved in some form of activism to change cultural beliefs, HIV being an excellent example. Multifamily discussion groups are particularly useful for conditions associated with stigma and societal prejudice. By facilitating contact among families, they alleviate isolation and promote a normalizing process that helps restore family pride and dignity (see Chapter 4).

Individual, Family, and Illness Life Review

From a life-cycle vantage point, a central task of later life and in terminal illness is to develop and share one's life narrative as a coherent account that represents a synthesis of one's life and provides perspective. King and Wynne (2004) describe *family integrity* as a developmental striving toward meaning, connection, and continuity within the multigenerational family system. Two key aspects of shared meaning-making involve passing on individual and family legacies to the next generations and resolving or accepting past losses and relational conflicts. Walsh (2016a) has described the value of a *family life review*, which complements and expands an individual life review. Here, family members or couples can share accounts of their life together as a way to integrate individual life narratives into a fuller collective account that incorporates multiple perspectives and subjective experiences of their shared lives over time. Sharing satisfactions and disappointments along with different perceptions of hopes and visions expands the family narrative, enhances shared empathy, deepens bonds, and fosters healing of relational wounds.

Individual, couple, and family life reviews can be very therapeutic with progressive or life-threatening conditions, in approaching the end of life, and after a final loss. I routinely propose a session in which families can do an *illness-focused review* of their personal and collective experiences (see the extended case example in Chapter 17.) This is particularly useful for families that have been burdened for years by a condition in which painful experiences often overshadow the whole of the relationship, including life before the illness. A review facilitates expanding the story to include other aspects of their lives, which puts the illness experience into a larger perspective. This review is often best done well after the immediate mourning period following a final loss. This process helps to reaffirm core beliefs, to strengthen the positive ones acquired through the ordeal of a serious illness, or to revise an illness story laden with destructive or shameful beliefs. When family members share their illness stories, they frequently offer each other suggestions for reworking their narratives in a more positive direction.

Rituals

Rituals are the primary means by which families maintain, store, and convey their identity and core beliefs (Imber-Black, 2012; Imber-Black, Roberts, & Whiting, 2003). Rituals provide stabilization and continuity over time; can facilitate transitions around critical events and a transformation of beliefs; and are particularly important with chronic disorders, where they can be used therapeutically to facilitate change or healing.

There are four kinds of family rituals: (1) *daily routines and regular patterned family interactions*, such as mealtime or bedtime rituals and weekend activities; (2) *family traditions*, such as birthdays, anniversaries, annual vacations, and reunions, which are unique to each family and solidify and convey family identity; (3) *celebrations*, such as Thanksgiving and religious holidays, which serve as cultural symbols connecting families with their larger group identity; (4) *life-cycle rituals*, such as births, retirement, weddings, funerals, and memorials, as well as the healing rituals associated with unexpected life events, such as illness. If the family or community is seen as influential in either the illness cause or the healing process, rituals that incorporate different system levels might involve an extended network of friends, neighbors, coworkers, faith congregations, or a community vigil.

Rituals and routines are easily neglected or interrupted with illness or loss (see Chapter 10), when a family is overwhelmed and consumed by immediate illness-related demands or grief. When a member with physical or cognitive impairment is unable to maintain his or her previous roles or participation in family rituals, we can encourage families to transform rituals or to create new ones that keep the ill member included in family life. Neglecting rituals can reflect a deeper despondency. Family members may believe they have failed in their efforts to conquer a condition, which gets expressed as "we have nothing left to celebrate." Encouraging families to preserve rituals or transform them in positive ways helps them to sustain adaptive empowering beliefs.

A serious illness and threatened loss can heighten awareness in a family that each gathering and ritual may be their last together. Clinicians can promote the timely creation and use of rituals involving celebration, inclusion, and appreciation. For instance, a reunion can invigorate family members, affirm and strengthen their bonds, reconnect estranged members, and revitalize energies in supporting the ill member and key caregivers.

Rituals are also useful in painful situations of unacknowledged or stigmatized loss, as experienced in a miscarriage, infertility, or a suicide, in which members may distance themselves and a loss may not have been adequately marked (Werner-Lin & Moro, 2004). Practitioners should be cautious not to minimize the significance of the loss and should explore its impact for a couple or family.

In one case, a young couple, Sandra and Phil, had endured two ectopic pregnancies, as well as a lengthy fertility workup and interventions over a 2-year period. Because the physician detected no apparent physiological problems, he encouraged the couple to continue their efforts to have a child and emphasized that the odds were in their favor. This fatigued couple, however, had not taken sufficient time to mark their losses or allow a sufficient respite period.

After their loss issues became apparent, the therapist encouraged the couple to take a vacation together to reaffirm their strained relationship. He suggested that before going, they create a ritual to mark the losses of the two ectopic pregnancies. This idea resonated strongly with Sandra, while Phil was reluctant, wanting to forget the past "failures." The therapist reinforced her need to mark these losses and encouraged Phil to support her. She asked him to quietly join her and participate more actively if he felt like it, to which he readily agreed.

Based on some images in her recent dreams, Sandra designed a ritual in which she would release two roses (one representing each lost pregnancy) at the Chicago waterfront as the tide was going out. Symbols of letting go (the tide), of precious lives (the roses), and of healing (water and gentle waves) were central to her ritual. She also read a brief eulogy for their lost children as the tide took the roses away. Phil was spontaneously moved to speak about his own sense of loss. The ritual, held just before departing for their vacation, enabled them to renew their relationship.

This case highlights the usefulness of rituals in helping families endure chronic conditions, honor and transform a painful experience into something positive, and appreciate life beyond the illness or loss. Clinicians can suggest the idea of a ritual and encourage couples or families to design it to fit their own beliefs, symbols, and culture. They can support the need for personal rituals and be flexible regarding the degree of involvement of members. Because rituals are specific to a certain place and time, they facilitate family members' sharing of strong emotions with lower anxiety.

Many dread a family gathering after a significant loss, feeling "It's not the same without her," or "It will be too sad." But when clinicians can encourage families to find symbolic ways to remember and honor their deceased loved one through stories, photographs, toasts, and remembrance rituals, studies find that the pain of the physical absence is eased and loss can be transformed into deep, continuing bonds that facilitate healing.

The Health Belief Fit among Family Members

Health care providers should not assume that all family members share one set of beliefs and act in unison. It is valuable to consider the interaction among family members' beliefs and those of health care providers and systems (see Chapter 17). To what degree do family members view the family system as the healing unit that requires unified agreement or that welcomes different viewpoints? How much do family members feel the need to stay in sync with prevailing cultural or societal beliefs or with family traditions? Family values are strongly influenced by cultural norms and multigenerational family beliefs, yet given the diversity in contemporary family life and our rapidly changing society, families need to respect multiple perspectives among members, especially across the generations.

Family beliefs that balance needs for consensus with diversity and innovation maximize flexible options. The guiding principle "We can hold different viewpoints," welcomes diversity. New and creative ways to approach issues may be needed in situations of protracted and shifting illness challenges. A flexible approach gives a clinician greater latitude to work separately with the patient or other family members without mobilizing family resistance. However, where consensus is the rule and individual differentiation may imply disloyalty, paying attention to the entire family is essential. In culturally attuned ways, it is useful to help families negotiate their differences and to support the separate needs and goals of each member.

Time-Phase Issues

The fit of beliefs evolves over the course of a disorder. Normative cultural differences among family members' health beliefs may emerge into destructive conflicts during a health crisis or a transition, as in the following case.

James and Carla have been married for 8 years. James was raised in a highly intellectual, scientifically oriented European American family. Carla grew up in a traditional Puerto Rican family. When Carla's aging father had a recurrence of cancer, he decided to turn to traditional indigenous healing practices alongside standard oncological treatment. Carla, as a daughter, who understood and embraced traditional Western medical beliefs, felt that it was important to support her father's preferences. James, however, ridiculed Carla and her father's beliefs as "hogwash." This precipitated a serious marital crisis.

The cultural differences between Carla and James had been manageable over the years, yet the power of a health crisis, bringing to the fore basic beliefs and practices, derailed a previously functional marriage. This chasm, based on beliefs about treatment and healing, could easily tear the marital relationship apart and create a rift between their families. When clinicians respectfully affirm such cultural differences, it helps family members shift from blaming or depreciating to respectful accommodation.

INTEGRATIVE MEDICINE AND HEALING PRACTICES

Increasingly, patients and families coping with chronic conditions seek and utilize complementary medicine as part of their "system" of health care and healing strategies. The burgeoning interest in integrative medicine is a response to the overuse of technology, the lack of access to health care, and the inadequacy of traditional Western biomedical approaches in treating chronic conditions. Initially termed "holistic medicine," then "complementary and alternative medicine" (CAM), integrative medicine is person centered and healing oriented. It values collaborative practice in contrast with the orientation of the traditional biomedicine, which is focused on treatment and cure by the physician as expert. One of the core tenets of integrative medicine is that healing is an active multidimensional process, that attends to the whole person—body, mind, and spirit—and that considers all aspects of life, including environmental influences (Rakel, 2012; Weil, 2004). Making use of all appropriate conventional and CAM therapeutic approaches, integrative medicine programs increasingly include a relational and family component of care.

The field has expanded beyond the National Center for Complementary and Integrative Health (*https://nccih.nih.gov*) to the Academic Consortium for Integrative Medicine and Health (*www.imconsortium.org*), which strives to advance the principles and practices of integrative medicine in a rapidly growing number of academic institutions in North America. A National Center for Health Statistics Report (Clarke, Black, Stussman, Barnes, & Nahin, 2015) shows that yearly over a third of adults in the United States use some form of complementary health approach, particularly adults who struggle with chronic pain conditions and those who are medically uninsured. Some of the most commonly used CAM therapies include acupuncture, biofeedback, diet-based therapies, homeopathy, massage, meditation, movement therapies, natural products, traditional healers, and yoga.

Unfortunately, integrative healing strategies are often marginalized in standard Western medicine, leaving patients and families with two parallel, disconnected healing tracks. Providers sometimes respond dismissively when patients share their interest in or information about alternative healing approaches, often because of unfamiliarity with them. Besides being a missed opportunity to optimize patient health care, such dismissiveness can be very stressful and alienating to families. Inquiry and curiosity about a patient's or family's use of nonstandard approaches shows an interest in and acknowledgment of their potential value. This facilitates a respectful collaboration and the integration of diverse beliefs and healing practices.

Largely because of growing consumer demand, health systems increasingly offer integrative medicine programs or refer patients to community resources. Just as with behavioral health, optimal collaboration includes integrative care (e.g., acupuncture, mindfulness meditation, nutrition) as part of routine care with expert practitioners providing these approaches in a coordinated, or ideally collocated, way with primary or specialty care as part of a unified health care team (see Chapter 18).

Meditation and specifically mindfulness-based stress reduction (MBSR) approaches have proven extremely valuable adjuncts to chronic-illness treatment planning (Didonna, 2009; Ledesma & Kumano, 2009; Ludwig &

Kabat-Zinn, 2008). MBSR training is available in many hospitals, clinics, and stand-alone programs nationwide and internationally. Online e-learning programs are also widely accessible. Such techniques are useful to both patient and family members (see case example in Chapter 17). They can be incorporated into individual, couple, and family therapy and have been combined with other therapeutic techniques, such as mindfulness-based cognitive behavioral therapy (MCBT). I have found it useful sometimes at the beginning of a session to help relax and focus the provider, patient, or family. This is particularly beneficial during an illness crisis or high-stress periods. These approaches can also help with health care provider stress and compassion fatigue (see Chapter 17).

PART III

PHASE-RELATED ISSUES AND SPECIFIC POPULATIONS

PRACTICE GUIDELINES

CHAPTER 9

Helping Families with Anticipatory Loss and Suffering

The anticipation of loss in physical illness can be as challenging and painful for families as the actual death of a family member. It touches the existential knowledge of their own mortality that they may want to deny (Becker, 1973).

Scant attention has been given to the process of families' anticipation of *future* loss and suffering and how that experience evolves with illness, individual, and family development. Most literature on loss has focused on *anticipatory grief* in terminal illness, when loss is imminent (Rando, 2000). It has not addressed the "if" aspect of threatened loss and has narrowed the "when" to the last phase. When diagnosed, most illnesses are uncertain (Mishel, 2014). The issues are the *degree* of uncertainty and *when* loss might become salient. What is overlooked are the enormous challenges to families living with uncertainty, while needing to sustain hope. I term this experience *anticipatory loss*.

Encompassing both uncertainty and threatened loss, it refers to living with possible, probable, or inevitable future loss in the context of illness and disability (Rolland, 1990, 2004). It also includes acknowledging and adapting to genetic risk information (see Chapter 15; Rolland, 2006a). This chapter offers a systemic relational framework that addresses the interweaving of family efforts to sustain hope, to cope with varying degrees of uncertainty, and to prepare for loss over the course of an illness.

Research on anticipatory grief has focused primarily on its effects on parents with terminally ill children and on key survivors (e.g., partners) of terminally ill adults (Doka, 2002; Rando, 2000; Stroebe & Schut, 2010). Studies have yielded inconsistent findings about the value of having time to anticipate death. Further, research has documented a broad range of effective coping strategies to deal with loss over time that are grounded in diverse cultural norms and that cast doubt on traditional progressive-stage theories of loss (Kübler-Ross, 1975). The family systems literature has concentrated on the mourning processes after death and the impact on the family of prior unresolved losses (Bowen, 2004; Walsh & McGoldrick, 2004, 2013).

Anticipatory loss includes the mutual influence of family processes with

1. Family members' threatened loss of the ill member.
2. The ill member's anticipation of losing his or her family.
3. The ill member's expectation of disability, suffering, or death.

It encompasses the patient, the family's relationships with the patient, the patient's role functions, and the sense of intactness of the family unit. The impending loss of the intact family unit is the level most easily overlooked, despite its importance. A family member's lament that "we will never be the same" is one expression of this kind of loss. Families that emphasize high cohesion or small families with a sole parent or an only child are more likely to anticipate the loss of the intact family unit if a condition worsens, especially if the ill member has had a central role.

The *experience of anticipatory loss* involves a range of difficult emotional responses that may include separation anxiety, existential aloneness, denial, sadness, disappointment, anger, resentment, guilt, exhaustion, and desperation. There may be intense ambivalence toward the ill member, vacillating wishes for closeness and distance, and fantasies of escape from an overburdened or unbearable situation. Families often become hypervigilant and overprotective, especially when a chronic illness involves long-term threatened loss. Members may repeatedly rehearse the process of loss and imagined scenarios of family suffering and hardship. A patient may dread becoming a burden to one's partner or family and experience the guilt-laden fear of future caregiving and financial strain. Premature distancing can occur when family members are torn between their wishes to sustain connection and their need to "let go" emotionally of an ill member whom they expect to die. Although all relationships involve the existential dilemma of choosing intimacy in the face of eventual separation or loss, life-threatening illness heightens this awareness.

Yet, overemphasis on anticipatory loss can itself become emotionally disabling if it is not counterbalanced by ways of harnessing the experience to enhance the quality of life. Clinicians can be very helpful by assisting families in achieving a healthy balance. For illnesses with long-range risks, families can maintain mastery in the face of uncertainty by (1) acknowledging the possibility of loss, (2) sustaining hope, and (3) building flexibility into family and individual members' life-cycle planning that conserves and adjusts major goals. Clinicians can help families agree about the conditions under which further family discussion would be useful and which members would be appropriate to include.

A close brush with death can lead family members to develop a better appreciation of their loved ones and a sharpened perspective on life that clarifies priorities (Walsh, 2016b). A heightened sense of being alive and an appreciation for "routine" daily events is common. Actively creating opportunities can replace procrastination for the "right moment" or passive waiting for losses to occur. Threatened loss, by emphasizing life's fragility and preciousness, provides families with an opportunity to heal unresolved issues and develop more immediate, caring relationships. For illnesses at a more advanced stage, clinicians can help families emphasize quality of life by defining goals that are more readily attainable and that enrich their daily lives and relationships. To foster a resilient narrative, it is essential to keep in mind and highlight these positive opportunities for families.

The FSI model clarifies how the meaning of potential loss evolves with the life-cycle passage (Rolland, 1987a, 1990, 2004, 2006a, 2016). The salience of anticipatory loss varies, depending on members' multigenerational experience with actual and threatened loss. It also differs with the kind of illness, its psychosocial demands over time, and the degree of uncertainty about prognosis.

The quality and degree of anticipatory loss shifts with the developmental phases of illness. In contrast to families in acute grief near death, families face seemingly incompatible psychosocial tasks earlier on. They try to sustain vital membership for a person who is expected to or may become disabled or die, while simultaneously striving to maintain family integration by reallocating the ill member's role functions. It is essential to distinguish a family's awareness of the *possibility* of loss at an early point in the illness, from an increasing *probability* of loss with illness progression, and from the expectation of *inevitable* loss in the terminal phase. It is also vital to assess concerns about *disability* and *suffering* regarding physical, cognitive, and functional losses as distinct from *death* (see Table 9.1). Patients and families often express their greatest fears about helplessness in the face of uncontrollable pain and suffering.

TABLE 9.1. Anticipatory Loss in Context

1. Kind of Illness (including genetic risk):
   - Possible vs. Probable vs. Inevitable Loss
   - Threat of Death, Disability, and/or Suffering
   - Physical and/or Cognitive Disability
2. Phase of Illness or Genetic Risk
3. Phase of Family and Individual Development
4. Multigenerational Experience with Illness and Loss
5. Belief Systems

ILLNESS TYPE AND TIME-PHASE ISSUES

The psychosocial types and phases of illness provide a time line of potential nodal points of loss, including disability and death.

Time-Phase Challenges

Families begin to develop their own time lines at initial diagnosis. As described in Chapter 3, early discussions with health care providers about the nature of the disorder, its expected course and prognosis, and prescriptions for management constitute a "framing event." As families face threatened loss through disability and/or death, they must learn to live over the long term in limbo with ambiguities. Efforts to resist acceptance of an illness's chronicity may reflect a wish to avoid acceptance of living with uncertainty or "with death over their shoulders." Having to cope with threatened loss for an indeterminate period makes it harder for families to define both present and future structural and emotional boundaries, as well as to engage in life-cycle planning.

Helping families establish functional patterns early on in an illness promotes optimal coping and adaptation. Encouraging open discussion about threatened loss counteracts denial and distancing among family members. A "what if" inquiry helps families bridge the gap between hoping for a positive outcome and the possibility of treatment failure and begin to actively plan in case their hopes are not realized. Essentially, this is hoping for the best, yet preparing for the worst. This is particularly important in the chronic phase when a disease is progressing and the transition to a terminal phase is likely.

In the initial crisis phase of lung cancer, for example, the patient and family may have specific fears related to future complications or intractable pain. Yet, physicians typically do not discuss possible complications at the time of diagnosis. If they were asked, they could reassure the patient that in more than 95% of cases such pain can be well controlled without compromising the patient's cognitive functioning. The tendency of the health care team, the patient, and the family to emphasize hopefulness and successful treatment inhibits discussion of potential complications and concerns. Typically, I ask the patient and family members if there are specific forms of suffering that worry them if treatment does not go well, and I suggest raising any concerns with key providers. A provider can simultaneously express optimism about the treatment plan, while allaying any fears about possible future complications—"I am very hopeful about your treatment plan. However, if you had a major recurrence, significant pain could occur. But, almost always, it can be well controlled, without significantly compromising your quality of life."

Facing a serious loss can shatter a family's belief that life-threatening illnesses happen only to others. A family's loss of a sense of control can be a debilitating experience, leading to frenetic or immobilized behavior. In this period of intense uncertainty, families need to reestablish a belief, even if illusory, that they have some control of the situation. Assisting them in prioritizing tasks and taking direct actions such as gathering information about the illness, attending support groups, and learning about community resources is useful in helping them reestablish a sense of mastery. Patient and family involvement in self-help support groups for particular disorders should be encouraged. Educating families about significant versus minor physical symptoms may avert unnecessary alarm. Helping them distinguish the expected emotional roller coaster from their fears of "craziness" can lower reactivity at this stage.

The Internet can make it easier for patients and families to gather information in the initial crisis phase and to connect to online support groups. Those groups may include people in the chronic phase who are more experienced with a condition and have adapted well. Since some websites provide incorrect or unhelpful information, when possible, I provide suggestions. Also, patients and family members who are dealing with complications of advanced disease and severe psychological distress disproportionately visit and post comments on websites. Reading such comments can terrify families in the initial crisis phase.

Individual family members may hear the same discussion through very different historical and cultural filters, which can lead to conflict with the health care team or with other family members. Beliefs about the likelihood and timing of further disability and death strongly influence the relationship rules established in the face of threatened loss (Olkin, 1999).

In one family, the husband had a benign skin cancer removed and was reassured by the dermatologist that he need not worry about the growth. Marital conflict developed over the ensuing weeks because his wife expressed growing terror about a possible fatal recurrence; wisely, the couple sought help. During the initial consultation, when I inquired about prior experiences with illness and loss, the wife tearfully revealed that in her adolescence her father had died within a year from malignant melanoma, discovered 6 months after being reassured by his physician that his tumor was "benign." That traumatic loss led her to distrust her husband's prognosis and fear losing him. Although he knew that his father-in-law had died from cancer, he had been unaware of the kind of cancer or the misdiagnosis. Once he understood the reasons for her fear, he was able to be supportive.

After this consultation, I contacted the dermatologist to share the wife's history and asked if he could do a quick check of the husband before 6 months passed rather than the planned routine 1-year follow-up to address the wife's psychosocial needs and avert unnecessary suffering. In hindsight, if the dermatologist had initially inquired, "Have either of you ever experienced anything similar?" the wife's account might well have prevented a marital crisis, reduced her suffering, and perhaps curtailed mental health care needs.

Generally, it is best to have the couple or family members share any expectations or catastrophic fears about the anticipated course and outcome so that divergent viewpoints are acknowledged openly. A mutual dialogue avoids escalating cycles of conflict or distancing that the family may fail to understand. If strong and tenacious differences exist among family members, at a minimum a clinician can facilitate mutual acceptance of divergent opinions about a prognosis.

Chronic Phase: Ambivalence, Shameful Thoughts, and Feelings

The *chronic phase* presents different dilemmas for families. Exhaustion and ambivalence are common, as financial and emotional resources may become depleted. The emotional tide of anticipation can be fraught with enormous guilt and shame as families sometimes replace a fear of death with a wish for it.

During a period of increased suffering, the patient may express the wish to die and end the ordeal. One woman with unremitting severe pain shouted at her husband, "If I have to feel like this every day, then I wish I would die. I wish you could feel what this pain is like for 5 minutes!" At a moment of exhaustion and exasperation, a caregiver may think or exclaim, "Yes, I wish you would die so I could be free to move on with my life." The patient, who is physically and psychosocially shackled, is implicitly sanctioned for having such thoughts. It goes with the rights and privileges of being a patient. Family caregivers may feel as psychosocially burdened as the patient but be ashamed of having such ambivalent thoughts or openly expressing them. Often, these thoughts are expressed in ways that under other circumstances would be labeled pathologically cruel. Most of us can reveal such thoughts only within our closest relationships. Here, heightened emotions and reactivity are sometimes inevitable. Family members need to understand and forgive themselves and each other for hurtful comments made in the heat of the moment. They can be helped to become aware that this situation occurs when the patient expresses anger at his or her plight, anger that may be communicated to other family members as "You are fortunate to have your health, and I am jealous."

Shameful thoughts and feelings are a major impediment to openness. Explaining in advance that having intense and seemingly "irrational" feelings of anger, ambivalence, death wishes, or escape fantasies is typical can help counteract feelings of secrecy, shame, and guilt on the part of well family members.

The fundamental issue here is that the caregiving burden is underappreciated because being physically burdened with disability and possible death cannot be readily compared with anything else. One solution is to suggest that the patient and caregivers live in somewhat separate and distinct worlds, each with its own burdens. The caregiving burden might then be considered to have equally valid currency. This helps address the imbalance that fuels survivor guilt.

In my experience, it is rare for patients and families in the chronic phase *not* to entertain escape fantasies and thoughts of wishing an end to the ordeal. Because of the shame associated with open acknowledgment of these feelings, I often introduce this subject by making a statement such as, "I haven't heard anyone mention a wish to have this over with; maybe you will be the family to make Ripley's Believe It or Not!" Or if the patient has made a comment along these lines, I may say, "It seems okay for Bill to voice his frustration, but I wonder if the rest of you feel, like many families, that they shouldn't have such distressing thoughts about someone they love dearly." The provider's introducing and normalizing such thoughts with this kind of statement frequently lowers the family's shame and anxiety level enormously. Even if family members have not had such experiences, a professional's inquiry can serve a preventive, normalizing function. The issue of what the family needs to do about its exhausted state and ambivalence remains, but the pejorative meanings attached to such toxic thoughts are alleviated, allowing for more open and productive dialogue. If these emotions remain buried, they can contribute to survivor guilt. In fact, sometimes they can be the seeds of interminable grief reactions that surface years later.

Clinicians need to distinguish the normative mixed feelings that arise in an extended ordeal from a preexisting conflictual relationship that has become heightened by the prospect of a possible loss. This is best assessed by thorough inquiry about the couple's or family's relationships before the onset of the condition.

Medical care for life-threatening illnesses is often provided in specialty clinics, where patients and families coping with similar disorders may develop significant relationships, even in the clinic waiting rooms. Even if patients keep to themselves, they can be acutely aware of other patients who arrive on the same day to see the same physician. A progression, relapse, or death of another patient can trigger fears of "Will I (we) be next" and deflate family morale. A clinician who informs a clerical assistant in a waiting room that another patient should be scheduled for a series of diagnostic tests can rekindle terror among other patients who are already well aware that new tests may signal serious trouble ahead. Rather than minimize this issue, it is useful for clinicians to inquire about such clinic contacts and offer family support or consultations.

The Expected Illness Course

Progressive diseases, such as Alzheimer's, involve numerous losses. Illnesses vary in terms of the balance between expected physical and cognitive disability. With Alzheimer's, the timing of these losses is variable, but the inevitable deterioration is not. Neurocognitive impairment involves a range of deficits that interfere with participation in family life. Family members may anticipate and grieve each milestone, such as loss of memory of shared experiences or even recognition of loved ones (see Chapter 16).

At key illness transitions, family role functions may need to adapt to a new phase. Clinicians should be sensitive to those points that may require major changes for the family, such as transferring financial management to an adult child. The timing of these crises usually involves a race between increasing disability and each family's resources and ability to keep up with the demands, without reaching its limits. Often the most serious crisis occurs when a family has reached a point of exhaustion and confronts decisions about altering caregiving plans, roles, and rules. Loss at such crisis points involves grieving for the biological decline of the ill member and for family core beliefs, such as never needing outside assistance or never putting a loved one in an institution.

One family tried at all costs to preserve their deteriorating father's role functions in order to keep intact his pride and their strong belief in his mastery. As his disability increased, it became more and more difficult for the family to deny, through elaborate facades and cover-ups, that the father was no longer the same person. Successful adaptation to loss required acceptance of what could not be changed. The family was encouraged to revise a rigid and narrow definition of mastery to embrace a dignified and normal view of bodily decline. Giving up restrictive and unworkable beliefs in this situation involved family grieving. However, their collective suffering was alleviated when family members could redefine mastery in terms of a healthy family process rather than outcome.

When a family member's cancer is in remission, tremendous fear often surrounds a possible recurrence. Every ambiguous symptom and appointment with the physician arouses more apprehension. The loss of the first remission may shatter a family's hope for a cure, bringing their worst fears to the surface. Medically, it means that the best treatment has failed and that further attempts are less likely to succeed. The ambiguous boundary between remission and cure stokes embers of anticipatory loss indefinitely.

Even 20 years after treatment for cancer, a vague symptom can immediately rekindle fears of recurrence and death. This boundary is also blurred because, in many life-endangering conditions such as cancer, the 5-year survival point has been reified as a "medical cure." This nodal point in the illness, although highly arbitrary, can easily become a psychological parting of the ways between the medical team's view of a cure and the family's continued concerns about a recurrence. Families can experience the 5-year landmark with sharp ambivalence. Joy can be mixed with a sense of abandonment by the medical team. The family can feel left alone to deal with real ongoing uncertainty. Health care providers may cloak their own anxiety about failing and losing a patient by using this 5-year definition of cure to label a particular case a success no matter what the future brings.

Clinicians can help a family at this juncture by inquiring about and validating the normalcy of experiencing a range of conflicting emotions. Stopping regular checkups with the cancer specialist, appointments once so-dreaded, suddenly can be experienced as an anxiety-filled loss. Clinicians need to be sensitive both to mutual separation issues and the distinctions between providers' comfort with a statistical medical cure and the actual, ongoing uncertainties for patients and their families.

Relapsing illnesses, such as asthma or heart disease, can flare up or cause sudden death, and issues related to anticipatory loss hover between the front and back burners. In the event of such crises (e.g., with angina, a heart attack, or hemophilia), families may become preoccupied with anticipated loss. Families most fear crises that arise suddenly, without warning, and require an immediate response to avert catastrophe. One woman with longstanding diabetes abruptly experienced severe episodes of hypoglycemia, resulting in a loss of consciousness. She and her husband then developed the fear that at any moment an episode could endanger the safety of their small children or end her life.

Frequently, family rules change to protect against life-threatening situations. For instance, when a parent has had a heart attack, the family norm of open communication may shift to conflict avoidance to protect against a potentially fatal recurrence.

For example, after a heart attack and as a precaution, the physician may advise a family to maintain a calm emotional climate ("Try not to upset Jeff") and to refrain from sexual activity; although sometimes only the well spouse is told this. Not infrequently, a time frame for these precautions is not clearly specified. This kind of information, conveyed in an intensive or cardiac care unit, is often not communicated verbally by the hospitalist or cardiologist to the primary care physician or entered into the patient's electronic health record. Also, it may not have been clearly decided which health care provider will reassess and update the patient and family on these kinds of "life-preserving" precautions. This leaves a couple or family with major ambiguities as to when it will be safe to resume sexual relations or express upset or anger. The husband may feel a need to reassert his intactness as a man and to master his own fears about death by performing sexually. The spouse may feel protective and decline the husband's sexual advances not because of a basic change in her desire or attraction, but because she fears losing him through a fatal recurrence. An escalating cycle of conflict or avoidance can result in which the husband experiences his wife's protectiveness in refusing sex as rejection or as a confirmation of his weakened state. In a circular fashion, he may double his efforts to have sex with his wife, which increases the wife's anxiety that her husband needs monitoring and increases her protective behaviors.

This cycle can lead to violence, starting an affair, or the husband turning to other forms of physical exertion, sometimes recklessly, to prove his wholeness. The driving force behind these kinds of interaction is unacknowledged fears of death, coupled with a lack of sufficient professional guidance. In such contexts, what is typically labeled a caregiver's controlling behavior needs to be reinterpreted as a part of an interactive cycle representing an attempt to master threatened loss.

Patterns that are developed early in a chronic disorder can have a major impact on the entire family system and profound effects on other relationships, especially between parents and their children. The following case highlights this point.

Bob, in his early forties, sought psychotherapy for help with repeated problems of commitment to relationships with women. He feared that marriage would rob him of his freedom and his zest for an adventurous lifestyle. He viewed his "controlling" mother, who monitored his father's actions and refused to allow him to engage in the sports and traveling he loved, as the source of his concerns.

In family systems-oriented individual therapy, the young man came to realize that what he viewed as his mother's "controlling" behavior had begun with his father's heart attack (when he, the son, was 5 years old), and was part of a relationship bargain that preserved his father's sense of masculinity and kept him alive. The father denied the seriousness of his condition, failed to comply with doctors' orders to cut back his activities, and threatened to run off on impulsive and risky adventures. He tacitly put his wife in charge of controlling his behavior and thus could maintain a macho bravado and blame her for setting limits on him (actually for him). I pointed out that his mom was actually a "hero" who had arguably saved his father many times from potentially life-threatening behaviors. Had the health care team met with the couple soon after the father's heart attack, they might have been able to interrupt this pattern and help the father accept his condition and the need to take responsibility for his own health and, with it, his family's well-being. This template for relationships, driven by unacknowledged and unresolved fears of loss, became an impediment to intimacy for the children.

This case demonstrates the importance of inquiring about multigenerational legacies related to illness and loss. For this client, understanding the connection between his father's serious heart condition and his parents' interaction about the disorder was necessary to address his own problem with intimacy. Previous therapy had not succeeded in altering—only, in fact, reinforcing—his view of his mother because it left out essential parts of the story.

THE FAMILY LIFE CYCLE

A family's experience of threatened loss can best be understood through a developmental perspective, particularly in multigenerational encounters with threatened or actual loss and the timing of life-threatening illness within the individual and family life cycles (Rolland, 2004, 2016).

The Past: Multigenerational Issues

Multigenerational information related to previous family encounters with death, disability, threatened loss, and living with ambiguity are particularly important (McGoldrick et al., 2008; Rolland, 2004; Walsh & McGoldrick,

2004, 2013). Other forms of uncertainty or loss, such as poverty, migration, divorce, violence, abandonment, or dangerous occupations, for example, military service or law enforcement, provide valuable information.

Past unresolved, traumatic, or unexpected loss may generate catastrophic fear for family members confronted with impending loss. This may be expressed in a heightened preoccupation with one's own or other family members' physical health. Physical symptoms, especially those without a clear, immediate explanation, can unleash a torrent of fear that history will repeat itself. As such, it is important to distinguish between issues of unresolved loss and sensitization based on a previous ordeal. The latter is akin to the long-term sequelae of posttraumatic stress. Other people, with a history of traumatic loss, will deny the existence or significance of clear bodily symptoms as a way to assert control over profound fears. Some may respond to a loved one's illness, or even the possibility of one, by distancing, emotionally withdrawing, or separating. One man who had lost his first wife to breast cancer started an affair and filed for divorce from his second wife within weeks of her surgery for breast cancer despite her good prognosis.

Sometimes a preoccupation with anticipated loss concerning oneself or a family member can begin at the same point in the life cycle at which a significant family member has died, especially if the loss was untimely, unexpected, or traumatic.

Sam, a married man with small children, developed somatic symptoms at the age of 40. He was convinced that they indicated serious heart disease. Several thorough medical workups revealed he was in excellent health; but he remained skeptical, and his symptoms kept increasing. During an initial consultation, when I inquired about past experiences with illness and loss, Sam revealed that when he was 9 years old, his father had died suddenly in his forties of complications of rheumatic heart disease in childhood. At that time, Sam, his brother, and his mother arrived at the hospital only to find out his father had died unexpectedly.

After the funeral and over the years, Sam and his mother almost never discussed his father's death. When he turned 40 and had children at almost the same age as he was when his father died, Sam felt he had entered a health danger zone.

Sam had been sensitized to the possibility of sudden, untimely loss, which in his mind would begin at 40. Failure to discuss his father's death had left buried many unresolved issues about the loss. This only heightened the intensity of Sam's anxieties, and at turning 40 triggered his own fears about death and abandoning his family. My reassurances that complications of rheumatic fever had nothing to do with a genetic predisposition to heart disease could be heeded only when these underlying issues were addressed in therapy. The timing and intensity of Sam's symptoms were heightened by the fact that his oldest son was the same age as he was when his father died unexpectedly.

When unexplained symptoms are interpreted as psychosomatic, it is worth screening for past sudden or traumatic losses that might be connected to the current physical complaint. Often, these somatic "time bombs" are largely out of the person's awareness until he or she approaches or reaches the relevant life-cycle phase. Yet, these associations are typically not unconscious, and therefore accessible to a health care provider's inquiry.

Present and Future Timing with the Life Cycle

Anticipatory loss poses different challenges depending upon how it fits with current or future hopes and dreams. For instance, a family launching a 19-year-old daughter must shift gears developmentally to pull together when she develops a potentially fatal brain tumor. The daughter not only must refocus her energies onto dealing with her cancer, but also must face the implications of living with a life-threatening condition while aspiring to be a young adult, focusing on making career plans or plans for having children. The parents may need to alter or indefinitely put on hold their postlaunching phase personal and relationship goals and cope with possibly giving up their dreams for her future.

Major life-cycle plans can be blocked by the threat of loss. For young couples, anticipatory loss may intersect with hopes of child rearing and career development. Preparation for disability and death, not normally on the horizon, must be considered. The hard fact is that the family life cycle may be permanently altered and possibly abbreviated. One young woman with small children, whose husband's car accident left him quadriplegic and with a TBI, confided, "I see a long difficult road ahead raising our kids and caring for my husband, who will have a very limited role as a parent to our kids."

Life-threatening or severely disabling illnesses that coincide with family planning are particularly poignant. For the well spouse, the desire to have children may remain an active dream because he or she is physically capable of having a child, but is blocked by the spouse's illness. The ill partner may become more permanently absorbed in a life-or-death struggle. As time passes, this discrepancy can powerfully alter the sense of unified goals and togetherness (see Chapter 14). One husband lamented his wife's cancer. "It was hard enough 2 years ago to absorb the fact that even if Jackie was cured, her radiation treatment would make pregnancy impossible. Now I find it unbearable knowing that her continued slow, losing battle with cancer makes it impossible to pursue our dreams like other couples our age."

Off-time loss may occur quite suddenly due to trauma, such as an automobile accident. With advances in organ transplantation, families in which a member has survived such a trauma but ultimately succumbs to brain death may be offered the option of donating their loved one's organs and tissues. While these losses are generally sudden, families still experience anticipatory loss as they may have hours or days before their loved one is officially brain dead. Clinicians need to be mindful of the immediate needs of these families, by providing accurate information regarding prognosis and the meaning of brain death, allowing families to say good-bye to their loved one, and giving them the time and privacy to make the decision as to whether to donate his or her organs (Holtkamp, 2000). Many families find it healing to make contact with organ-recipient families and to know that although their own loss is painful, they and their loved one have helped to save another life.

Life-Cycle Transition Periods

Families in life-cycle transitions may be more vulnerable to the emotional upheaval generated by anticipatory loss. For example, if a family is launching young adults when the mother is diagnosed with cancer, the threat of her death may influence young adult members in transition to alter life decisions in ways that compromise personal independent strivings. Here, it is important both to know the interplay of personal developmental plans with expectations for family loyalty and to be aware of important differences across cultures.

As families with long-term threatened loss experience normative life-cycle transitions, there may be a resurgence of anticipatory loss that they thought they had "worked through." The following case shows how a very positive celebratory family transition can stir up "old" feelings.

A family presented for treatment when the younger daughter, Andrea, was about to graduate from college. Her older brother, Tom, age 25, had developmental disabilities related to damage sustained at birth during a complicated forceps delivery. His disability involved some mild right-side weakness and learning difficulties, particularly with mathematics. Despite his disability, with persistence, a substantial commitment by his parents, and the help of professionals, Tom was able to attend college, but had been struggling to finish for 7 years. Most of his age peers had moved on and were settling down in careers and/or committed relationships.

Andrea's impending graduation was a marker that forced more open acknowledgment and acceptance of Tom's being passed by his sister, something all family members had dreaded for years. Although she was always superior academically, this was the first time that Andrea "passed" him publically. It heightened Tom's sense of inadequacy and of being left behind and his fear that he would never be able to master adulthood. It rekindled his mother's unjustified feelings of guilt surrounding his delivery and both parents' feelings that if they had done enough, their son would not experience suffering.

This event enabled the parents to work through a deeper level of acceptance of their own heroic efforts and to let go and allow their adult son to handle his own suffering. It provided an opportunity for Tom to address more fully the part of himself that linked self-esteem with performing equally with others in all areas. He needed to learn to accept his limits and work around them without sacrificing his self-esteem.

At these transitions, developmental tasks of the next life phase may need to be altered, delayed, or given up when they become unrealistic or impossible to achieve. Each transition may generate intense grieving over opportunities and experiences that were anticipated but must now be relinquished in a more final way. Family members often need to mourn the loss of certain future hopes and dreams. For instance, when a mother learns about her son's diagnosis with a terminal cancer, she must mourn the loss of anticipated experiences, which might include school graduations, her son's marriage, and her own grandparenthood. Clinicians can inquire about losses related to future life phases and explore options for alternative positive experiences.

Issues Related to Childhood versus Adult Onset

Threatened loss affects families differently, depending on the age of illness onset.

Childhood-Onset, Congenital, and Inherited Disorders

A child's socialization and identity are shaped by the interplay among developmental milestones, limitations, and future illness risks. In coping with serious childhood conditions, parents and extended family lose their normal hopes and dreams for their child. With clearly fatal illnesses, parents become aware that their child will suffer a relentless decline. Yet, research finds that most parents choose to love the child fully and cherish the child's every ability and small joy. The key is to help parents find this both-and stance—loving the child amid the sorrow.

With many inherited disorders, family beliefs about mastery and the rules for social interaction have been shaped over generations to be in sync with anticipatory loss (Rolland, 1994, 2004, 2006a). For example, in hemophilia, life-threatening bleeding episodes can be triggered by trauma, intense affect, or extended periods of stress. Because sudden death is an ever-present possibility, parents may teach affected children a fine-tuned form of mastery over their bodies that is juxtaposed with a fear of social interaction, whereby emotions are carefully monitored in the interest of self-preservation. Anticipation of loss guides this interweaving of belief system and developmental processes.

Individuals with a hereditary or childhood-onset disorder bring the developmental experience with threatened loss to their adult relationships. Such couples may begin their relationship either with the possibility of loss overtly acknowledged or covertly overshadowing their commitment. It is important for clinicians to facilitate communication about the impact of possible disability and premature death in areas such as intimacy, child rearing, career plans, and division of labor, so that the couple can develop the flexibility necessary to adapt to the added strains. These couples also need to discuss subjects such as disability and life insurance, advance directives, and wills, issues that healthy young couples often postpone.

In long-term illnesses, such as diabetes and hemophilia, concerns about future loss become embedded in life-cycle planning in more subtle, covert, and sometimes devastating ways, as illustrated in the following case.

Greg, a 45-year-old man with lifelong hemophilia, was referred for severe depression. The severity of his condition required the use of crutches. He had divorced his wife 3 years earlier, and his only daughter had just left home for college.

Evaluation revealed that his mother's family had a 200-year history of hemophilia, with scores of affected members. A brother had died in childhood following a traumatic injury, and only one member with hemophilia had lived beyond age 50.

When asked about how he had imagined his life from childhood, Greg stated that at age 8, after his brother's death, he decided that if he could survive the higher risks of trauma in childhood, he had enough time to marry and raise children, but given the statistics and his lengthy family history, life beyond 45 seemed unlikely. After 40, he began to view his life as "pre-dead." He had no vision or plans for his life beyond 50, except an anticipation of death.

This case demonstrates how a person can structure his entire life course to conform to an expectation of disability and death at a particular life phase. The timing of Greg's divorce coincided with a vaguely conscious plan to spare his wife's having to deal with his becoming a burden and dying, and gave him control over the end of the relationship. His daughter's launching left him alone with his depression, suicidal thoughts, and hopeless outlook.

Greg's story highlights the danger of anticipatory loss becoming a runaway process and the need for a preventive clinical framework. Greg's version of anticipatory loss, developed as a child, was inevitable and timed, rather than possible and uncertain. Also, the runaway process accelerated at his most vulnerable point in the life cycle. An earlier intervention might have predicted the time of highest risk by taking stock of how his multigenerational experience influenced his personal illness time line. It would have enabled him to plan for life after 40 in a way that acknowledged the possibility of disability and early death, but did not preclude meaningful life goals and relationships within a context of heightened uncertainty. This case highlights the need to ask ill children their beliefs about how their condition will affect their life expectancy.

Adult-Onset Disorders

A key issue with adult-onset disorders is the need for the patient to alter fundamental beliefs, hopes, dreams, and expectations to accommodate actual loss and threatened further loss. When a condition predates an intimate relationship, the patient has more opportunity to adapt first individually. This can help couples cultivate more congruent expectations as their relationship develops from the beginning. If a diagnosis occurs after marriage, couples must alter their original relationship understandings to accommodate actual or possible barriers to their hopes and dreams.

Serious illness that occurs early in a couple's relationship is particularly stressful because the partners are still establishing their partnership. If the onset occurs later in the family life cycle, a firmer relationship base can help counter any strains. If dysfunctional patterns exist prior to the illness, the threat of loss may drive the couple further apart.

However, there are significant risks in starting a relationship during the initial illness crisis phase. It can foster a permanent caregiver–patient relationship that precludes a balanced partnership. Also, an ill person may develop a relationship with someone vulnerable to becoming a rescue-oriented caregiver because of unresolved family-of-origin issues; examples include a person who grew up as a rescuer in a family with alcoholism or was a child caregiver for a parent with a disabling chronic disorder.

Stress Points of Anticipatory Loss for Couples

The type of illness and time frame of anticipated loss influence how a couple responds to threats to their life plans. With an illness like diabetes, the possibility of disability or a shortened life span is often a distant concern. A person with diabetes may accommodate to potential complications through denial and minimization.

As a couple's relationship becomes more intimate, the well partner will need to be educated about diabetes. The well partner's fears may be expressed by hovering over the partner with diabetes, questioning his or her dietary habits, and being overprotective about any behavior that could indicate hypoglycemia. The individual with diabetes may respond angrily, "You are treating me as my parents did. It took me years to get them off my back." The need for the well partner to master his or her fears is confused with earlier parental control issues, which were also related to threatened loss. The ability of the ill individual to educate the well partner can be blocked by fears about deterioration, abandonment, and death. These are sensitive subjects for both partners. Clinicians need to be aware that often issues related to impending loss are obscured by pronouncements such as, "It's my illness and I'll handle it myself." It is helpful to convey to such couples that this normative learning period is time limited.

Another common stress point occurs when decisions about having children need to be made. Often such couples' ambivalence about having a child is directly related to issues of anticipatory loss that have not been openly acknowledged. Risks of pregnancy complications must be considered for both an ill mother and the unborn child. Other fears include (1) genetic transmission to offspring, who will carry the burdens of anticipatory loss; (2) anticipation of loss of a dreamed-for child, who may contract the illness at some point; (3) anticipation of illness complications that interfere with effective parenting; (4) fears that the ill parent might not survive to rear children to adulthood; and (5) associated financial and psychosocial burdens for the surviving well partner. Frequently, fears have been exaggerated by a failure to receive or seek accurate information (e.g., about the risk of genetic transmission of diabetes). It is very useful to offer couples and families prevention-oriented consultations that are timed with such life-cycle transitions.

A third stress point in diabetes occurs at the time of the first complication, as in the case of one young couple, in which the wife had been living with diabetes since childhood without any complications. When doctors discovered a small asymptomatic hemorrhage in one eye during a routine checkup, an emotional crisis ensued. All of her fears about the well-known circulatory complications of diabetes that had remained suppressed since childhood came flooding back. Fears about going blind, painful neurological complications, possible amputations, and heart and kidney failure preoccupied the couple at a time when they were considering long-term plans. A brief couple's treatment helped both partners discuss their fears, affirm their commitment to the relationship, and build greater flexibility into future plans. Previously the wife worked as a video technician, a position in which good eyesight is critical. After this crisis, she decided to apply for a job developing and administering a new visual arts program at the regional high school. This job allowed her to use her professional skills in a new, creative way that was less dependent on her eyesight.

BELIEF SYSTEMS

As discussed in Chapter 8, a family's beliefs about what and who can influence the course of events are fundamental. When a family member feels responsible or is blamed for a disorder involving threatened loss, any illness exacerbation or disease progression can cause these issues to erupt into a full-blown family crisis.

In one case, a mother who both blamed herself (because her own mother had diabetes) and felt blamed by her husband for her teenage son's diabetes was unable to set limits on her son, who was flagrantly nonadherent about his diet and his insulin injections. She believed that her possible genetic contribution and full-time career were the primary reasons that her son developed diabetes and was doing poorly medically. Her husband, who had always been uncomfortable with their dual-career marriage and felt chronically neglected and competitive with his wife's career, concurred with her self-blame. These beliefs were unknown to any of the providers involved and only surfaced during direct questioning in a consultation when the son was hospitalized for a life-threatening episode.

Clinicians should help families obtain clear medical prognoses and management guidelines. Ambiguities may blur behaviors that can affect the odds of a tragic outcome, increasing the likelihood of blaming attributions whenever disease progression can be linked to errors of omission or commission. Women are more prone to blaming and shaming attributions because of societal role expectations defining them as primary family caregivers.

For childhood disorders, parents and siblings (especially those close in age to the ill child who may be strong sibling rivals) are at heightened risk of feeling guilty for being well, for not suffering, or for not experiencing the stigma of a disability. Parents may ruminate about possible negligence as a causal factor. For some members, especially siblings, this feeling can be expressed as a general somatic preoccupation or catastrophic fear of suffering the same fate. In a family whose child's apparent influenza turned out to be leukemia, the mildest respiratory symptoms in another family member can trigger family panic. Family members may become overprotective of all their children.

Larger System Values

In the United States, male, middle-class values that emphasize individual achievement, stoicism, and mastery have historically prevailed. We live in an era that promotes personal responsibility and effort as the road out of adversity. From national policy making to popular psychology, there is a tendency to localize problems in the individual or family. These societal values can interact powerfully with belief systems in a family facing threatened loss.

Societal Stigma: The Example of HIV-Related Conditions

HIV-related conditions dramatically illustrate how the process of family coping with anticipatory loss and bereavement can be compromised by societal stigma, fueling shame and guilt. Condemning attitudes toward gay sex or drug use attached to HIV/AIDS (Doka, 2002) can victimize families and rival with unresolved family issues as a potential cause of complicated grief. Threatened loss associated with stigmatized conditions is often experienced in a context of secrecy and isolation. Clinicians can help to dispel such attitudes by promoting positive rituals, as well as facilitating community support for patients and their families.

Epidemic conditions, such as HIV and the Ebola and Zika viruses, have unique and challenging aspects. Families often experience multiple losses and have friends or family members who are living through various phases of the condition and coping with anticipatory loss. Clinicians need to be sensitive to the waves of threatened disability, death, and bereavement surrounding families in high-risk communities. People must cope sometimes with their own fears of decline and death concurrently with the potential loss of a partner or another member of their family or community. One or both parents may be confronted with their own diagnosis at the same time that they learn that their child is affected. Clinicians need to build extended family and community supports for nurturance of orphaned or affected children and for planning for their future needs.

CHAPTER 10

Helping Families in the Terminal Phase

When death is inevitable, the boundary between the chronic and terminal phases is often hazy. Medical technology and the aggressive use of treatments may reverse or delay these transitions. While it is possible to induce multiple cancer remissions, such persistent medical interventions designed to prolong life can be difficult to distinguish from attempts to reassure a dying patient that all is not lost.

This chapter will focus specifically on challenges for families coping with the terminal phase, which can last days, weeks, or months. Fatal illnesses, such as ALS, or amyotrophic lateral sclerosis, are known to be terminal from the time of diagnosis, but still have a chronic phase that varies in length. The timing of the terminal phase of such conditions is somewhat arbitrary. For many types of cancer, a widespread metastatic recurrence that is not responsive to further effective treatments may herald a terminal phase. For other types, it begins when caregiving demands necessitate a referral to hospice care.

Medical training often fosters ambiguous communication to families, prompting doctors to be cautious about revealing bad news surrounding the prognosis. This "let's wait and see" attitude may generate heightened anxiety and uncertainty that confuses a family about the phase of the illness, as illustrated in this case.

Tom and Lydia were referred for consultation when Lydia was rehospitalized for a recurrence of lymphoma and their daughter, Alison, suddenly refused to visit her mother in the hospital. Although three prior recurrences had been "easily" treated, this time multiple treatments had not worked. With a highly optimistic physician and a stable illness course, the family had never openly discussed the possibility of death. The daughter's behavior signaled a needed change. Although Lydia felt worse and thought she might be dying, her oncologist maintained that she was "doing well" and proposed a number of additional treatments (which I viewed as long shots). My discussion with the oncologist revealed his steadfast belief that continued aggressive treatment would be undermined by talking about death with the family. The family's loyalty to their physician prevented them from transitioning to the terminal phase of anticipatory grief. It was only when Lydia was in a coma in the intensive care unit, 48 hours before her death, that the physician agreed to finally discuss her dying with the family.

LIVING DURING THE TERMINAL PHASE

In the terminal phase, the main question is the amount of time left to prepare for death and survivorship. Bereavement issues come to the forefront in this phase and continue into the grief and mourning period after death. The family's challenge in the terminal phase is in certain respects isomorphic with a clinician's involvement in a time-limited treatment that requires setting immediate objectives and making plans for termination.

Adaptational Tasks

Chapter 3 introduced several basic family adaptational tasks that begin in the terminal phase and continue after the patient's death (Walsh & McGoldrick, 2013). These tasks are outlined in the following list and are discussed in more detail in this chapter.

- *Sharing acknowledgement of the impending loss.* Each family member will grapple in his or her own way with confronting this reality and making meaning for themselves and the family unit. In most cultures, this acknowledgment is facilitated by direct contact with the dying member.
- *Sharing in the process of anticipatory grief and addressing any unfinished family business.* This task underscores the importance of having open communication and a problem-solving process that promote family resilience in dealing with loss. It comprises having clear, consistent information, emotional sharing and support, and collaborative problem solving.
- *Supporting the terminally ill member.* This task includes helping the survivors and dying member to live as fully as possible in whatever time remains. Also, clinicians can help families transition from hoping that the ill member won't die toward hoping for loved ones to be nearby and spend precious time together. For the dying member, the most important needs are controlling pain and suffering, preserving dignity and self-worth, and receiving love and affection from family and friends (Gawande, 2014).

- *Beginning or continuing the family system reorganization process.* One challenge for family members is oscillating back and forth between tending to the immediate needs of the dying member and the emotional processing associated with dying, and moving forward with the necessary family reorganization and adaptation to new roles (Stroebe & Schut, 2010). This oscillation may be easier with longstanding progressive diseases that involve gradual increased disability and shifting of responsibilities.

- *Reinvesting in other relationships and life pursuits.* Sometimes, a spouse or partner begins another relationship. The reasons are myriad, including the exhaustion and need for nurturance with a protracted ordeal, such as with ALS, or wishes to escape the intensity of the experience with a dying spouse (see Chapter 13 on couples).

Clinicians can help families distinguish the need to accept that death will occur from the more difficult task of making peace with the many losses—the loss of their loved ones as well as the loss of their hopes and dreams. When families are coping with anticipatory loss in the final phase of an illness, the quality of time spent with a dying member becomes a high priority. Perhaps more than at any other phase, families function best when they can create an atmosphere in which their needs and emotions can be openly expressed without fear of resentment or disapproval. Clinicians can explore both a family's fears about the process of dying and the impact of the death itself. As discussed in Chapter 9, the anticipation of increased pain and suffering is often more upsetting than death itself, especially in longstanding progressive disorders, where the anticipation of death has been rehearsed many times.

Individual and Conjoint Meetings

Depending on the circumstances, I have used different combinations of individual, family, and couple sessions throughout an illness (see Chapter 4). This approach is especially relevant to terminal illness. Depending on cultural norms and the patient's personal preferences, the dying member may need private sessions to process issues related to existential or spiritual concerns and "making peace" with his or her own life. Part of the farewell process involves the dying person coming to terms with death's finality and parting with all they have known. For a spouse and family, some aspects of preparing or reorganizing are easier without the dying member's presence. Conjoint couple and family meetings can focus more on the farewell process for specific relationships. This includes possible repair and affirmation of relationships.

Meaning-Making: Existential and Spiritual

The narratives that families develop over time during the illness experience have major implications for meaning-making in the terminal phase (see Chapter 8).

Attributions about who or what caused the illness, the perceived treatment success or failure, and the quality of life and relationships since the time of illness onset all converge in the terminal phase experience of creating meaning. The meanings that families make profoundly affect family members' bereavement and grief (Nadeau, 2008; Neimeyer, 2001; Stroebe & Schut, 2010; Walsh & McGoldrick, 2004). The family's coconstruction of a narrative about the dying member and his or her illness is key to positive adaptation, independent of the individual narratives they create. Clinicians need to facilitate the family's own process, rather than offer their own interpretations. Possibly troublesome explanations, such as blaming others for the impending death, deserve sensitive clinical attention and exploration (see Chapter 8). Some sources of blame can include the perceived negligence of family member(s) or health care provider(s) or larger societal problems, such as poor access to health care. When relevant, an acknowledgement of larger system inequities is important.

For most of us, whether we are religious or not, dying raises existential questions about the meaning and significance of life, not just for the dying member, but his or her loved ones as well. Lorraine Wright described how suffering invites both the patient and family into the spiritual domain (Wright & Bell, 2009). As death approaches, families often transition from a reliance on medical treatment toward a greater reliance on belief systems and spirituality. Many cultures provide rich traditions, rituals, and ceremonies to help families prepare for and deal with this major transition. They can provide solace and strengthen a transcendent sense of purpose.

As discussed in Chapter 8, it is vital to inquire about families' spiritual beliefs and practices. The spiritual meanings of death are very diverse. For instance, death can represent God's will and not be something for humans to plan or determine. Any religious and cultural differences within a family should be explored. If these differences are not acknowledged, they can be a source of distancing or intense conflict, especially with a dying member. Where possible, creatively combining traditions or rituals can be very helpful. Important existential concerns and spiritual issues may surface for a dying member. Do members believe in an afterlife? The vast majority of Americans do. Belief in a spiritual afterlife, offering transcendence over death, has been a core principle of most religions and cultures for millennia (Hood, Hill, & Spilka, 2009). Most people don't believe that death is final, but is rather a passage to an afterlife or spiritual realm, such as heaven, or to being reincarnated. Contemplating the passage of the dying member to a heavenly realm and reuniting with deceased loved ones and ancestors can be a great source of comfort.

Continuing Bonds

Traditionally, death has been viewed as a final separation to be accepted. From a relational perspective, death ends a life but not a relationship (Walsh, 2009). Thinking increasingly has shifted to the idea of adaptive mourning. This involves transforming the relationship with the dying/deceased person from a physical presence to continuing bonds through spiritual connection, memories, deeds that honor the dead, and stories that are passed through kinship networks and across generations (Klass, 2009; Neimeyer, 2001; Stroebe, Schut, & Boerner, 2010; Walsh, 2016b). In many cultures, deceased family members continue to have a real presence and to play active roles in family life. Surviving members talk to the deceased person and communicate their continuing love and inner thoughts (Parkes, Laungani, & Young, 2015; Rosenblatt, 2013).

Life imprint is one therapeutic strategy used in grief work (Neimeyer, Burke, Mackay, & van Dyke Stringer, 2010) that can be used in the terminal phase and can include the dying member. The principle involves inviting family members to reflect on and record the durable legacy of the dying member in their lives. This remembrance can involve recognizing and honoring the dying person's distinctive gestures and verbal expressions; ways of speaking or relating to others; and his or her values, life's purpose, and major life pursuits. This process identifies and clarifies "imprints" from the dying member that one wishes to retain as a resource in the future. These imprints can help family members during the upcoming period of grief and mourning after the death. In a family session, members can share their respective thoughts, promoting increased closeness among the surviving members and the dying person. Encourage family members to let their loved one know that he or she will not be forgotten and what positive forms the remembrance will take. One example would be saying something such as, "Every time I go to Truro Beach on Cape Cod, I will order the lobster rolls we loved and remember the wonderful times we spent together."

Retrospective Life Narrative

One simple yet meaningful idea involves encouraging the dying member to reflect on and share his or her life story with loved ones. This process can facilitate a sense of life coherence for the dying person. The story that is imparted to family members and close friends can become a treasured family heirloom to be passed on to succeeding generations (Walsh & McGoldrick, 2013; King & Wynne, 2004). It is even more rewarding if surviving members participate in the process by conducting or participating in interviews, based on what they are curious about. With modern technology, there are myriad options for recording the narrative and incorporating photos and earlier videos. Ideally, a life narrative is something that families can do with any parent or spouse. Overall, this process can be extremely meaningful for the dying member and family during this period.

Unresolved Relationship Issues and Possibilities for Repair and Healing

Heightened awareness of unresolved relationship issues often occurs in the terminal phase; it can be very distressing and become intertwined with caregiving efforts. For instance, a family member who feels extremely guilty about not having been a good parent, son, or daughter hopes that caring for a dying member can serve as restitution for earlier misdeeds.

Teresa Rando (1984) has beautifully stated that "Suffering is pain without meaning" (p. 343). Dying and healing can coexist. The terminal phase can offer a precious opportunity for families to heal old wounds like relationship cutoffs and to find caring and love that can lessen the suffering. Clinicians and families need to avoid thinking that it is too late to address such issues. When the dying member is too debilitated or effective communication is not realistic, clinicians can help family member(s) normalize the experience and let go of old issues and disappointments, while acknowledging the positive in a relationship. At other times, clinicians can encourage and facilitate members' dealing with unfinished business by openly talking with other appropriate family members. Whenever possible, clinicians should offer family systems-based consultations directed toward emotional and relational healing. The following case illustrates the possibility of relationship repair by working systemically with one family member during a terminal phase.

Mary, a 43-year-old married, working-class, devout Catholic, sought individual consultation after her mother, Anne, was diagnosed with advanced metastatic lung cancer with painful bone metastases. Anne lives alone and is a retired factory worker. Since Mary is the only daughter, Anne sought Mary's help when she went into the hospital for 2 weeks of palliative surgery and radiation treatment. Mary believes, as a daughter and a Christian, that she should "be there" as a caregiver for her mother, regardless of the quality of the relationship.

Mary has been estranged from her mother since leaving home as a late adolescent, having infrequent contact over the years. Her parents, who had a very conflictual, abusive relationship, divorced when Mary was 16. Throughout her childhood and adolescence, Mary remembers her mother as being remote, hostile, and self-absorbed. Leaving home after high school graduation, Mary took a clerical job, got married at 19, and has three terrific young adult and teenage children. She is a devoted wife and parent, keenly aware of not wanting to repeat her family-of-origin experience. She has never discussed the past with her mother, yet harbors feelings that somehow she warranted the neglect. Her mother has been critical of Mary's "lack of strictness" in parenting. Mary asserted that despite the strain of caring for her mother (who is "demanding"), she would not "abandon" her as she felt she was "abandoned" when growing up. Mary had never seen her mother in such pain and so vulnerable and clearly fearful of death.

My strategy during this initial 6-week phase of intensive medical treatment and recovery was to support Mary in her tireless efforts to provide care for her mother. During the extended time spent together at the hospital and then at home, Anne increasingly began to welcome Mary's caregiving efforts. In turn, Mary found herself feeling, uncharacteristically, some empathy toward her mother. Few words were exchanged during this period, but the experience altered the climate between them.

With Anne now becoming more independent and using these positive changes in the emotional climate as a starting point, I coached Mary to ask her mother more about her background. Mary learned for the first time that Anne, born in Poland during World War II at age 8, had witnessed her father being shot in front of the family home by German soldiers, leaving her own mother bereft and raising five children. Anne's mother never recovered emotionally, necessitating Anne, the oldest, to assume major parenting responsibilities for her siblings under dire circumstances. After the war, Anne was sent to the United States to live with relatives, separated from the rest of her nuclear family for some years. Mary was stunned by her mother's "opening the door" to her past and witnessing Anne's obvious emotional pain. For the first time, Mary could see her mother's extraordinary resilience. Unsolicited, Anne expressed remorse for her shortcomings as a mother, asking Mary's forgiveness. Over the ensuing 6 months before Anne's death, Mary and Anne grew closer, with Anne enjoying time with Mary's family and community of friends.

Shame-Based Secrets: Sexual Abuse

With a final separation looming during the terminal phase, family members, including the dying person, can feel an urgency to reveal and deal with past secrets, such as sexual abuse. A wish to go to one's grave with a less-burdened heart may motivate a dying person to admit to long-denied abuse of another member. This "better now than never" admission affords an opportunity for some degree of relational repair and healing. Under limited time pressure, faster and more substantial progress can often be achieved in even a few meetings.

Sometimes, the abused member has been put into the awkward and painful position of caregiving for the past perpetrator who is dying. In one case, a daughter, tending to her dying father, was viewed by the visiting nurse as doing an inconsistent and careless job of managing her father's care, such as bathing and feeding him and changing his clothes. When the nurse asked the daughter in a private conversation if there was something amiss, she reluctantly and with shame revealed being sexually abused repeatedly by her father as a child and early adolescent. The nurse empathically responded, "I am amazed that you are able to provide any hands-on care at all."

This case highlights the value of clinicians asking individual family members at the time of initial contact whether anything could interfere with his or her caregiver role. Once the member has admitted to past abuse, either as the perpetrator or victim of abuse, consultation with the other involved family member may be appropriate. When both individuals are amenable to dialogue, negotiating potential individual and conjoint sessions with a clinician who has trauma expertise can be discussed.

Family System Reorganization

One of the most challenging issues in the terminal phase is for the dying person to witness other family members gradually take over important family roles. For most, it can be a relief that others can manage prior responsibilities, for instance, that a spouse can handle finances and raise children on his or her own. For elders, it can be a source of pride in "passing the torch" to the next generation. However, for some, it can be very distressing. One man with terminal cancer felt devastated when he had to turn over to his oldest son the management of the family business that he and his now-deceased brother had begun over 40 years earlier. When families avoid the need to reallocate functions that the affected member can no longer handle, scapegoating of the patient sometimes results or tensions escalate between other family members. In one family, a conflict escalated between the husband and his mother-in-law as each tried unobtrusively to cover up for the disability of the wife, whose progressive dementia impaired her management of normal household responsibilities. They fought not only because of their shared grief, but also because neither could bear to tell the wife that her dementia had reached a point where someone else had to take over. The grief associated with this process can be lessened when family members communicate to the affected member how much he or she is valued and loved, qualities that transcend physical limitations.

It is useful to affirm the family's need to prepare for practical realities. An avalanche of medical bills incurred during a terminal phase can be daunting for all survivors, and they typically require prompt attention. In such situations, immediate pragmatic help is needed. A breadwinner father may need help in learning how to care for small children when his spouse is dying. In families in which traditional gender-based roles are the norm, wives facing the loss of a spouse can feel terrified about having to manage financial matters.

Palliative and Hospice Care

In the terminal phase, palliative and hospice care are often initiated as part of the overall health care approach. Both types of care are recognized as a medical subspecialty by the American Academy of Hospice and Palliative Medicine. Yet, it is important to distinguish between the two.

Palliative care is "whole-person care," designed to relieve symptoms, such as pain, fatigue, and suffering resulting from a disease, and improve the quality of life. It is delivered by a team, which may include a physician who specializes in palliative medicine, a nurse, a pharmacist, a mental health professional, a dietician, volunteers, and others. *Patients can receive palliative care at any phase of a serious illness*, whether the condition is potentially curable, life-threatening, or incurable. Palliative care can be given concurrently with regular medical treatment. It remains seriously underfunded and is often not considered a health care benefit.

Hospice care is a specific type of palliative care designed mostly for terminally ill persons, and it is usually limited to those who have a prognosis of 6 months or less to live. Increasingly, hospice care can also be provided for certain types of chronic conditions (e.g., severe and persistent pain). It can continue as long as necessary, when a physician certifies that that patient continues to meet eligibility requirements. It usually cannot be given along with curative or aggressive treatment like chemotherapy.

Hospice care is considered the model for quality, compassionate care at the end of life. It involves a team-oriented approach to expert medical care, pain management, and emotional and spiritual support expressly tailored to the patient and his or her loved ones' needs and preferences (Lattanzi-Licht, Maloney, & Miller, 1998). The patient and his or her family are considered the unit of care. At the heart of hospice and palliative care is the belief that each of us has the right to die pain free and with dignity, and that our families have the right to receive the necessary support (King & Quill, 2006).

Hospice services range from hospice nurse visits every few days in a patient's home to around-the-clock palliative and supportive care. Many hospices offer complementary therapies, such as healing touch, meditation, and aroma, music, and pet therapies. Most hospice programs take place in family homes as patients increasingly express the wish to die at home in familiar surroundings and in the company of loved ones. Hospice care also is offered in freestanding hospice centers, hospitals, nursing homes, and other long-term care facilities. It is covered under Medicare, Medicaid, and most insurance plans.

Palliative Care Provider–Family Member Conflict

In the terminal phase, the arrival of a palliative care clinician can sometimes create a dysfunctional triangle with the family. The following case highlights the value of an early assessment and recognition of family relationship difficulties, in this instance, at the time of referral to hospice. Alternatively, family consultation or therapy could have been offered earlier to address the mother–daughter relationship issues.

A hospice nurse entered a home where a daughter was caring for her elderly, terminally ill mother. Although the nurse was medically necessary, the daughter was extremely resentful of her attempts to exercise any control. She was clearly an unwelcome guest in the eyes of the daughter. The nurse became exasperated as the interactions between the two became increasingly contentious. As the clinician described the case, it became clear that this daughter had never felt affirmed by her critical mother, who, she thought, favored her two sisters.

As sometimes happens, the primary caregiver is a sibling who has felt rejected and still seeks approval from an aging parent. The adult child envisions the caregiving situation as a final attempt to get what he or she needs from the parent. Often this situation does afford a real opportunity for reconciliation and relationship repair between family members. In this case, the mother had not responded to her daughter's efforts. The arrival of the hospice nurse signaled that time was running out. It also represented for the daughter a reenactment of old conflicts in which she had witnessed her siblings being favored and interfering with her attempts to get close to her mother. Just as she had done repeatedly while growing up and as an adult, she fought with her perceived rival (now the nurse) rather than express her feelings of rejection directly to her mother. Although the nurse knew pieces of the story, she had not recognized how her presence fit systemically into an unresolved family issue.

I suggested to the nurse that during the next home visit she begin by affirming how much the daughter had done for her mother and also sympathize that sometimes it is hard not to be fully appreciated (a feeling with which a home health care nurse can easily identify). This led to an immediate softening on the daughter's part, who then confided to the nurse that she had relationship difficulties with her mother. After this joining of forces, the sharing of roles could be negotiated more smoothly. In addition, the nurse was included in the system in a way that potentially enabled her to intervene with regard to the daughter's issue, help her accept the limits of her relationship with her mother, or include a family consultant.

THREE TERMINAL-PHASE PERIODS

In the terminal phase, the patient, family, and professional caregivers become a close group, working together and separately through three different periods: (1) arrival, (2) here-for-now, and (3) departure. Naturally, the length and nature of these periods varies tremendously. I find them useful in identifying what issues a family is dealing with in the terminal phase and in helping to guide and prioritize family challenges and tasks.

The Arrival Period

In the arrival period, families typically are depleted from their protracted efforts to save a member's life. Clinicians need to help the patient and family accept the fact that from now on, medical interventions are intended to maximize comfort rather than cure.

Often, initiating hospice care involves a transition to new health care providers. It is not only a time to discuss and process stopping aggressive treatment, but it is also an opportunity to acknowledge the meaning and value of the relationships among providers, patients, and families and the journey they have taken together. Often this process is too brief or is bypassed altogether. This can be very hurtful to the patient and the family, heightening a sense of abandonment or even failure, thereby complicating the transition to the terminal phase. Clinicians need to contend with their own feelings of connection and loss with such families and make time for a mutually satisfying termination process. Patients and families (and sometimes the health care team) can benefit from consultation(s) that address both the transition to new health care providers and from medical treatment to palliative care.

This transition is fraught with possibilities for blame, shame, and guilt. The family may blame the medical team for failing to provide a cure, especially if physicians have earlier given an overly optimistic prognosis. Or the patient and family members may blame themselves or each other for having lost the battle with the disease, particularly if they are guided by a strong sense of personal responsibility and control, as in the following case.

Sally, 52, had metastatic breast cancer for 4 years and became terminally ill. Fiercely independent and a tenacious "fighter" throughout her life, she had vowed to control and cure her illness in the same way as "exceptional" cancer patients she had read about in popular literature. She also wanted to distinguish herself from her mother, who poorly managed her bipolar disease while raising her children. Sally deeply resented her for having died a "broken" person in a nursing home after she sustained a TBI during a psychotic manic episode. When Sally developed brain metastases and became cognitively impaired and unmanageable at home, her husband and adult children were left with no alternative but to hospitalize her. Family members were burdened by intense guilt because they knew that Sally would die in an institution like her mother. Family therapy focused on unlinking the sense of failure from the inevitability of death. The inability of Sally's mother to control her mental illness needed to be differentiated from Sally's valiant struggle with cancer. Also, it was important to affirm all family members' courageous efforts.

Clinicians can function as guides for families, helping them gently relinquish their hopes for a cure, initiate a humane plan for palliative care, and develop a pathway for the experience of death. This includes being mindful about a family's cultural values regarding end-of-life norms and rituals. Our task is to join with the family at a time when members are preoccupied with a final separation. In an inpatient facility, such as a hospice or nursing home, clinicians need to sensitively orient patients and families dealing with impending loss to this new, unfamiliar setting.

Families coping with a loved one's approaching death can easily lose a sense of control, because of myriad, continual caregiving demands, taking on new roles, emotional upheaval, and various changing needs. They need help to regain a sense of mastery over this painful process. Involvement of all family members, including children, in some aspect of caregiving normalizes the process of dying, provides a sense of control through participation, and counteracts feelings of anxiety and helplessness. Children, in particular, adjust better when they can do something—draw a picture, make a card, or pick flowers for a loved one—rather than feeling helpless on the sidelines.

While I try to convey respect for family members' limits, I also communicate that the processing of painful feelings and achieving closure is very natural and important. Painful feelings are more tolerable when families can be encouraged to experience joys and pleasures despite the inevitable loss.

Reading together and recounting good family times are just a few examples. One family, whose father was dying from a brain tumor, sang songs from cherished past family vacations. The father, who had difficulty speaking as a result of the tumor, led the songfest from his bed as a conductor joyfully waving his arms and pointing. Constant or relentless sorrow can interfere with these positive experiences. It is very useful to help families see how they can stay involved with the dying member, even during a gradual process of saying good-bye.

Complex Feelings

Family members often experience heightened feelings of anxiety, guilt, and anger in this phase of an illness. Increased anxiety can be due to more frequent and intense thoughts about a final separation from the dying member, feelings of helplessness to control the outcome, and ruminations about one's own mortality. As the dying member deals with anger and disappointment about unfulfilled personal dreams and expectations, family members, as well, commonly experience distress about dashed relationship dreams and expectations for the future. Guilt feelings of loved ones in the terminal phase are related to issues, such as escape fantasies, being repelled by the wasting away of the dying person, having some respite or enjoyment, and anger or resentment toward the dying person because of added new burdens. These guilt-inducing feelings can prevent members from feeling sadness and grief. Normalization of these common feelings helps family members get to the fundamental terminal-phase emotions of sadness and loss. Individual and family consultations may be needed if these feelings are compounded by longstanding unresolved relational problems. A baseline family consultation earlier in the illness or at the time of entry into palliative or hospice care can help the provider distinguish between normative feelings and the expression of underlying, unresolved family issues.

In the context of the intense strains of coping with end-of-life challenges, outbursts of anger and frustration are common and expected. However, these outbursts may be experienced as shameful in families with controlled emotional styles, especially if they are directed at the patient. Where possible, clinicians can support family members by normalizing angry feelings and reminding them of their extraordinary efforts and their instinctive caring for each other.

The Terminally Ill Child

Research shows that loss of a child is among the most devastating experiences that families endure (Stroebe, Schut, & Finkenauer, 2013). The impending death of a child deprives parents, siblings, and grandparents of witnessing the unfolding life of that child and their hopes and dreams, including important milestones and celebrations.

As discussed earlier (Chapter 9), children who have life-threatening conditions are often aware of that reality. Frequently, communication between a child and other family members has become blocked over time because the parents have reassured a child that he or she will do "fine" when the child has inquired, either directly or indirectly, about the possibility of death (see Chapter 11 on childhood illness). This response more likely reflects the parents' fears about being devastated if that outcome were to occur. In turn, the child learns not to communicate such concerns. Unfortunately, this pattern can easily continue into the terminal phase, when the child desperately needs to talk about his fears with his family. In one instance, a teenager who was terminally ill with leukemia shared his fears of dying with a close friend, but said that his parents couldn't talk about it because they felt devastated. His emotional support came from his closest friends. Sadly and ironically, after he died, his parents told others, "He was so brave. He never talked about how sick he was!" It is important to establish healthy illness-related communication patterns early in an illness, especially if loss is possible. Clinicians need to combine inquiry about cultural norms with educating parents about the age-appropriate emotional and communication needs of children.

Parents of seriously ill children often find the transition to the terminal phase one of the most difficult. Clinicians need to keep in mind that parents' resistance to turning over care to professionals may represent not only profound grief, but also guilt at not being able to save their child. It is very important to help parents participate in the terminal care of their child in any possible way. During this phase, siblings frequently become distraught because of the added attention being given to the dying child and the increased responsibilities they may have to assume as part of family coping. The inward pull and focus required to attend to a dying child is especially difficult if the terminal phase becomes prolonged. Parents may need help in maintaining a balance between their devotion to a terminally ill child, siblings, and work responsibilities. It is extremely beneficial to call on extended kin, such as grandparents, if they are available.

The Here-For-Now Period

In the here-for-now period, attention is narrowed to a "living-in-the–present" experience. This period may be nonexistent if the patient's health rapidly deteriorates, or it may last days or months. The challenge is to live as fully as possible in the time left. Families may need assistance in redefining hope with the terminally ill member as present focused, not future oriented. Besides enjoying the here-and-now moment by listening to music, for example, conversations may include reminiscing together and asking the dying member to participate in discussions about the family's future (e.g., reorganizing roles or celebrating important future family nodal events, such as a graduation), being mindful that longer-term future plans will occur *without* the dying member. This is distinct from having conversations about being together in the afterlife or reassuring the dying member that he or she will be there "in spirit."

The patient and family need a mutual understanding of unpredictable mood swings and the courage and strength to "live in the moment." The patient hopes that family members will be compassionate about his or her variable responses to pain and its relief, and provide reassurance that he or she will not be abandoned while still alive. It is unfortunately all too common for European Americans to avoid any contact with a dying person that might be painful. Some say they are too busy; others say they would rather remember the person as he or she was. Workplaces and coworkers may shift assignments to others without talking it over with the terminally ill employee. One physician with terminal cancer was well enough to keep working, but his superiors and colleagues avoided all contact with him, referred new patients to other doctors, and treated him as if he were already dead.

It is useful to encourage the dying person to contact other important family members and friends in order to see them once more, when possible, and to say their good-byes. It's not uncommon for those who are dying to search for relatives or friends who have been important at some point in their lives, but with whom they may have had little or no contact. One man wanted to contact a cousin whom he had not seen in many years, but who had been a close boyhood friend. He wanted to share his life journey, hear about his cousin's, and convey the importance of their earlier friendship.

Exhausted family members may need assurance that the dying member's effort to withdraw from the struggles of daily life is not a rejection of the family or a rebuke for their not having done enough. Clinicians play a critical role in helping family members stay involved, while also pacing themselves for handling a final separation from the patient. One colleague observed that new hospice clinicians often leave within a year. He believed, for multiple reasons, that these clinicians found it difficult to develop the delicate balance needed between attachment to and the inevitable loss of the terminally ill patient. Clinicians can learn not to expect or need another meeting. Proactive professional psychoeducational training and peer or group support are essential in fostering this skill (see Chapter 17).

Life Celebrations

Once death's imminence is clear, clinicians can deal more openly with practical arrangements, such as planning the funeral, ensuring understanding of the dying person's will, and resolving unfinished relationship issues. Clinicians can facilitate families' active participation in gatherings that include the dying member to celebrate his or her life.

Cleo, a married African American woman in her late fifties, had a second recurrence of ovarian cancer. After giving it much thought and discussing it with her family, she decided to forego further aggressive treatment, return home to receive palliative hospice care, and spend her remaining precious time with her family and friends. With Cleo's input, the family organized a fabulous life celebration for her on Mother's Day. The guiding premise was to celebrate Cleo's life while she was alive, rather than wait for the traditional memorial services that would be held when she passed away.

In another case, Phyllis, a Jewish woman in her eighties, who was widowed for many years, was diagnosed with a rapidly progressive neurological condition. Born in Hungary, she had emigrated as a child to the United States with her family, when they fled the Nazis. Her family of origin had been very musical, and she had sung and performed in the theater. In many ways, her own children and grandchildren had "lost touch" with their ethnic traditions. In the face of a progressive terminal condition, Phyllis decided to wear some of the clothes from the older generation that were in storage, sing traditional songs, and tell stories about her family's ethnic and religious roots. Family members gathered to watch and videotape the event. It was incredibly meaningful to everyone, and honored her own and a previous generation's life story and immigrant experience.

Funeral-Related Planning

Planning for funeral rituals, burials, or cremation is essential and may include choosing favorite music or writings for the funeral service and selecting a cemetery location, a headstone and inscription, and where to spread cremation ashes. Active participation by the dying member in any of these decisions supports a sense of control over the dying process and the respectful honoring of preferences. It also helps offset a source of conflict and potential guilt among family members.

Bequeathing special possessions while the dying member is still alive can be a very powerful and meaningful way for him or her to connect with friends and family. At Thanksgiving, a cousin of my father who was coping with terminal cancer gave me a ring that had been in his family for several generations. This gift gave us an opportunity to express our feelings about our relationship over the years and enabled me to hear more about our background and important family stories that I had never heard.

Encouraging families to take an active role in developing meaningful rituals counteracts the dominant culture's commercialization of this important milestone. In times of acute loss, a stunned family may turn the process over to professional funeral directors, which can result in an impersonal memorial service. It is helpful to ask the dying person how he or she would like to be remembered, what favorite music or readings should be used at the funeral, and how he or she would like others to express their sympathy or remembrance, for example, with flowers or donations to a favorite cause.

The Departure Period

In the final departure period, the patient lives in a world of diminishing concerns that center on controlling pain and suffering and having contact, when possible, with meaningful people in their fading hours. As family members share their last contact(s), they face the challenge of being survivors. A desire to be with a spouse or child in the person's final hour cannot eliminate the experience of separation and transitioning to a different way of remaining connected over time.

It is useful to inform family members about the dying process itself. Family members need to understand that the patient's withdrawal is not rejection or abandonment, but a natural and necessary part of the dying process. This can be perplexing or hurtful to friends and family who were closest to the dying person, and who may have fantasized a final death scene in which beautiful and meaningful words were to be exchanged.

The transition at death is a solitary journey that must be made by each of us alone. For some, fears of separation from loved ones and facing death alone may rival the fear of uncontrolled suffering. It is crucial that family members not pull away emotionally. Since hearing is the last sense to deteriorate, even when the patient is in a coma, the presence of family members and talking to the patient can be helpful. It can be very comforting to mention this to family members who may not have had the opportunity to speak with the dying member. This is particularly true for members who live far away and are arriving to say good-bye.

Clinicians can provide vital information about the physical details of the natural dying process. Several days before my father died, he stopped eating or drinking fluids. Despite knowing otherwise as a physician, I tried to get my father to take liquids though a straw. The hospice nurse noticed this and gently reminded me that refusing to drink was a natural part of his dying and that if I were to succeed in getting him to take fluids, it would actually cause discomfort. That's all I needed emotionally to let go of my attempts and more comfortably settle into just being with him. Normal and nonpainful changes in breathing, which can seem like air hunger, are other common examples.

Sometimes, dying persons will cling to life because they do not want to cause the deep pain of loss to the surviving family. If family members notice this, it is acceptable for them to give permission for the dying member to "let go" and die.

The death of a patient whose long debilitating illness has heavily burdened family members can bring relief as well as sadness. This is quite common after protracted ordeals, such as Alzheimer's disease, in which the affected member may have died psychologically for the family much earlier (see Chapter 16; Boss, 2011). Relief over death, even when it ends patient suffering and family caregiving and medical financial burdens, can trigger strong guilt reactions that may be expressed through symptoms such as depression and family conflict. Clinicians can help family members accept as natural their mixed feelings about the end of a loved one's suffering.

Geographic distance of some family members can foster imbalances in their readiness to let go, leading to a crisis. The following case is an illustration.

A father with a longstanding blood disorder and a history of kidney failure rather suddenly developed a respiratory complication that resulted in coma. Despite the medical team's best efforts, it became clear that the situation was irreversible. The primary physician, in consultation with the wife (who had health care power of attorney), a son, and a daughter, who lived locally, reached consensus to stop respiratory support and allow the father to die. However, a second son, who lived far away, arrived and declared that he would sue the hospital and health care team if they proceeded. The son's demands resulted in a family uproar outside the intensive care unit (ICU). In response, the health care team adopted a legally informed "defensive medicine" approach, continuing to provide life-sustaining care.

In consultation with the son, I learned that he had had a complex and conflictual relationship with his father, which had never been addressed. He was not prepared to say farewell to his father, especially with so many unresolved issues. His geographical distance compounded the problem. Having had little contact with his father, he had been removed from dealing with his physical difficulties and frail condition for some years. In a series of consultations over several days, I first helped the son shift from anger to disappointment about his unmet needs. I then coached him to speak to his father about the things that he had hoped for in their relationship. I told him that his father would quite likely be able to hear, but not respond. Doing this freed him psychologically to say good-bye and join the rest of the family in their readiness to let go.

In hindsight, these issues could have been identified and potentially addressed in an earlier family consultation, thereby averting a wrenching crisis as the father lay dying. Social media technology, such as Skype, can be extremely valuable in bridging geographical distances and fostering crucial dialogue, especially for family members who are unable or cannot afford to travel.

The dominant American orientation toward taking action and solving problems often makes us uncomfortable when there is nothing more we can do. Simply being with, sitting beside, holding hands, and/or listening to favorite music with the dying person can be extremely comforting. Relatives or close friends who are too busy to come to a dying person's bedside may simply be uncomfortable with facing loss and the prospect of their own mortality.

Sometimes, visiting a hospital room or intensive care unit full of equipment and a patient laden with tubes can terrify a child. Clinicians can suggest flexible alternatives, such as making a special card or speaking to the dying person by phone, Skype, or email. I make a clear distinction between this form of participation during a terminal phase and my recommendation for all family members to be present at a funeral or memorial service. However, we should not assume that a visit to an ICU would be scary for a child. In one situation, a parent had to fight the hospital staff to allow her 8-year-old son to say good-bye to his beloved grandmother who had been his full-time caregiver while the mother worked. Years later, they all agreed that it was very important and meaningful for him.

Deathbed disappointments and complicated grief can be lessened when family members are urged not to procrastinate, but to communicate their affection or to deal with unresolved issues earlier. Doing so also eases family members' concerns, enabling them to take needed respite as death approaches. When it is too late to address unresolved issues, clinicians can encourage an expression of regret for past hurts. We need to be mindful of the wide range of personal and cultural ways of saying good-bye to help families through this process (Rosenblatt, 2013).

ETHICAL AND LEGAL ISSUES AT LIFE'S END

The complex web of ethical and legal dilemmas surrounding decisions about control over life and death is one of the most difficult areas for clinicians and families.

Advance Directives (Living Wills)

In the United States, the Patient Self-Determination Act of 1991 stipulates that all patients admitted to hospitals and nursing homes be given information concerning advance directives in areas such as any desired limits of treatment, including do-not-resuscitate orders, and designating the person who has the authority to make decisions for the patient in the case of severe incapacitation. It is essential that clinicians encourage an open dialogue among family members and involved health care providers. As described previously, these discussions need to be revisited as the illness experience and family feelings or circumstances change. Sometimes, patients change their minds about what illness complications they earlier thought would be acceptable to live with (e.g., in ALS, the paralysis of muscles that controls eating or breathing). Others find positive meaning and satisfaction with the limitations, for example, being wheelchair bound, that they previously thought would be intolerable.

Early, informed family discussions regarding the patient's wishes about lifesaving measures and effective means of pain control can alleviate some of the anguish. Initiating discussions about whether and when to enact a do-not-resuscitate (DNR) order is often difficult for clinicians as well as for families. However, in these conversations patients and family members can ask detailed questions that help them make informed decisions (Lynn, Schuster,

Wilkinson, & Simon, 2007). Some urgent clinical indications for discussing end-of-life care may include individuals talking about wanting to die, individual or family inquiries regarding hospice care, recent hospitalization for a progressive illness, severe suffering and a poor prognosis, and imminent death.

All states provide standardized forms that typically cover the limits of aggressive and life-sustaining medical care. Individuals can create a personal document that is more explicit about such things as life support in the context of a vegetative state, or an incurable, progressive disease that causes intense suffering. Because most forms are not personalized and do not address nonmedical aspects of compassionate care, consumer-based organizations have developed alternative forms to standard advanced directives that can legally supplant the standardized versions.

An excellent example is the Five Wishes, created by Aging with Dignity (*www.agingwithdignity.org*) and used by more than 20 million people. It meets the legal requirements for an advance directive in most states and can be attached to legal forms in other states. The Five Wishes address the following:

1. The person I want to make care decisions for me when I can't.
2. The kind of medical treatment I want or don't want if I am close to death, in a coma and not expected to wake up or recover, or have permanent and severe brain damage.
3. How comfortable I want to be (e.g., what type of pain management, favorite music, or religious or other readings I want).
4. How I want people to treat me (e.g., do I want faith- or community-group involvement, to die at home if possible, to have my hands held, and to be talked to, even if not responsive).
5. What I want my loved ones to know (e.g., family and friends to respect my wishes even if they disagree, that I forgive family members for when they may have hurt me, that I would like family members to make peace with each other if they can before my death).

Because each wish includes questions that address the quality of familial relationships, the process of discussing and completing the Five Wishes can serve as a stimulus for healing relationship wounds and generally deepen family bonds.

Since death or severe incapacitation can strike loved ones as well as the patient at any time, I encourage all adult family members to complete an advance directive. I also recommend that family members, especially spouses or partners, engage in this process together. It is vital that a living will be shared and discussed among all family members, other key caregivers, and the primary care physician (Rolland, Emanuel, & Torke, 2017). This discussion ensures that the health care proxy understands and agrees to honor the patient's wishes. A significant disagreement may need processing in a couple or family consultation. If the designated member is unwilling or unable to honor a person's wishes, then it is better to designate another family member who is willing to do so. I advise that advance directive decisions be revisited periodically, ideally at regular intervals, but particularly at crucial transitions in the illness and in individual or family life cycles.

Cultural beliefs can complicate the completion of an advance directive. In one case involving a Filipino family, the father, with severe cardiovasular disease (including a heart attack and stroke) and renal failure, had been in a coma and on a respirator in the ICU for several weeks. Medically, there was no hope for recovery. The physician looked to the family for guidance about the father's wishes. Family members explained that they had turned down a request to complete an advance directive before the father's surgery. In their culture, to speak about such things before surgery would "jinx" the outcome. At a minimum, an early knowledge of this family's cultural values would have allowed the health care team to incorporate that awareness and think proactively about how those values would interact with the illness trajectory and possible medical crisis points. Also, having a conversation with the family facilitates exploration about whether they might be flexibile about particular cultural norms before such emotionally wrenching decisions need to be made.

It is important to check that the patient and family members understand the distinction between a DNR order and an advance directive. A DNR refers to medical attempts to resuscitate a person when the heart or breathing has stopped. A living will or advance directive refers to life-sustaining treatments, which in a terminal illness can include tube feeding, artificial nutrition or ventilation, kidney dialysis, transfusions, or antibiotics. When confronted directly with an end-of-life situation, families may need to consult with a professional to help clarify a hazy understanding of the technical issues, as well as the psychosocial implications for the entire family. One of the most difficult situations occurs when there are strong differences among family members about how long to sustain life, often because the patient has not dealt with advance directives or a DNR and now is unable to communicate his or her wishes. When a patient's wishes are known beforehand, health care providers can help guide families as to the right time to honor an order in their situation.

It is essential to learn who has been designated as health care proxy with power of attorney. This is the person chosen to ensure that the patient's end-of-life wishes are honored if he or she is, for example, in a comatose state and no longer able to make such decisions. Ensuring that the loved one's wishes are carried out is most complicated when he or she either does not want life support initiated in the first place or wants life support to be terminated under certain hopeless circumstances. Clinicians need to be mindful that often the family member who has agreed to honor these wishes finds that making the actual decision is much more difficult than anticipated. On one hand, family members may not want to prolong or witness suffering. On the other, they do not want to lose a beloved family member. Some may feel they are "killing" their loved one. This underscores the importance of involving and supporting all key family members and the medical team in the process. As one physician remarked in trying to comfort a family, "It's the disease that's killing your dad, not your decision to honor his wishes."

Euthanasia: Assisted Dying

Individuals or families may explore issues such as euthanasia or physician-assisted suicide (usually by prescription medication) when they are inquiring about end-of-life care. The issue of euthanasia is highly controversial. Whatever our personal feelings and religious moral convictions may be regarding this subject, we should remember that families in hopeless situations often discuss assisted dying and sometimes do take matters into their own hands, acting in shame and secrecy. Over two-thirds of Americans believe that when patients and their families desired it, doctors should be allowed to "end the patient's life by some painless means." Highlighting religious differences, a Pew Research Center study (2013) found that black Protestants, white evangelical Protestants, and Hispanic Catholics overwhelmingly disapprove of assisted dying, while white Catholics, mainline Protestants, and the religiously unaffiliated strongly approve. In terms of race, whites are more accepting than blacks (Werth, Blevins, Toussaint, & Durham, 2002), who have lower levels of trust in the medical establishment.

In 1994, Oregon enacted the Death with Dignity Act, making physician-assisted dying legal in that state. The Act stipulates the requirements and safeguards that must be adhered to before a physician can assist a patient's dying with a prescribed lethal dose of medication. The patient must be of sound mind when making the request in writing. Two doctors must confirm a diagnosis of a terminal illness, meaning the patient has no more than 6 months to live. Two witnesses, one of whom is not a doctor and is unrelated to the patient, must confirm the patient's request, and that patient must make a second request after 15 days. Patients must be referred for counseling if a mental illness is suspected. A number of states, including Washington, California, Montana, Vermont, and New Mexico, have similar statutes. Hospitals, doctors, and pharmacists may opt out of the program, but doctors are required to inform terminally ill patients about this option.

In an Oregon study, the most frequent reasons for choosing assisted dying are loss of autonomy, dignity, and the ability to enjoy life (80%); being a burden to family members (30%); and inadequate pain control (22%) (Okie, 2005). For many patients, just knowing that the option is available is a source of great comfort. In 2013, of 122 patients who obtained lethal drugs, only 71 actually used them; the others died naturally without using the pills. For many, it increased the likelihood of dying in the comfort of their homes with family and friends becoming more involved.

In the Netherlands, patients with terminal conditions, their families, and physicians have been able to negotiate the terms for ending life for more than 35 years. One man with terminal cancer articulated most poignantly the issue of an individual's right to choose a peaceful end to unbearable suffering:

> I don't see the point of suffering for nothing. . . . Initially, the fear of death and the unknown sucked away so much of my energy. When I was assured that I was allowed to hold my life in my own hands until the last second, then this energy that I had used for this fear was set free to use for fighting the cancer. . . . My energy was set free by the real human attitude, not moralistic one, of my doctor. . . . I felt that I had always been responsible for myself and that the last part (of my life) should be included. (*Choosing death*, 1993)

In recent years several national organizations have emerged to serve the unmet needs of patients and their families. Compassion & Choices is a nonprofit organization in the United States that advocates improving patients' rights and choices at the end of life (*www.compassionandchoices.org*). It provides free consultations about advance directives; referral to hospice and illness-specific support groups; adequate pain and symptom management; and safe, effective, and legal methods for aid in dying. Also, it has an advocacy Action Network that seeks to strengthen advance directives and laws that mandate palliative care training for health care providers. Many states and cities have developed End of Life Care Coalitions consisting of consumers and palliative care providers. Their mission is to improve the care of dying patients through educational and outreach resources.

Professional Values

Health care providers should be cognizant of the complexity of medical, legal, moral, and spiritual issues regarding the acceptable limits of aggressive medical care and assisted dying. It is crucial to be mindful of our own personal and professional ethical positions about these issues in order to sustain a sensitive and collaborative relationship with families who may be guided by different values. This is particularly significant when there is disagreement among family members. If a clinician voices an opinion prematurely or too forcefully, there is a risk of imposing his or her values on families, shutting down a family process that needs to continue. Our role is to facilitate a family's ability to discuss various options and arrive at their own decisions. In one case with end-stage widely metastatic liver cancer, a family member asked the oncologist, "What can be done to end Mom's suffering? It's unbearable to all of us." The physician's comment, "You need to keep your head up and be positive," was experienced as shaming and dismissive, and it severely damaged a family's relationship with providers and the health care system they work within.

When contentious divisions exist within a family, it can be problematic if a clinician sides with one part of the family. All of us can have potential professional limits beyond which we feel that we are violating our own religious and ethical beliefs. In such cases, I think it's best to sensitively inform the family, without implying what they should do, and recuse oneself from this particular aspect of decision making.

In states without any legal statutes regarding assisted dying, physicians often contend with personal values that do not have legal liability protection, as illustrated in the following case vignette.

A man with a terminal form of cancer, who was admitted for possible brain and bone metastases, informed the consulting psychiatrist and the oncologist that if medical tests confirmed widespread disease, he was going to go home and commit suicide. He was not clinically depressed. Further, he said that he and his wife, who had no children, had discussed this fully and with other close friends and family members. He had no psychiatric history and had led a satisfying personal and professional life. The two physicians felt torn. On one hand, they were aware of both the mental health laws pertaining to suicidal patients and that the state did not sanction assisted dying. On the other, they both felt that patients with terminal illnesses involving great suffering should have control over how and when they chose to end their lives. In this instance, the two physicians decided not to document the patient's comments, leaving him and his family with final control over the decision. Fortunately, this man's medical tests were normal.

CLINICIAN SELF-CARE

Our own experiences and values specifically related to threatened loss, end-of-life issues, and fears about our own mortality can become activated and sometimes compromise our clinical effectiveness (see Chapter 17; McDaniel, Hepworth, & Doherty, 1997). As we come to accept the limits of our ability to control the uncontrollable and increase awareness of our own experiences with loss, we can work more sensitively with the life-and-death challenges facing the families we serve. It is very beneficial for clinicians to have some type of professional peer forum to discuss difficult cases and common ethical dilemmas.

CHAPTER 11

Chronic Conditions in Childhood and Adolescence

Serious illness or disability in the young is one of the most difficult of all human experiences to accept. The profound sense of unfairness makes it one of the most challenging for families to master (Rolland & Walsh, 2006). In the United States, the prevalence of childhood chronic illness and disability has increased dramatically, doubling over the past two decades to over one in four children (nearly 18 million) (Van Cleave, Gortmaker, & Perrin, 2010). Obesity now affects over 17% of children (Ogden, Carroll, Kit, & Flegal, 2014), a number that has tripled since 1994. Because childhood obesity has reached epidemic levels, other chronic diseases, such as type 2 diabetes, are increasing rapidly. There has been a significant rise in childhood asthma, as well as in diagnoses of behavior and learning disorders, such as ADD/ADHD (CDC and NIH, 2013).

With advances in medical technology, children who are born with illnesses like cystic fibrosis (CF), hemophilia, or sickle cell disease, or acquire conditions, such as leukemia or kidney failure, are living into adolescence and adulthood (Halfon & Newacheck, 2010). Pediatric cancer remains the leading cause of illness-related death in childhood (Heron, 2012). However, in situations where life can be prolonged, ongoing concerns about recurrence and important delayed effects in cardiac, endocrine, and neurocognitive functioning remain (Robison et al., 2009). In short, both the good and the bad news associated with serious conditions impose psychosocial burdens that must be borne by families (Compas, Jaser, Dunn, & Rodriguez, 2012).

A burgeoning research literature demonstrates the impact of childhood chronic illness on the family (Barlow & Ellard, 2006; Cousino & Hazen, 2013; Kazak, 2006; Leeman et al., 2016; Long & Marsland, 2011; Patterson, Holm,

& Gurney, 2004; Rodrigues & Patterson, 2007) and the role of family functioning in disease status (Alderfer, Nausaria, & Kazak, 2009). Pediatric illness research also shows increased family resilience and posttraumatic growth (Barakat, Alderfer, & Kazak, 2005; Picoraro, Womer, Kazak, & Feudtner, 2014) including with developmental disabilities (Greef & Nolting, 2013). Yet, research is almost completely absent on the efficacy of family systems-oriented programs offered at the time of diagnosis.

When a child develops an illness or disability, the family faces several basic challenges, including the following.

- The need for parents to keep the child safe often conflicts with the affected child's need for increased autonomy. It can be challenging to achieve a balance between protecting the child and promoting exploration and "acceptable risk."
- The child needs to be integrated into his or her own peer group and be allowed to play in ways that are age appropriate and consistent with reasonable safety.
- Ill and disabled children need to be reassured about their intrinsic value and guided to develop life-cycle goals that promote self-esteem, hopefulness, and a positive sense about future possibilities.
- Over time, affected children need to be encouraged to take an increasingly major role in their own care. Because parents often develop a sense of pride and self-worth through caring for an ill child, as the child becomes more competent, the parents may experience some sense of loss. Parents often need permission from professionals to tend to their own adult needs and relationships.
- When parents have significant strains or conflicts in their relationship before a child's health problem becomes known, attention to those issues may be displaced by focusing on the affected child, which often increases family dysfunction.
- Families, out of necessity, must learn how to interact and assert themselves effectively with many other systems within the broader social ecology that may be discriminatory or inadequately structured to deal with the special needs of ill or disabled children, their siblings, and parents. Important examples include the educational and legal systems and the workplace environment.

CRISIS-PHASE ISSUES

Psychosocial Typology of Illness

Diagnosis of a chronic disorder marks the beginning of a protracted journey that includes grief and often anticipatory loss, particularly for parents, who must mourn the loss of a physically healthy child and, sometimes, their future hopes and dreams for the child. Educating the parents about the disorder's psychosocial demands over time in relation to child and adolescent development can give them a better sense of control. Progressive and life-threatening conditions are the most taxing because parents have to live with the uncertainty of their child's survival to the next developmental phase. If the child survives, what will then be the extent of his or her disability, and how might it interfere with specific developmental milestones (Jessop & Stein, 1985)? A progressive condition that imposes ever-increasing limits on a child's normative development is on a natural collision course with development toward more independence. Constant-course disorders, such as cerebral palsy or deafness, present relatively fewer ambiguities.

Because physical activity is so important in children's play, disorders that affect physical abilities and motor skills (e.g., muscular dystrophy or blindness) or involve deformities are often the most disruptive. These conditions inhibit a child's natural exploration and learning processes and limit the options for spontaneous play and creative expression. In the short run, such disorders interfere with the formation of peer relationships more than do life-threatening diseases. Other children may avoid the ill child because he or she cannot keep up with them or because they fear the physical differences. Sometimes they ridicule a child with disabilities. In relapsing conditions, the affected child and siblings need reassurance that a flare-up does not indicate progressive deterioration or a life-endangering crisis will occur.

The Influence of Family Beliefs

The meaning given to a child's illness has profound implications for the family's well-being. What are the parents' beliefs about what is a "normal" child? Clinicians can help them think of a *child with asthma* as just that rather than as an *asthmatic child*. This distinction fosters an acceptance of a condition as one aspect of a child's being. When an illness comes to represent everything about a child or a family, it becomes more devastating and overwhelming and sets the stage for dysfunctional adaptation, especially family communication. The child's illness can become a source of resentment, guilt, blame, and hopelessness. When these feelings occur, parents may dutifully provide care, but give up on the child psychologically on a deeper level. This fosters feelings of rejection, inadequacy, and being a burden in the affected child.

Families adapt best when they maintain a sense of balance between coping with the child's illness and the rest of family life, especially the needs of other children. Having flexible rather than stereotyped ideals about competency helps maintain this balance. Supporting affirmative family meanings and narratives can initiate a successful long-term process. The notion of keeping a condition in its place (Steinglass et al., 2011) helps all family members see the affected child as a competent human being who has specific limitations and prevents them from falling into extreme patterns, such as denial.

From this more balanced position, parents can expect an affected child to meet reasonable developmental goals. To the extent possible, the child needs to be a contributing member to the family's daily life. Sharing some family responsibilities enhances the child's self-esteem.

Guilt, Blame, and Gender Issues

Under duress, couples' gender roles can easily become distorted (see Chapter 14). In dual-career families, a mother may sacrifice her job and possibly her career to stay at home to take care of an ill child. A mother's taking a few days off in an initial health crisis can easily develop into a long-term arrangement when a frank discussion about future caregiving needs is bypassed. Added financial pressures, coupled with the fact that fathers generally earn more than mothers, may result in a pragmatic decision that has lasting relationship implications. Social policies that limit workplace flexibility regarding family medical leave only exacerbate this problem.

Parental self-blame, especially for mothers who are held primarily responsible for their children's well-being, increases the likelihood of overprotective patterns. To offset self-blame, a parent may be unreasonably demanding of her or his own time and energy. Parents are especially sensitive to professionals' comments that can be construed as implying neglectful behavior. One woman remembers the pediatrician asking "Why didn't you bring Billy to me sooner?" as a condemnation of her as being an inadequate parent responsible for her child's diabetes. This kind of framing event is a serious risk to healthy parenting and child development. As discussed in Chapter 8, illness beliefs that entail parental guilt are best addressed in the initial crisis phase.

When an infant or small child becomes ill or dies, both parents, but especially the mother, are prone to blame and guilt. Because infants are so dependent and vulnerable, parental feelings of responsibility for them are at a peak. Conditions such as SIDS, which have less-clear etiologies, prompt parents to wonder who was at fault. Each parent may feel unlovable and unable to express love toward the spouse at this time. Early intervention can help prevent interminable grief and unending cycles of recrimination that contribute to the high divorce rate among such couples.

In one case, a family was referred because the mother was seen as being overprotective of her withdrawn 5-year-old son. The family background revealed that an older son had died of a high fever in infancy. The husband and his mother had blamed the wife, saying that if she had been more attentive, the deceased son would have received medical attention sooner and been saved. The beliefs expressed in this story resulted in the husband's withdrawing from the marriage and intensifying his ties to his biological family, while the wife withdrew into her next pregnancy and vowed to protect the replacement child, who was now symptomatic. In the face of a tragic and ambiguous loss, blaming the mother was a gender-biased reaction that filled a vacuum. In four brief therapy sessions, the couple explored the interplay of the prior loss, its connection to the presenting issue, and unresolved gender roles in the parents' marriage stemming from each parent's family-of-origin cultural traditions.

Control Issues

One of the most painful aspects of a serious childhood diagnosis is the parents' sense of loss of control over protecting their child from physical harm and suffering. Clinicians can help families redefine mastery and mitigate feelings of helplessness by identifying controllable aspects of their situation, such as gathering information about their child's illness and participating in caregiving. If the initial crisis phase requires intensive hospital care, clinicians can minimize parental feelings of helplessness and inadequacy by seeking ways to include them in the caregiving process. Inviting a parent to remain in the hospital room overnight and to seek advice about the child includes parents in the process at the outset. When providers display respect for parental knowledge and preferences, it empowers the parents, helps establish effective collaboration, and reduces the chances of resistance and withdrawal that often compromises treatment adherence.

COMMUNICATION

An open acknowledgment of a child's condition by all family members promotes flexible communication that is age appropriate for the child. Although children's ability to understand the nature of a serious condition is linked to their stage of cognitive development, a substantial body of research documents that children as young as age 5 have a real comprehension of the seriousness of their condition and are eager to talk about it. Even younger children display clear reactions to parental strain related to life-threatening illness. Children's reluctance to ask direct questions is correlated with parental anxiety that leads to protective patterns of communication within the family, and their reticence to talk freely is often related to their parents' discomfort about discussing their disorder. Yet, a child's open discussion of their illness with parents is positively associated with well-being (Barlow & Ellard, 2006). Patterns of closed communication are associated with a heightened sense of isolation in children. Secrecy promotes children's fantasies, which typically are terrifying and lead to a profound sense of aloneness.

Fundamentally, I believe children are entitled to an understanding of their conditions. The level at which children understand CF and the amount of detail they may need will change as they cognitively mature. If a child has a disorder with avoidable life-endangering risks, he or she must begin to deal with the possibility of death from an early age. Death is not an abstract issue from which a child can be completely protected. There is no substantial evidence that facing death or serious personal risks in childhood leads to pathological development. Murray Bowen (2004) commented that he never saw a child hurt by exposure to death, but only by the anxiety of other surviving family members. In fact, many of the most resilient adults I have met are those who had to cope with serious health conditions in childhood. They developed an increased sensitivity to children who have personal struggles and to life's preciousness and fragility, which enhanced their lives and relationships. They learned that growth is possible during and in the aftermath of traumatic experiences (Barakat et al., 2005).

Lack of communication is a major risk factor when a child has a health problem (Barlow & Ellard, 2006; Seligman & Darling, 2009; Weihs et al., 2002). Often the affected child and siblings are curious but his or her parents discourage inquisitiveness, turning it into fear by deflecting invitations to answer questions and concerns. As they do regarding sexuality, children will ask questions about chronic conditions when they are ready for an age-appropriate answer. One child with cancer asked his parents whether he might die. The parents response "No, you'll be fine" served more to protect parental fears about displaying their feelings than protecting the child. A response such as "Yes, it is possible. But the doctors have very good treatments for your cancer and are very hopeful" honestly acknowledges the illness by name and the possibility of death, but does so in a hopeful context. Families can be helped to learn that avoiding use of a cancer-related word, such as *leukemia*, is not wise; referring to the illness by name is not the same as saying, "You are going to die."

Psychosomatic and Triangulation Patterns

Early studies have found that with childhood and adolescent chronic disorders, such as diabetes, an affected child's condition is responsive to dysfunctional family processes (Minuchin et al., 1978). More recent research (Wood, 1993; Wood et al., 2008) with childhood gastrointestinal conditions, such as Crohn's disease, has shown that marital dysfunction and triangulation are the most significant family processes.

As discussed in Chapter 4, an ill child can become triangulated into preexisting unresolved conflicts of other family members, most notably between the parents. Children from a young age can learn to use their condition to express their feelings and manipulate parents and siblings, especially with illnesses marked by life-threatening crises and that are very responsive to emotional factors. Many children with asthma describe how they can induce an attack. Adolescents with diabetes can hold their parents hostage, using their illness as a weapon in battles for control.

Not infrequently, illness onset can set in motion a dysfunctional structural shift in a previously healthy family. For example, if a mother is designated the sole primary caregiver without parental negotiation, the added burden can foster strong resentment toward the father. This is particularly true for disabling conditions that require extensive caregiving. Such a family may gradually develop significant dysfunction stemming from flawed structural and communication patterns originating in the initial crisis phase. Over time, such illness-generated patterns in a family can become indistinguishable from a family with preexisting dysfunction. Prevention-oriented consultations are essential.

DEVELOPMENTAL ISSUES

The psychosocial demands of childhood chronic disorders interact continually with normative developmental goals. New illness narratives emerge as the child and family encounter each developmental phase. Different psychosocial types of conditions create their own unique and challenging pattern. A major therapeutic goal is to help families find a workable fit between normative developmental goals and what the disorder allows at each phase of development.

Distinguishing standard developmental issues from those caused by an illness is a common family challenge. For instance, age-appropriate rebelliousness and oppositional behavior are common in adolescence. At the same time, any chronic disorder can normatively cause anger and irritability that may be expressed in oppositional behavior. Some conditions, such as diabetes, can physiologically cause intermittent irritability and oppositional behavior as a consequence of hypoglycemia. It can be very confusing for parents to know how to interpret such behaviors and intervene properly. If hypoglycemia is the cause, then getting sugar into the child is essential. If irritability signifies trouble coping with chronic illness, then addressing the illness's effect on the child will be most helpful. If the behavior is related to individual development, providing guidance on normative adolescence is paramount.

Often normative and medical influences are interwoven and need to be approached from that perspective. Some parents find it very difficult to relinquish control over the daily testing and necessary restrictions required in an illness like diabetes. These parents may benefit from a developmentally focused consultation to better understand their role in facilitating a child's earlier transition toward managing his or her disease.

Child Temperament

A child's temperament significantly affects responses to his or her own or a parent's illness (see Chapter 12). The degree of inhibition in a child's approach to unfamiliar situations, such as illness, and his or her level of reactivity in terms of physical or emotional distress, are key variables (Zentner & Shiner,

2015). Asking parents how a child has coped with past life challenges affords some insight into temperamental style and how a child might cope and adapt to a chronic health condition. For example, a shy, unadventurous child may have a relatively easier time adapting to the restrictions of hemophilia than a boisterous, very physically active child. Conversely, with a disability or illness not susceptible to life-endangering exacerbations, an active child, who is eager to explore unfamiliar situations or push the limits of rehabilitation, may be a good fit with maximal physical functioning over time. By extension, the restrictions on a parent who suffers from chronic fatigue may be an easier fit with a temperamentally less active than more active child.

Determining Reasonable Developmental Goals

One of the most frustrating issues for parents is determining reasonable developmental expectations for a chronically ill child. It is useful to ask about each parent's understanding of which developmental milestones will be unaffected or delayed, subject to alteration, or unachievable. How are the parents' views similar or divergent, and how do their perceptions dovetail with the providers' perspective? The psychosocial typology and time phases can provide providers and parents with a common language for these discussions. It allows clinicians to frame future-oriented developmental questions that are relevant to specific disorders. For instance, in addressing parents and their teenage daughter, Sally, who has CF, a clinician might inquire:

- How does each of you think about Sally's plans after high school, given the ongoing disease management and possible complications of her illness?
- Is there anything you think she cannot or should not do?
- How do you envision Sally assuming control of managing her illness? Are there any aspects of disease management that concern you?
- Sally, what is your perspective on managing your condition in light of your plans after high school?
- How does this fit with any advice you have already been given by health care providers?

Often parents are aware of a complication that will affect a future developmental goal, and the question becomes if, when, and how to communicate it to the child or adolescent. In one case, I consulted with parents of a 5-year-old daughter who had been cured in infancy of a cancer near the pelvis (neuroblastoma). The treatment had required radiation of the pelvic region, which precluded normal reproductive development. When asked when and how they would discuss this complication with their daughter, the couple became very emotional and argumentative. One parent felt that the history of cancer should be openly discussed and that the daughter should be forewarned before adolescence. The other felt that she should not be told about her cancer experience and its complications, but left to discover her own reproductive limits. They had never discussed this issue together. My own bias was toward openness; but at this stage it was essential, first, for each parent to express his or her opinion and feel understood before professional advice was offered.

Developmental versus Medical-Management Goals

Ambiguities about whether developmental goals can be achieved, to what degree, and with what physical consequences are inherent in many conditions. Some illnesses, such as hemophilia, can worsen under stress and lead to a life-threatening recurrence. One adolescent boy had a nearly fatal bleeding episode while cramming to get good final grades so that he could be accepted to a more competitive university. His drive to succeed academically was motivated largely by his wish to please his father, whom he felt he had disappointed because of the physical limits imposed by his illness. Because parents may differ on what are acceptable risks, decisions about whether an affected child should be involved in activities such as sports can be highly conflicted. One parent may adhere to a somewhat conservative philosophy, while the other may believe in "going for it" despite moderate risks. Some disorders, such as hemophilia or severe asthma, require strict limits to achieve medical control. In these situations parents can often be too permissive in setting limits because they try to compensate for the illness-related restrictions the child must endure.

Early consultations can identify the origins and meanings of these important parental differences, which can become an ongoing source of child-rearing conflict. Family behavioral consultations can help parents more fully discuss and understand their differences and aim for a mutually acceptable compromise that is consistent and in collaboration with the health care providers' viewpoint.

Assessing the quality of life both in terms of acceptable medical management and normative developmental goals is an ongoing process for parents; often one must be compromised for the sake of the other. Obtaining accurate biomedical information about the illness course and the risk factors involved is essential in weighing pros and cons. Any ambiguities about what activities can make a disorder worse can fuel intense, conflictual family interactions. As part of an initial assessment, it is always important to ask both the adults and the children about what level of risk they each understand as acceptable.

Parents often set aside their own personal goals because of a perceived or actual need to be the child's caregiver. This can lead to poor self-care for the adults, including a neglect of the marital relationship and, sometimes, job and educational needs. Collaboratively consulting with parents can facilitate determining an appropriate level of caregiving, exploring other caregiving resources (e.g., extended kin, community members), and helping them achieve a healthier balance between caring for the ill child and other individual and relational goals.

An important question is whether, when, and how to include children and adolescents in deliberations about balancing medical management and psychosocial development. Although parents make decisions about various trade-offs, children, at any age, deserve an explanation about their decisions. Actual participation in the decision-making process is more complex, particularly with adolescents. A chronic disorder can seriously impede the natural movement toward central developmental tasks of autonomy and independence. Generally, when children have been overprotected, they respond in adolescence either by remaining fearfully dependent or by vigorously defying parental control. When parents establish early on a pattern of including chronically ill children in disease-related discussions, then in adolescence a more natural, less reactive, gradual transfer of decision-making authority can occur.

Adolescence and Transition to Early Adulthood

Anticipatory Loss

During a child's adolescence and the transition to early adulthood, a powerful resurgence of anticipatory loss often emerges. Potential limitations, unrealistic hopes, and issues of permanent dependence come to the fore in the context of the major developmental goals. These goals can include lessening of parental controls, preparing to leave home, and setting up a new, independent life structure in which the "center of gravity" with one's family of origin is rebalanced. A realistic appraisal of independent living is often necessary. The possibility that a young adult will remain permanently dependent and need family support raises developmental challenges for the parents, who typically look forward to the time when child-rearing demands are ending and individual or couple's goals can be pursued more freely.

Autonomy and Dependency

Normative parent–adolescent control issues can become more complex because of disability-related dependence and threatened loss. Adolescents have a great need to be like others their age, to belong to a desired peer group, to feel strong, and to develop "dreams" about their future. These normative adolescent strivings can collide with fears of dependency and threatened loss. The experience may be heightened because normal cognitive development enhances the adolescent's ability to look into the future and contemplate loss.

For adolescents with illnesses such as cancer, diabetes, or cerebral palsy, powerful fears may emerge for the first time about living independently, about infertility, and about genetic transmission that may affect perceived or actual possibilities for intimacy and a family life. These concerns need to be clarified and adolescents need encouragement in modifying either-or thinking and developing positive alternatives. Teens can learn, through family and individual consultations, that personal agency and mastery is a human quality that transcends physical capabilities.

Adolescents confronted with life-threatening conditions can use denial and an attitude of invincibility as a defense against feelings of despair. Those with diabetes can threaten not to take their insulin injections, disregard dietary restrictions, or claim to forget them, with immediate and dire consequences. Such behaviors are a powerful way to deny or to express anger about having to cope with a chronic condition and deny all its possible ramifications for the future. Self-destructive behaviors can reflect fears about being unable to take care of oneself because of the chronic illness. Acting out is one way an adolescent can express ambivalence, forcing parents to monitor health behaviors more closely and apply stronger limits.

As the following case illustrates, family therapy can help address the multiple issues being communicated through such behaviors.

Charlene, a 17-year-old African American teen, and her parents were referred after Charlene returned home before the end of her first semester on scholarship at college. Her type 1 diabetes, previously well managed since it was diagnosed at age 9, was out of control, and Charlene had made several trips to the emergency room in diabetic ketoacidosis. She had become neglectful of her diet, often skipping meals, eating sweets indiscriminately, and consuming excessive alcohol. She had also become obsessively concerned about being too heavy. Going to college had been the first time Charlene was away from home and fully in control of managing her diabetes care.

She was the first in her family to leave her working-class neighborhood for college, with dreams of financial success and a better life. On initial consultation, it became clearer that her parents and siblings had noticed her somewhat increased anxiety and more lax diabetes management during her last year of high school. But, when asked, Charlene had maintained, "Everything is fine. I can handle my own life!" Everyone was extremely proud of her academic talents, seeing her as the prime hope for the family "moving up" in the world.

Her mother, Sarah, who had grown up with her own sister's diabetes, had meticulously managed her daughter's diet over the years. Sarah's sister, who had been nonadherent for many years, died several years earlier of complications of end-stage renal disease and owing to lack of access to a possible kidney transplant. Consistent with the family's general style of not talking about difficult feelings, Charlene and Sarah had never spoken about the meaning of Charlene's aunt's diabetes and demise in relation to Charlene's own diabetes. Both had intense and unspoken fears. Sarah worried that without excellent diabetes control, her daughter could experience the same fate as her sister. As Charlene approached leaving home, her anticipatory loss-related fears became more conscious. This was heightened by her own dependence on her mother's watchfulness and concerns that she would not be able to manage her own care adequately. These fears were compounded by Charlene's feelings of pressure to succeed for the whole family and making up for her parents never having the same opportunities when they were young adults. Both parents had worked very hard to make a better life for the next generation. All these issues came together in a "perfect storm" during Charlene's developmental transition to young adulthood at the point that she left home.

Family therapy focused on these various issues. Charlene took a medical leave from college and remained at home until the following fall. This hiatus allowed time for Charlene to gradually assume full control of her own diabetes care and for the family to process these underlying issues and themes. In hindsight, prevention-oriented psychosocial consultation(s) earlier in adolescence might have helped avert this crisis.

Parents' reactivity to an oppositional adolescent can represent their own anger about a perceived lack of appreciation for their tireless efforts to help the child master the illness. Adolescents can interpret these normal feelings as signs of being a burden and a disappointment to their parents. In a vicious cycle, this interaction can further fuel conflictual and self-destructive behavior. The situation is further complicated by adolescent tendencies toward impulsive, immediate gratifications, by difficulties with adopting a long-range perspective, and by peer pressures to engage in risky behaviors. In adolescents coping with a progressive or life-threatening condition, these normative features of adolescent behavior can be taken to extremes because of underlying feelings of despair about the future. All family members need affirmation and, when possible, normalizing of their struggle at this phase of the life cycle. Prevention-oriented consultations for the ill adolescent and the family in early-to-mid adolescence can help allay concerns regarding these common experiences, as well as identify higher-risk families that could benefit from brief or more intensive family treatment.

Multifamily discussion groups are a valuable, cost-effective way of providing developmentally geared education, of problem-solving common issues, of networking families at the same transition points, and of identifying families experiencing significant dysfunction (see Chapter 4). Both the diabetes and CF programs that our Center for Family Health collaborated with developed very successful adolescent and transition-to-adulthood services that included 1-day multiple-family discussion workshops. Pragmatic psychosocial information about shared challenges given to the entire group was combined with discussions in small breakout groups dealing with special topics, such as effective communication, negotiating independence, exploring romantic relationships, and sibling issues.

In cases that present with these issues, clinicians need to be cautious about blaming parents for faulty child-rearing patterns of overprotection or inadequate limit setting. Often with life-endangering disorders, the family may have had early, almost fatal experiences with a child that sensitized them. Health professionals may have reinforced a cautious approach in the crisis phase without considering the psychosocial impact over the long haul. In genetically transmitted disorders, such as hemophilia, multigenerational legacies of traumatic loss may underlie beliefs in the need for protection. When there are ambiguities about appropriate cautionary measures, a family consultation with the primary care provider can be extremely helpful in establishing suitable limits.

All family members can experience tremendous ambivalence in this developmental phase. Older adolescents may feel a need to prove they can keep up with peers. Parents may want to protect the affected adolescent from experiencing limits and disappointment. The real letting go at this phase is about letting adolescents assume responsibility for their own life and potential disappointments, while finding their niche in the world. Parental guilt at this phase represents a combination of several issues. One of them, most commonly experienced by mothers, is resurgence of the feeling that "this condition was my fault." Parents may unrealistically define adequate child rearing by confusing protection from suffering with the more adaptive goal of helping children bear life's inevitable suffering.

Siblings can feel guilty about succeeding or surpassing their affected brother or sister. Key developmental points that can arouse such emotional reactions include that of a sibling leaving home and embarking on an independent life, or beginning a serious intimate relationship. In some instances siblings and parents may block their own achievement or abandon their own life ambitions out of "wellness" guilt or an attempt to protect the ill adolescent from emotional pain. When parents address any of their own feelings of blame, shame, and guilt, they also help healthy siblings and the affected adolescent move ahead developmentally. Realignment of the old parent–child relationship will maximize the adult child's ability to assume responsibility for his or her own well-being.

Transition from Pediatric to Adult Services

With improvements in health care, an increasing number of individuals with child- or adolescent-onset conditions are transitioning from pediatric to adult services (Pai & Ostendorf, 2011). This transition coincides with and is embedded in the affected adolescent's developmental transition to early adulthood, in which young adults generally assume responsibility for their own disease management more fully. It is a transition for the family system as well, and its emotional impact is frequently underestimated. This manifests in several ways. The chronically ill young adult does not follow through adequately, which results in missed appointments with new health care providers; lowered medication adherence; increased clinical symptoms of the disease, such as breathing difficulties with asthma; abnormal metabolic signs, such as increased blood pressure, or increased blood glucose levels in diabetes; and mental health difficulties, such as anxiety or depression.

One pediatric CF program emphasized celebration. In essence, the mindset was, "You have done well with your illness and are now graduating to adult services." The experience of loss for the young adult and parents was underplayed. Yet to the child and family, the pediatric health care team had become a second "life-saving" family since the child was diagnosed in infancy or early childhood. The relative lack of acknowledgement of the loss can complicate and undermine the transition. Further, in a large city, the transition is limited not only to changing providers, but also frequently involves a transition to a new health care system altogether.

Family systems-based consultation(s) in preparation for, during, and after the health care transition can improve the process, and the clinician's mindfulness to the following interwoven transitions is important.

- The patient and family's transition from pediatric to adult services.
- The patient's transition from adolescence to young adulthood.
- Family life-cycle transitions to the launching young-adult phase and to the parents' changed relationship as a couple.
- Pediatric and adult services providers coordinating with each other during the transition.

Collaboration between the child and adult services is vital to success. Optimally, this includes an appointment with the pediatric and adult providers together to initiate a "warm handoff." With larger specialty services, such as oncology, endocrinology, and respiratory conditions, the use of multifamily psychoeducation workshop formats at this transition can be very effective.

CHALLENGES FOR SIBLINGS

Particularly with life-threatening and disabling disorders, siblings can easily become forgotten family members. Resentment about not receiving as much attention as an ill sibling, guilt-ridden fantasies about how they might have wished for or even caused their brother's or sister's condition, fears about the death of the affected sibling, and concerns about their own or their parents' vulnerability are just a few of the typical experiences of healthy siblings that require therapeutic attention (Barlow & Ellard, 2006).

Research on the impact of childhood illness and disability on sibling relationships shows mixed results. On the one hand, meta-analytic reviews of existing research (O'Brien, Duffy, & Nicholas, 2009; Vermaes, van Susante, & van Bakel, 2012) continue to find that siblings are at heightened risk of internalizing (e.g., anxiety or depression) and externalizing (e.g., oppositional behavior or aggression) behaviors; having negative self-attributes (e.g., low self-esteem); and experiencing a range of individual, peer, family, and school-related problems. Also, data show that greater disease severity or having a fatal illness is correlated with siblings' increased psychological risk and lower health-related quality of life (Limbers & Skipper, 2014). On the other hand, some investigators cite positive influences on variables associated with better sibling adjustment, such as resilience, self-esteem, empathy, prosocial behavior, assertiveness, increased family cohesion, an expressive family environment, and the health of the mother (Alderfer et al., 2014; Barlow & Ellard, 2006). A growing body of research shows the effectiveness of broad-spectrum psychosocial services (Hartling et al., 2014) and specific family-oriented programs for well siblings (Lobato & Kao, 2005).

Younger siblings, in particular, usually need answers to and support in handling their most basic questions.

1. How did my brother or sister get ill?
2. Did I have anything to do with causing it?
3. Will this happen to me or someone else I care about (my parents, teachers, and close friends)? Is it contagious?

Because of embarrassment and fear, conditions that have visible symptoms are often the most disturbing to siblings. Like adults, children adapt best when they can develop narratives that promote a sense of competence and mastery. Direct and clear information and supportive reassurance from parents are the best preventive medicine for well siblings.

Guilt

Siblings sometimes believe that angry feelings toward a brother or sister caused the illness. Such beliefs, when unexpressed, can cause feelings of guilt and a need to be punished, expressed as withdrawal, depression, suicidal ideation, self-destructive and aggressive behavior, and declining school performance. Parents can inadvertently reinforce such feelings if they do not allow a child to express guilt feelings or are too quickly reassuring. Parents may falsely assume that talking about the illness will upset siblings and encourage lingering unease. Avoidance of this kind protects parents from their own self-blaming thoughts. When sibling guilt is not openly addressed, a child can harbor fears, such as of losing control of his or her anger and physically harming someone. Especially when working with younger children, it is important to elicit any such magical fantasies so that they can be explored and clarified.

Anger

Caregiving demands and parental preoccupation with the needs of an ill child are the most common causes of well siblings' anger. During the transition to the chronic phase, families need to review the psychosocial demands that can be expected. For instance, will illness course and caregiving demands be constant, periodic, or increasing? In this context, parents can discuss effectively balancing the needs of well siblings with those of the ill child. If there will be predictable periods of intensified focus on the ill child, parents can plan ahead to provide additional supports for the well siblings (e.g., from grandparents or other members of the extended family or community). Also, families can plan special times that compensate for medically demanding periods, thus reducing feelings of discrimination. Sometimes well siblings become angry and feel rejected in the aftermath of a health crisis. Children need to be reassured that they are important and that everything is all right again. Unfortunately, exhaustion, depression, and financial pressures may undercut parents' ability to give quality time to their healthy children. Extended kin can be a valuable resource in giving special attention to siblings by taking them for a day or weekend to give parents needed respite.

Life-threatening disorders that require constant monitoring affect siblings more powerfully, fostering greater jealousy and conflict. It is useful to consider whether any role asymmetry will diminish or grow as a result of a disease as the ill and well sibling pass each developmental milestone.

The willingness of siblings to accept and care for each other can become an increasing source of conflict as they enter adolescence. The desire for independence can make both siblings resentful about these roles. Natural adolescent concerns about body integrity and image can heighten fears about vulnerability for the well sibling and humiliation for the affected sibling when they need to interact in giving and receiving care. Parents often do not take into account the complex concerns of well siblings and, because they place greater trust in their maturity, assign increasing caregiving responsibilities to them as they get older. An awareness and sensitivity to a family's cultural norms is essential. In some families, a well sibling might be expected to accommodate any life-cycle goals to the present and future caregiving demands of their affected brother or sister.

Sometimes guilt and anger merge. Particularly in situations in which a child has a serious disability, such as intellectual limitations, or dies, a well sibling may be designated to make up for the loss. A family's inconsolable grief can become displaced in a romantic fantasy of heroic proportions to be lived out by a sibling. This tremendously burdensome task can never be fulfilled, as this case vignette illustrates.

A highly competent pediatric resident entered individual therapy with intense feelings of guilt and anger toward his brother with a severe developmental disability and his parents. During the initial visit he exclaimed, "No matter what I do, I never feel I can do enough to make everyone happy." His father's seeing the disabled son as a source of shame compounded the situation. His career choice, to become a pediatrician, was motivated partly by his deep desire to overcome his own guilt and shame by "rescuing" other children with chronic disorders. Meetings with his family of origin helped enable him to experience feelings of self-worth and accomplishment in his personal and professional life. The consultations included a separate meeting with his parents to understand and come to terms with their sense of shame and experience of stigma in their community over the years.

Somatic Preoccupations

A sibling's illness shatters children's beliefs that serious health problems and death only happen when a person is old. They can lose their sense of immunity. Siblings often develop fears or phobias that even the smallest symptom may be serious. Parents can counteract this tendency by giving clear explanations of the affected child's condition and differentiating it from the usual acute childhood illnesses. Also, siblings can develop negative attitudes and fears about doctors and hospitals. Such feelings can be compounded by having overheard parents' complaints about physicians caring for the ill child.

Well siblings may develop somatic complaints, such as sleep and appetite problems, headaches, and abdominal pains. Typically, these represent anxiety about becoming ill. Often such complaints coincide with changes in the status of the affected child's disorder. In some families somatic symptoms may become a dysfunctional way of expressing a need for attention. A well sibling may feel that physical complaints are the only valid form of currency that can compete with a chronic disorder. The following vignette illustrates this point.

> Mr. and Mrs. C. presented with behavior problems in their 12-year-old daughter, Sue, who had severe asthma and crippling juvenile rheumatoid arthritis that required the use of crutches. Sue's asthma was volatile and led to increasing visits to the emergency room over the past year, including visits for two life-threatening episodes. Mrs. C. had chronic back problems that flared every few months, necessitating days or weeks of bed rest. Mr. C., who worked at a desk job, had chronic bronchitis and emphysema that limited his energy and ability to do more than basic household chores. The couple had a chronically conflictual relationship in which physical complaints were regularly used during disagreements as a lever to gain control and sympathy. Their 7-year-old son, Jimmy, was presumably fine.
>
> During the initial assessment, I asked Jimmy, who had been very quiet up to that point, how he got attention with all these serious physical problems in the family. Jimmy got up, grabbed his sister's crutches, and demonstrated how well he could use them. His parents confirmed that during periods of family stress, he would take the crutches and walk around the house and neighborhood using them in front of the rest of the family and neighbors. This behavior usually coincided with conflict between Mr. and Mrs. C. or with Sue. Jimmy then said, "If things get really tough, I do this." He went to the center of the room on the crutches, feigned extreme pain (like his mother's), dropped the crutches while grabbing his throat with both hands as if gasping for air and coughing (like his sister and father), went into a dramatic "death twirl" such as he had seen in the movies, dropped to the ground, and lay motionless.

This case highlights the power that physical symptoms can exert over family life. Jimmy as a small child had learned how to get attention, gain control, and deflect conflicts between other family members by means of physical symptoms. Since adequate family communication was missing, his tactic also gave him a way to try to master his fears of becoming ill or disabled.

The timing of this particular crisis coincided with the ill daughter's becoming an adolescent. This life-cycle transition was superimposed upon unresolved family problems, including struggles for control over physical problems, power struggles among family members, dysfunctional communication patterns, and parental conflict and exhaustion. Often, a well sibling like Jimmy will protect his parents by distracting them through acting out. Healthy children sometimes feel excluded and different from the rest of the family because they do not have physical symptoms, a process that is frequently not a conscious one. In this case, some of the key problems addressed during treatment included the following.

1. Addressing the parents' marital difficulties, especially the issues related to dysfunctional, blocked communication; gender and power issues; and mutual nurturance.
2. Strategizing pragmatically for times when the parents' and daughter's illness symptoms were exacerbated. This included planning for additional caregiving support from extended kin, their fellow church members, and community professional resources.
3. Initiating a dialogue with the parents about anticipatory loss concerns and related sensitive age-appropriate communication with each child.
4. Helping parents effectively collaborate with their daughter about age-appropriate expectations and rules.
5. Coaching the parents about the needs of well siblings.
6. Planning enjoyable nonillness-related family activities and special times.

DEVELOPMENTAL DISABILITIES: CHALLENGES IN ADULTHOOD

Developmental disabilities, such as cerebral palsy, Down syndrome, and autism, present profound and unique challenges to families as the affected member enters adulthood. Social services supports and school-based individualized educational programs provided to children are mostly not available after age 18, leaving families with added caregiving responsibilities that extend open-ended into the future. Family planning for the immediate young adult period is not sufficient. Although many of these conditions are not life threatening and typically allow a normative life span, effective medical treatment to control or alter the disabling aspects is minimal. This limits the options for effective collaborative health care models for such adults and their families.

An individual and family life-cycle lens can be very valuable in these situations. The following case highlights many of the ongoing life-cycle challenges for all family members.

The S. family was referred by their longtime rehabilitation medicine physician. Nancy, age 28, has had cerebral palsy since birth. With severe spasticity, she was confined to a wheelchair and required extensive caregiving with all aspects of daily living. Her parents, Stan and Marjorie, were in their mid-sixties and had lovingly and tirelessly provided caregiving since infancy. Stan had developed heart disease over the past 5 years, and it was beginning to limit some of the care he could give to Nancy. Nancy's sister, Marybeth, age 32, with whom Nancy is very close, had lived at home until 2 years ago. She finally got an apartment and was exploring a promising long-term relationship. This family's individual members' and collective resilience over the years was extraordinary.

Nancy was highly intelligent, but had limited verbal ability. Despite her disabilities, she was outgoing and thrived in high school, but since then had remained at home and, with her parents' help, was taking online courses and remaining in contact with friends through social media. Her extreme spasticity and verbal limitations had constrained her independence and career and relationship options. Most of her childhood friends had moved on in their lives, starting careers, entering relationships, or marrying and starting families. She had become increasingly isolated and depressed over the past few years, perceiving few choices. In particular, she worried about her long-term living and caregiver options.

Normative, overlapping life-cycle issues were apparent for each family member and the entire family system. Nancy's personal development largely came to a halt in early adulthood, and now approaching 30, she was discouraged about her future. She worried about her father's heart condition, which is both life-threatening and potentially life-shortening, and about both parents entering later life with their own looming caregiving needs. Given both Nancy's constant-course illness and her father's heart disease, all family members were aware of the complexity of planning their futures. Because the family had had a stable and mostly unvarying life structure for 30 years, Marybeth's move to an apartment being the first major change, they avoided direct discussions about the inevitability of having to consider future changes. Anticipatory loss was a major concern. My therapeutic approach benefited from being mindful about the interaction of a life-threatening illness in a parent (that also affects the couple) entering later life with a highly disabling constant-course condition in a young adult and with a well sibling in early adulthood with career and relationship aspirations.

Consistent with their personal values, all family members encouraged Marybeth to pursue an independent life, rather than dedicate herself primarily to the huge task of caring for her sister. When asked about family traditions regarding caring for other family members, the parents made a clear and very useful distinction between more time-limited, less-intensive caregiving for an elder with less-disabling disorders and the lifelong commitment to caring for a sibling with massive, daily caregiving needs. Also, they were attuned to the ways Marybeth had limited some of her life choices to be available to the family through her early adulthood. Marybeth planned to remain close by to help with managing family finances, when needed, and talking with her sister's health care providers, but not to provide the daily caregiving required for Nancy and perhaps eventually for her parents.

My consultations took place in their home and had two main goals: (1) to enable both Nancy and her parents to become more involved in meaningful community activities and (2) to begin family discussions about future living and caregiving arrangements for both Nancy and her parents separately and as a family unit together.

One aspect of the conversation involved eliciting each person's version of the family narrative about Nancy's condition, situating that narrative within the broader family story, and highlighting the resilience that had sustained them in the past and could be tapped into looking ahead to the future. Our discussion included realistic plans for each family member and for the family unit. Initially, their collective fear was that any change would destabilize a precarious functional balance and worsen the situation. Hence, they had kept their thoughts to themselves and hoped that nothing "bad" would happen. My view was that change was inevitable, that not speaking openly was vitiating everyone's spirit, and that if they explored some positive options, which took into account both constraints and resources (Madsen, 2011), a new, perhaps more satisfying, life might be possible for all family members. Stan said that this perspective was very "powerful" in getting the family unstuck and moving forward positively.

A second focus of therapy was pragmatically gathering information about options for community involvement and living arrangements, further family discussion about these options, and then trying some out. The family, largely through their church, began volunteering at a soup kitchen for the homeless, at an animal rescue shelter, and at a local elementary school. With the help of several agencies, they explored group home possibilities for Nancy and assisted living options for Nancy, Marybeth, and Stan as a family unit. They networked with other families to explore the development of an intentional community for families coping with similar disabilities in an adult member. This involved reconnecting with families from Nancy's childhood who were living in similar circumstances.

The family also began to explore the possibility of relocating to another region of the state in order to be closer to Nancy's extended family. The potential for decreasing isolation through living in a nurturing community with their extended family slowly emerged as the best choice. Making this decision required extensive discussions with family members, who lacked hands-on familiarity with the myriad intensive, ongoing caregiving issues.

Like many affected families, the S. family was extremely wary of considering more institutional options, which are inadequate and often poorly resourced. They accurately perceived that current institutional funding severely limits the possibility of receiving individualized caregiving plans, and that Nancy's natural agitation about living in such a place would likely be managed with long-term use of sedating psychotropic medication. They were also fearful that an adult with a condition like cerebral palsy is often not distinguished from others with severe cognitive impairment or chronic mental illness. These outcomes are disproportionately experienced by nonaffluent families or those lacking an extended family nearby or community resources for ongoing caregiving needs. Prevention-oriented psychosocial consultations during adolescence and in the transition to adulthood could have averted some of this family's suffering by starting their life-cycle transitions process significantly earlier.

CHAPTER 12

Parental Illness and Later Life Challenges

Parental illness that occurs during the child-rearing years and the needs of aging parents present formidable challenges for families. How can we optimally support family adjustment and well-being, meaning-making, reorganizing family role functions, and disease-care management?

PARENTAL ILLNESS AND DISABILITY

Over 10 million U.S. families have at least one parent with a disability. Major parental illness significantly alters the parent–child relationship. However, along with the losses and risks incurred, opportunities for acquiring resilience abound. Children can acquire self-sufficiency and self-assuredness. Those who are privileged and otherwise protected from adversity and loss can acquire a maturity about negotiating life's challenges and relationships that is normative in lower-income families and in most parts of the world. Many such children become extraordinarily perceptive and empathic. A guiding principle of any intervention is that parents are experts about their own children, whereas our role is consultative and being a resource. This chapter's first section focuses on the impact of a parent's illness on children and adolescents.

Communication

Ill parents struggle over how much, if anything, their children should be told about their condition. Obviously, in visible disorders, such as a spinal cord injury, or when home treatments like home dialysis are noticeable, some form of explanation is unavoidable. To counteract fear and anxiety, children need to be included in conversations early on and in age-appropriate ways. Research shows that children who are given specific information and opportunities to discuss a parent's illness experience less anxiety (Osborn, 2007). Similarly, findings show that adolescents prefer detailed information near the time of diagnosis and regular updates about treatment progress and prognosis (Grabiak, Bender, & Puskar, 2007). It is valuable to ask each parent the following questions.

- When you were a child or adolescent, how did you experience communication in your own family about situations of illness, crisis, or adversity? (Circumstances that involved their parents' or grandparents' illness or a similar kind of condition are most informative.)
- In your current nuclear family, how have you communicated about prior major family crises?
- How do those experiences inform your approach to your current illness with your own children?

Because of children's developmental differences, it is useful to set aside time to discuss the illness with each child separately, even if families are accustomed to meeting and talking over important issues together. I generally advise directly naming the disease (e.g., diabetes). Euphemisms such as "having too much sugar" can be confusing and make it difficult for a child to distinguish Dad's diabetes from common childhood illnesses and from the short-term risk of eating something sweet, such as an ice cream cone. Also, an accurate description helps counteract the tendency for children to be concerned that the condition is contagious (O'Donnell, Eddy, & Rauch, 2013).

Parents need to understand that children, starting at a young age, may seek information about a parental illness from the Internet or friends through social media. Since the accuracy and relevance of information from these sources vary enormously, parents should be coached to ask their children what they know and where they received the information, and to suggest appropriate resources. Parents and children can review and discuss the content and quality of condition-related Internet sites together. Speaking with their children's teachers is also sensible to apprise them of the situation as it evolves and to be informed about illness-related questions or concerns that surface in the classroom.

Beliefs and Blocked Communication

As discussed in Chapters 8 and 11, it is vital to ask each child about his or her beliefs regarding the cause and course of a parent's condition or treatment effects, such as hair loss from chemotherapy. A small child may feel that an instance of misbehavior and frequent crying caused his mother's cancer.

An adolescent may believe that numerous, heated arguments resulted in his father's heart attack. Parents and health care providers can reassure the child or adolescent that he or she is not the cause. A "You can't think that way" reassurance is typically not sufficient.

One case dramatically illustrates how unqualified reassurance about a major illness and a failure to discuss it further can cause serious emotional problems in a child. This problem may manifest itself as symptoms that are ascribed to something completely unrelated.

Mrs. L. called the child psychiatry clinic, concerned that her daughter, Janice, age 5, had been compulsively masturbating for the past 3 months, and that this was an indication of sexual abuse. When the child assessment revealed no evidence of abuse, the therapist inquired about other recent stressful events in the family. Only at that point did the mother reveal that her husband had had most of his stomach removed 9 months earlier because of stomach cancer, and that 6 months later he had been rehospitalized for further tests that proved inconclusive. When Mrs. L. was asked what the children had been told, she reported that after her husband's surgery they had told the children only that, "Daddy had a tummy ache, so the doctors removed Daddy's stomach so he'd feel better."

The therapist then inquired whether Mrs. L. was concerned about her husband's health. She replied, "Of course, I think about it constantly!" The therapist then asked if they ever talked together about these concerns, and if they would like to come in together to discuss them, to which Mrs. L. replied, "He won't come in. After the surgery he was adamant that he did not want to ever talk about it. He went back to work almost immediately and has insisted that everything is fine."

The clinician asked Mrs. L. if she thought this medical crisis had had any impact on the children, especially Janice. Mrs. L.'s response was, "Well, she doesn't tell me about any worries. But now that you ask, at dinner every night when we say grace Janice prays out loud for Daddy's stomach." No one in the family ever commented on this.

The therapist then suggested to Mrs. L. that her daughter's compulsive behavior might be her way of expressing her worry and confusion about her father's "stomach problem." She commended Mrs. L. for her desire to respect her husband's wishes about not discussing his cancer, but felt that her daughter's behavior signaled a need for more communication in the family. She coached Mrs. L. to tell her husband that the therapist wanted to talk to both parents first so that they could decide together on the best way to keep their children informed about their father's condition. With more open communication, the daughter's symptoms resolved rapidly.

The therapist later revealed to her supervisor that she had resisted the supervisor's suggestion to include the husband because her own husband had been diagnosed with cancer 2 years earlier and had made it clear that he did not want to discuss it. This highlights the need for clinicians to be mindful of presenting problems that may represent isomorphs of past or current concerns and communication patterns in their own families (see Chapter 17).

This case demonstrates the ability of children to sense danger and the threat of loss despite secretive or nonexistent communication. Ill parents need to confront their own vulnerability and despair about the possibility of not seeing their children reach adulthood. A spouse who is unable to acknowledge his or her own fears of loss may project worry onto a child through overprotective behavior.

One must not underestimate a child's need to hear about, understand, and come to terms with adversity. Children need to know they will be secure. Blocked communication only fuels anxieties. When age-appropriate, open communication is established, parents can inform children about realistic and exaggerated fears concerning a parent's condition. Catastrophic fears and fantasies held silently are far more destructive than realistic concerns that are aired and relieved by and with parents. Children can be reassured that they will be told about any important changes in the parent's condition. This reassurance can help children concentrate better, especially at school. Also, having some knowledge about the parent's condition allows them to participate in helping the parent in some way. This includes pitching in with household chores or age-appropriate assistance of a parent, as discussed in the next section on role functioning. Children are thus encouraged to see themselves as part of the "family team," countering any feelings that they only are an added burden to stressed parents.

Parents who have gone through an emotionally and physically taxing illness phase, such as the initial diagnosis, intensive chemotherapy, or rehabilitation, may be overwhelmed and exhausted. Severe fatigue can temporarily affect their sensitivity to their children's needs. In such circumstances, parents often need to meet separately with the clinician to help them first process the experience and decide what would be most helpful to express to their children. Also, parents need professional guidance concerning any residual effects of the treatments that may alter their ability to think clearly and concentrate for a period of time (e.g., "chemo brain"). The involvement of grandparents, extended kin, or friends and community members can be vital supports at these times.

Parent Illness and Child Attachment

Although a detailed discussion regarding the development of secure attachment is beyond the scope of this book, it is important to consider how a serious illness may affect the process (Davey, Kissl, & Lynch, 2016). A major physical or mental health condition can affect parents' emotional availability and responsiveness to an infant or toddler. The type of illness and its treatments, expected course, and uncertainties can inform discussion about proactive planning that involves other adults. It is always valuable to convey that children are inherently able to form nurturing, secure attachments with more than one adult. Reassurance may be needed that toddlers can incur normative separation anxiety that is not attributable to a parent's illness or treatments.

Role Functioning

Pattern of Psychosocial Demands over Time

Information regarding a condition's psychosocial demands over time can help parents decide on whether and to what degree they need their children to help with caregiving and other family responsibilities. Flexibly alternating such role functions is greatly facilitated when the whole family understands the expected course of a disorder. In relapsing conditions, in which disability is intermittent, it is easier and less risky to assign responsibilities to older children, because the time frame of such role changes can be restricted to the duration of a flare-up. Knowing the timing of treatments and length of recovery in advance reduces ambiguity and facilitates family caregiving that may involve children. Where possible, advance planning that includes other family members or community supports can provide some structure and predictability during a period of intense medical treatments and uncertainty.

With progressive, life-threatening, and severely disabling conditions, a parent's limitations are always present and continue to increase. In these situations, it is more likely that a lasting change in role functions may occur. Conditions that involve cognitive impairment are perhaps the most difficult, because a child may witness a parent reduced to a childlike state with a loss of the essence of the prior parent–child relationship. Sometimes, as in a fatal illness such as metastatic cancer, older children may need to assume certain responsibilities gradually to buffer the transition to life without one parent.

Balancing Illness-Related Roles with Normative Child Development

The key factor in balancing illness-related roles is determining how role changes are made. Are they sensitive to issues of fairness and the competing tasks of a child's or an adolescent's development? Have parents realistically assessed the need for role reallocation? In two-parent households, have parents first considered rebalancing responsibilities between themselves? In families governed by strict and traditional gender-defined roles, a consideration of these questions may be bypassed. If a mother becomes ill, her responsibilities may be automatically transferred to the oldest daughter, without first examining how the father and sons may do their part. If a father becomes disabled and homebound, the oldest son may feel pressured to drop out of high school and find work to support the family, rather than see his mother take a job outside the home. While keeping in mind a family's cultural values, clinicians can help the parents to renegotiate traditionally defined role functions to meet the condition's demands.

When children have to assume new responsibilities, families should be encouraged to discuss issues of balance, flexibility, and shared participation. Achieving balance means that if a child needs to care for a parent, it is important for the ill parent to remain a parent to the child nonetheless. One mother with a spinal cord injury maintained her role as listener and advisor to her husband and children, despite needing extensive caregiving support from them. To the extent possible, various responsibilities should be shared equitably among family members. It is important not to single out one child as the responsible caregiver, without giving the other siblings any responsibilities. Burdens can be shared and altered flexibly as life demands on different siblings arise. Equitable sharing reduces the chance of resentment and promotes family problem solving that will maximally preserve each member's individual developmental goals. Establishing time limits for added responsibilities, especially caregiving, can counteract a child's feelings of being trapped and permanently stuck in a parental role. How well parents can model handling imbalances in their relationship is a strong predictor of children's adaptation. As such, paying attention first to the parents' relationship helps the process of involving their children go more smoothly.

Grandparents and Extended Kin

Grandparents and other extended family members who live nearby and are in good health may be available to help. The inclusion of an adult's own parents in a major caregiving role needs to be carefully considered in terms of the rebalance of power this may imply. Such a solution may be inadvisable if it causes an ill adult child to feel infantilized, overly dependent, or dominated by a historically controlling parent, who may also be seen by the spouse as an intrusive in-law. On the other hand, it may provide a second chance to form a satisfying relationship if family members can rise to the occasion. One single-parent woman, in a yearlong recovery from a serious accident, reluctantly allowed her mother to move into the household and to cook and care for her and her children. This nurturance healed old wounds the woman had from having felt neglected in favor of her brother. Often adults are surprised that relationships can change dramatically in adulthood. When families consider this option, I encourage the parents to discuss the implications separately first, and then include the grandparents and the entire family unit. One important consideration is the likely future caregiving needs of the grandparent(s) and their own existing or potential illness journeys.

Crisis and Rescue Procedures

Children should be familiar with how to perform crisis or rescue procedures in an emergency. Frequently parents do not include children in these matters out of a desire to protect them and minimize their anxiety. Often this can have the opposite effect. One 7-year-old child whose mother had diabetes was terrified that he would be caught alone with his mother when she had a hypoglycemic reaction and might die while he stood by helplessly. In fact, this child had seen his mother, in an extreme reaction accompanied by an epileptic seizure, saved by an older teenage son's intervention. The younger child needed to learn what caused hypoglycemia; how to give his mother sugary foods; how, in an emergency, to administer an injection of glucose, which alleviates severe reactions; how to protect his mother if she had a seizure; and how to dial 911 and report a medical crisis. By comparison, most children at this boy's age with diabetes give themselves injections.

Other Child-Rearing Challenges

Anticipating that they may suffer an untimely death, parents with life-threatening illnesses may push their children too quickly toward independence. Conversely, they may spoil a child from feelings of guilt that they are not being good enough parents or that they will not be alive very long. This is especially common with conditions that require much self-care, wherein the illness demands conflict with those of parenting. This may also occur when a parent's illness is hereditary and the affected parent also feels guilty because of the future suffering that his or her children may have to endure. Especially when a condition is perceived as having been caused by neglect or a victimizing experience, parents may overprotect their children out of fears that the world is an unsafe place.

Adolescents

Adolescents may experience high emotional turmoil regarding their wish to be independent and their distress regarding a parent's chronic condition and prognosis. How do the biopsychosocial needs of a parent's condition interact with a family's cultural norms? Informed by the illness type and phase, a family consultation can be a very valuable way of exploring different parental cultural values and expectations for an adolescent approaching adulthood.

Lower-Income and Single-Parent Challenges

In single-parent and lower-income households, all the challenges of parental illness are greatly magnified. A sole parent may use a child as a sounding board because there may be no one else available with whom to speak. If the parent is significantly disabled, he or she will need to rely more on the children to assume a wide range of responsibilities. In these situations, children are apt to be reluctant to burden the parent with their own needs and therefore suppress them. Family consultations can help a parent decide on the limits of appropriate sharing and boundaries that are sensitive to the actual needs of both the parent and the child.

Children fear being orphaned by losing a sole parent. Thus, it is important to assess how a noncustodial parent or members of the extended family can become supportive and potentially involved. A clinician should inquire about ex-spouses and the nature of the relationship with the ill parent and children. Often, a cordial and effective coparenting relationship exists, insuring mutual assistance. Support can go beyond rebalancing time with each parent and also include cohabiting arrangements during high-stress medical periods. In one case, an ex-spouse moved into the family home for 6 months during a mother's flare-up and recovery period from fibromyalgia. Parents may need to explain to their children that this living arrangement is temporary and not a signal that they are getting back together permanently.

If the parent's condition is life threatening, the divorced couple may need to discuss contingencies for the well parent to assume fuller custodial care of children. Depending on the circumstances, similar discussions with grandparents and extended family members may be needed. Clinical consultations can facilitate these discussions.

In lower-income households, enormous financial strains may force an older child to drop out of school and go to work just to help the family survive. One second-grader, caught stealing food at a grocery store near school during lunch hour said, "My mommy is sick and needs food, so I bring her lunch every day." In these situations, rather than reflexively label the child as "the problem" and proceed with interventions from that viewpoint, it is vital to assess the underlying stressors that may include a family's major health condition. Here, the child's behavior needs to be situated within the context not only of a family's economic survival under duress, but also within the context of the threatened loss of a parent and witnessing a parent's suffering. A lack of access to adequate and affordable health care often compounds the strain.

AGING PARENTS AND CAREGIVING

Caring for aging parents is a significant challenge for families. It is always painful to observe a parent, who was once healthy and vigorous, become frail and dependent. Conditions that cause mental deterioration (see Chapter 16) or physical pain are perhaps the most difficult to bear.

The Status of Later-Life Caregiving in America

Family caregiving for elder family members is a growing major concern. Nearly three-quarters of disabled people rely exclusively on these informal caregivers (National Alliance for Caregiving & AARP Public Policy Institute, 2015;

Qualls & Zarit, 2009). Unlike many other countries that have national health care systems, long-term care is very limited in the United States or is not provided under most existing insurance coverage. Nearly 14 million Americans require long-term care, and their numbers will continue to rise. Family medical leave provisions barely begin to address the needs of families providing ongoing caregiving. The combination of an aging population and inadequate models of health care delivery place increased, and often, unbearable stress on families.

Based on research from the National Alliance for Caregiving & AARP (2015), nearly 35 million Americans provide unpaid family caregiving for an ill or disabled adult age 50 or older each year. Eighty percent of caregivers provide help 7 days a week, averaging 4 hours per day for over 4 years. A majority of family caregivers help with medical and nursing tasks, such as monitoring vital signs and managing machinery, often with insufficient skilled caregiving education. The value of the services that family caregivers provide for "free" was estimated to be a staggering $450 billion a year, twice as much as spent on homecare and nursing home facilities (Feinberg, Reinhard, Houser, & Choula, 2011)!

Nearly two-thirds of family caregivers are employed full- or part-time and are disproportionately from lower-income families. These caregivers have to make workplace accommodations, such as cutting back hours or taking a leave of absence, or they may be subjected to warnings about workplace performance or attendance (National Alliance for Caregiving/AARP, 2015). Further, caregivers in rural areas face the unique challenges of more limited access to primary and emergency health care, accessible transportation, and supportive services (Goins, Spencer, & Byrd, 2009). Almost half of LGBT elders care for either families of choice or families of origin, while contending with their own significant health disparities (Fredriksen-Goldsen, Kim, Barkan, Muraco, & Hoy-Ellis, 2013).

The Impact of Caregiving

There are conflicting data on the impact that caregiving has on families. Much research finds that caregiving takes an increasing physical and mental health toll on family caregivers over time (National Alliance for Caregiving/AARP, 2015), including increased mortality (Schulz & Beach, 1999), anxiety and depression (especially for spouses), and compromised immune system functioning. On the other hand, recent data show that manageable levels of caregiving can have positive health and psychosocial benefits (Roth et al., 2013), such as an enhanced sense of purpose, reciprocating for the care received as children, feeling appreciated, and helping sustain the well-being and identity of the family (Coon, 2012).

Several trends in contemporary society have heightened the challenge. Because of advances in medical technology, larger numbers of adults are living into their eighties, nineties, and beyond. As life expectancy has been extended, many more people in their sixties and seventies are still dealing with aging parents. Although most older adults remain healthy until advanced old age, many others are living longer with chronic conditions that can be medically controlled. This trend means that all of us can expect to deal with aging parents for a greater proportion of our adult years.

Although only 5% of the elderly live in institutions, the vast majority of people in later life have chronic health conditions that require additional medical expenditures and family caregiving. These additional financial and caregiving burdens often become the responsibility of adult children who also have the competing demands of child rearing and financial pressures (e.g., mortgages, college tuition) to bear. Clinicians should therefore inquire whether families are simultaneously caring for young children and aging parents with chronic conditions. Moreover, intergenerational caregiving has become more complicated because of families' increased mobility and geographic distance.

Adult Children

Families function best when adult children and their parents have discussed caregiving wishes and expectations. Timely family consultations that include aging parents early in an illness allow the whole family to weigh their preferences and options together. This permits taking into account the strengths and limitations of both aging parents and adult children, who can share feelings and concerns and arrive at solutions and decisions together. A normative filial obligation includes being responsible for both financial and caregiving support of parents in later life. Like discussions about wills, funerals, or advance directives, broaching this anxiety-laden topic is too often avoided and postponed, though almost everyone has usually given it some thought. Optimally, the possibility of having to care for aging parents should be considered and openly discussed at various junctures in the family life cycle, for example, at the time a couple makes a long-term commitment and, particularly, when they embark on family planning; when children leave home; or upon retirement. There are useful family-oriented guides for caregivers of aging family members (Jacobs & Mayer, 2016) and for clinicians who work with these families (Jacobs, 2006; Qualls & Williams, 2013).

When an elderly parent suffers neurocognitive impairment or dementia, physical caregiving responsibilities are compounded because the parent loses executive function capability and becomes increasingly frail and dependent. See Chapter 16 for a detailed discussion.

Intergenerational Patterns of Caregiving

Multigenerational patterns of caregiving are important. They provide insight into how loyalty is defined and shape how adults think about their own family. After my mother had a stroke, I became keenly aware, for the first time, that my parents could become ill and die, and that I was unsure about what caregiving they expected of me. My own grandmother had lived with my family until her heart disease worsened and she moved to a nursing home; this happened when I was an infant. Growing up, I began to realize that this arrangement had been complicated. I wondered whether it forced my mother to make a choice between caring for her mother and caring for me. I also wondered whether my father had felt that my mother's devotion to her mother and an infant left her with too little time to give him attention. Only when my mother had a life-threatening illness when I was a young adult did I ask questions about my past and what would be expected of me. On the basis of their past experience with my grandmother, both my parents strongly preferred an assisted living residence or a nursing home rather than moving in and "burdening" me or my brother and our families. Our discussion clarified family stories about caregiving for aged family members in previous generations and informed me about family preferences and expectations. It also brought my parents into a larger group conversation with my brother and sister-in-law and my nuclear family.

My personal experience rebuts a common myth that older parents never discuss such morbid issues. Often adult children mistakenly feel that they need to protect their parents from having this dialogue. Protecting them often fosters an unnecessary role reversal in which aging parents are viewed and treated as children by their own adult children. This prevents frankly discussing what the parents would want under different circumstances and creates anxieties and ambiguities. The reverse situation, where parents do not share their own decisions with adult children because they don't want to burden them, also can happen. They may also have difficulty acknowledging an inevitable transfer of responsibilities to the next generation. Either way, when such myths are challenged, an open dialogue between the generations is facilitated and a more balanced sharing of role functions occurs.

Involvement of Children and Adolescents

Family traditions concerning the involvement of children and adolescents in caregiving functions are important to acknowledge. In many families in which a parent needs to provide care for a grandparent, an older child, often a daughter, may be expected to keep the family from becoming overloaded by tending to younger siblings. She may quietly accept this responsibility without resentment, following a tradition of self-sacrifice for the collective well-being of the extended family. Clinicians need to question an arrangement in which family well-being comes at the expense of any family member or group, such as women.

For many children, witnessing an ill and aging grandparent is their first encounter with chronic illness, disability, and death. Eliciting memories of those experiences can help adults recall the impact on the family and the roles played by grandparents, parents, their siblings, and themselves during their own childhoods. Recalling past caregiving experiences can guide decision making about aspects of the experience they wish to preserve or do differently.

It is important to gather information from each side of the family, which can clarify differences in cultural norms or illnesses that required diverse kinds of caregiving. This inquiry lays the groundwork for collaboration and mutual accommodation.

Cultural Values and Traditions

Asking families about their cultural and ethnic caregiving traditions can reveal important insights. For instance, Latino and Italian American families traditionally have strong intergenerational ties to families of origin, in which caregiver well-being is secondary and often sacrificed for the sake of the ill member. In many Italian American neighborhoods, multiple-story homes are often built to accommodate three or four generations. Houses are often designed with an understanding that aging parents will be attended to by the younger generation in the same home. African American and Latino families may not live in the same household, but a rich and extensive network of shared responsibilities among immediate and extended kin effectively addresses the needs of aging parents. Family members may take turns phoning, visiting, or running errands for older adults. In both cultures, there is a strong reliance on family caregiving that is home based.

An awareness of ethnic and multigenerational traditions helps clinicians distinguish normative from dysfunctional patterns of caregiving. The United States is a very individualistic, youth-oriented society that often devalues older generations, but it is a myth that Americans do not care for their elders and dump them in nursing homes (Walsh, 2016a). Still, American culture differs from that of some other countries, such as Mexico, which has a reverence for and devotion to elders. Understanding cultural beliefs is essential for intervening skillfully. Attunement to the likely physical and psychosocial demands of a disorder over time clarifies the fit between a family's cultural values and the realities of the condition. Reinforcing adaptive cultural norms facilitates addressing those that may need to be further discussed by patients, families, and providers collaboratively, and adjusted over time.

Immigrant Families

In immigrant families, sharp differences regarding role expectations can emerge between the generations. The strains are more pronounced between older immigrants, who have more traditional values based on their cultures of origin, and the younger generation raised in the United States. For example, traditional East Asian families value harmony, filial piety, and treating elders with honor and respect. Cultural clashes occur when the younger generation departs from those norms. The need for family caregiving can amplify such differences and precipitate a crisis. Family consultations can address these normative changes, helping them achieve new mutual understandings that incorporate multiple cultural viewpoints (Lee & Mjelde-Mossey, 2004).

Gender and Caregiving

Women still provide approximately 60% of caregiving to older family members and friends (National Alliance for Caregiving/AARP report, 2015). Female caregivers spend 50% more time in caregiving than male caregivers do. Often, these are women at midlife who are working and still raising children. Many women will spend more time caring for an elderly parent than raising children.

Traditionally, women have been responsible for caring not only for their own parents, but also for the parents of their husbands. This longstanding role of women has become more complicated because of the increasing proportion of women in the workforce. There has not been a commensurate change in our expectation that women will be responsible for both child rearing and caring for infirm parents. Women in the child-rearing phase of life often are expected to handle up to three full-time jobs: paid employment, rearing children, and caring for their own and their husbands' aging parents. Problems caused by overload are inevitable, unless men share these responsibilities more equitably.

Providers can help families examine socialized patterns in which men are to be protected from pragmatic and emotional strains. Often an understanding has developed in families, particularly between mothers and daughters, that men cannot be relied upon or that they are incapable of nurturing. On the other hand, men may feel disproportionately strained by all the financial burdens they are expected to bear. There is a tacit agreement that if the father becomes ill, the daughter will help the mother, and that if the mother becomes ill, the daughter will tend to her and then take care of the father if he is left alone.

Women often present for treatment of anxiety, depression, or physical symptoms when their spouses' parents become seriously ill. This is most apt to occur when the husband has no female siblings and expectations concerning caregiving fall on the daughters-in-law. When this happens, it is important to convene both the husband and wife to initiate a dialogue. Ask couples how they decide about caregiving roles and about gender patterns in each person's family of origin. Rigid, gender-defined rules may need to be revised to avoid overloading one spouse and causing resentment and the deterioration of a marital relationship. Similarly, if a woman is drawn into imbalanced caregiving for her own parents, it is a useful strategy to convene other siblings for the purpose of discussing a shared responsibility for the ill or disabled parents.

Challenging Situations

Shifting Autonomy and Control to Caregivers

In many cases, adult children have to challenge a parent's judgment and take control of risky behavior. In our mobile society, driving a car is a symbol of independence and freedom. Older adults, especially men, often refuse to give up driving, even with seriously impaired vision, reflexes, and judgment, and may be unwilling to admit the danger. In one family, the sons had to take away the father's keys, only to find out that he had driven again using another set of keys hidden away. Next, they removed the car's battery; the crafty father called a service station to install a new one. With caring firmness and humor, rather than angrily rebuking him, they told the father that they appreciated his cleverness, while affirming their need to take further precautions. Regardless, having to give up driving can be a major loss, especially outside urban areas, where public transportation or community transport services are often insufficient. Forethought and planning for alternative means of transportation can help lessen the emotional difficulties related to this loss.

Giving an adult child the power of attorney over a parent's health care issues and personal property involves a loss of self-determination. Even in families that have made these arrangements in writing, the actual process of witnessing an infirm member relinquishing control can be far more difficult and emotionally wrenching. Since the ill member may disagree with the need to transfer control, fostering consensus and mutual support among all the adult children and their spouses can be enormously beneficial to the adult child who has legal authority.

The primary care provider and health care team can be immensely helpful at times when a family understands the need for a fundamental change, but the frail member feels that he or she can still manage a household, driving a car, and other daily activities. My father lived independently until 97, when cognitive impairment and general frailty made it impossible, even though he thought he was doing well. As safety concerns mounted, my brother and I apprised the physician, who suggested that one of us attend his next checkup. After the examination and some discussion, the physician gently but firmly suggested three options to my father—move to live with my brother or me (both of us lived at a distance), arrange for 24-hour care coverage in his home, or move to the local assisted living facility. After some follow-up conversations with other members of the family, my father decided to move to the local assisted living facility 2 days later. My father's respect for both the physician's expertise and neutrality were essential to the process.

As in my personal situation, the geographic distance between sons and daughters and their parents can be an issue when aging parents can no longer manage by themselves. Moving to another region of the country, or even 30 minutes away, can result in an elder losing longstanding friendships and community connections. The elder family member can feel isolated, and a son or daughter can experience an increased strain because they become the parent's primary social connection. Social media technology, such as Skype, can be tremendously useful in helping with these challenges.

The psychosocial typology and illness time-phases framework can facilitate family deliberation about these issues. If an aging parent has a condition that is progressive like dementia, increasingly disabling, such as arthritis, or can involve a sudden worsening, as in stroke, it can be beneficial to begin the process of finding a new living arrangement before a crisis develops. As discussed in Chapter 16, if the condition can cause growing cognitive impairment, including the affected family member as an active participant in these discussions early on helps prevent later conflict among family members.

Families with Young Children

A couple who has young children at the time a parent's health declines is particularly challenging. With increased life expectancy, this is common among people who have postponed childbearing or who have children in a remarriage. Just when their own family life cycle demands a focus inward on the intense demands of child rearing, a parent's decline from a disorder such as Alzheimer's disease may require extensive involvement with an increasingly dependent and childlike parent. The course of a progressive, dementing illness with a 4-to-5-year prognosis conflicts with child-rearing demands that will probably continue beyond the illness. Proactive family consultations that address the issue of likely unavoidable limits promotes planful strategies.

Pragmatic solutions may include home-based professional care, nursing home placement, or sharing caregiver responsibilities among siblings and other extended family members. Acknowledging the limits to caring for one's own parents or giving a higher priority to one's own nuclear family can present an excruciating conflict of loyalties. Although parents have borne the responsibility of rearing their children through to adulthood, it may not be possible for their adult children to care as extensively for them until their death. Almost certainly, the expectation is unrealistic if the responsibilities are loaded onto one designated caregiver. It may be more feasible, however, if all the adult siblings discuss and plan together how each of them can share the burden according to their abilities and limits.

The fantasy of being able to repay parents in this way (Boszormenyi-Nagy & Sparks, 1984/2013) needs to be tempered by the reality that certain types of disorders may entail psychosocial demands that are incompatible with home-based care or other life-cycle demands, such as child rearing. Beliefs about what constitutes sufficient loyalty need to be addressed as part of a process of defining limits. Otherwise, any choice will risk arousing feelings of shame and guilt that may later find expression in interminable grief or self-destructive behaviors.

Sometimes, family strains involving an aging parent remain hidden behind complaints or symptoms elsewhere in the system. A presenting problem is defined as one focused on a child or adolescent, when in fact an aging parent may be the central issue. Regardless of the presenting issue, inquiring about grandparents or aging parents is always useful, as in the following case.

Ms. H., a single parent with a full-time job, contacted the outpatient psychiatric clinic complaining that her 10-year-old son, Jim, was refusing to go to school and was difficult to control at home. The initial family consultation revealed that her son's problems had begun 6 months earlier when Ms. H.'s aging mother with advanced Parkinson's disease had moved in. Jim acknowledged that he frequently cut school and spent all day in his room, which was next to his grandmother's. Ms. H. tearfully described the burden of tending to her mother's advancing disease, which required around-the-clock attention. She felt especially anxious since her mother had developed serious balance problems and had fallen several times. Ms. H. worried that something terrible would happen to her mother while she was at work, and felt helpless about not being there to assist. In this case, it became increasingly clear that Jim's truancy was intended to fill the gap at home and to alleviate the limited caretaking resources available for the grandmother.

Family Enmeshment

Difficulties may also arise when there has been a history of enmeshment. An adult may have struggled during adolescence and early adulthood to become extricated from a dysfunctional family. Such an adult child may feel a tenuous hold on his or her own autonomy and independence. The onset of a parent's disabling or life-threatening chronic disorder that requires caregiving can rekindle powerful fears of becoming reentangled in the family web.

With this kind of family dysfunction, the aging parent may elicit guilt by communicating feelings of abandonment or betrayal by an adult child. Adult children and their spouses often experience increased marital tensions as a result. Intense conflict, characterized by mutual blame and guilt, can ensue between an adult child and aging parents. Sometimes the conflict can escalate into physically and verbally abusive behavior around caregiving interactions. Clinicians need to be mindful that any intervention with these families may be very difficult because of their entrenched protective patterns and suspicious views of outsiders.

Clinicians need to distinguish long-standing dysfunctional patterns from common situations in which overdependence has been fostered. Adult children may express fears associated with anticipatory loss by hovering over

Parental Illness and Later Life Challenges 237

an aging parent and taking away role functions the parent is still capable of handling. Often this coincides with the parents' own anxieties. This is most common in life-threatening conditions, particularly ones, such as strokes, that started with a serious health crisis followed by disability and the need for intensive care. Because of the fear and uncertainty surrounding a fatal recurrence, crisis-phase needs can easily become permanent unless professionals confer with the family about changing risks or caregiving needs. Proactive family consultations, timed with the transition to the chronic phase, can help prevent escalating caregiver responsibility that can lead to vicious cycles of helplessness, exhaustion, and resentment.

In some situations adult children assume polarized and extreme positions when an aging parent becomes ill. The following case poignantly demonstrates these tendencies.

Mrs. L., a 70-year-old widow, was hospitalized with multiple somatic problems exacerbated by symptoms of early dementia. She had two sons, Herb, age 44, and Tom, age 41. The sons reluctantly agreed to come in for a family interview. On the phone, Herb stated that, in his opinion, the hospitalization was merely a ploy for sympathy on his mother's part, an attempt to make him feel guilty for not being at her beck and call as Tom was. He said he had learned years ago that the best relationship with her was no relationship at all. In contrast, Tom, who had always been devoted to his mother since adolescence, had become increasingly responsible for her caregiving needs, particularly since her cognitive impairment had worsened. Yet the more helpful he became, the more dependent and helpless she became in managing her own life. At the point of hospitalization, Tom felt drained by his mother's growing neediness.

This case required two stages of therapeutic work. First, the overly responsible son was coached that he could be more helpful by challenging his mother to do more for herself. Herb, who was underinvolved, was asked to help his brother by taking on several specific, limited, caregiving tasks. Both sons were coached to communicate with each other and directly with their mother. They were warned that their mother might initially resist these changes and that they would have to be patient and understanding. Mrs. L., seeing her sons cooperating, began to show significantly improved functioning.

The second phase of treatment involved a conjoint family life review technique (see Chapter 8; Walsh, 2016a). This approach incorporates multiple perspectives of shared experiences that enlarge the family narrative and promotes empathy and healing of unresolved family members' wounds. In this case, using family albums and scrapbooks as a stimulus to elicit crucial memories, Mrs. L. and her sons were helped to explore and better understand emotionally laden and unresolved developmental periods in family life that were being reenacted as the mother's health had deteriorated. For instance, Herb and Tom's longstanding sibling rivalry was discussed and placed in better perspective.

Herb's rejection of his family became better understood once he recalled that during his adolescence, as the oldest son, he had felt terribly burdened by having to help his mother take care of his father, who suffered from emphysema caused by chronic smoking. He had had an intense conflict with his mother, which he handled by leaving home angrily, severing contact, and vowing to protect himself by remaining self-reliant and avoiding entangling commitments. His relationship with his parents, which had become frozen in his early adult transition, could now finally be discussed. His brother, Tom, had become the good son who inherited Herb's job, faithfully helping his mother with caregiving tasks until his father's death, and then watching over his widowed mother.

Both Herb and Tom had remained single—Herb, because of fears of any relationship commitments, and Tom, because of his ongoing caregiving obligations to his mother. Everyone's anger finally was aired at the father for smoking himself to death, without considering the impact of his serious illness on the rest of the family. Also, they all revealed having feelings of guilt that they might have been able to stop him. Herb and his mother were able to see that their conflict largely represented displacement of feelings that were not expressed directly to the father. Family therapy facilitated mourning together the loss of the father in the context of better understanding, reconciliation, and renewed caring among the surviving family members.

The Last Parent

When there is only one surviving aging parent, there is additional strain on adult children. Without counting on the likelihood of mutual support between two aging parents, it can feel harder for adult children to set limits on providing companionship, as well as caregiving. This situation touches on a powerful fear with which we can all empathize—that of dying alone or in an institution without the presence of family members.

The terminal phase of a last parent's illness can be particularly emotional for adult children. It signifies the impending death of the last member of the older generation, moving adult children for the first time into the senior position and making them the next to face the issues of aging and their own mortality. This heightened awareness may cause symptoms of anxiety or depression or a sudden preoccupation about one's own health and mortality. Such concerns may find expression in the adult child's marital relationship in distancing actions or increased dependency needs.

With greater longevity, many adults begin to deal with aging parents when they themselves are past the child-rearing phase. Although they are less encumbered by the conflicting demands of raising children, they may have their own health problems and reduced financial resources if they are retired. One man's own disability related to heart disease limited his capacity to help his aging mother, who had developed severe rheumatoid arthritis. Also, people whose own children are now adults may have planned for a golden period of greater leisure and independence from the heavy demands of early adulthood. An ill older parent can present an obstacle to such longstanding plans and become a source of resentment.

Professional Caregiving, Assisted Living, and Skilled-Facility Placement Planning

With improved medical care extending life and family members' living at a geographic distance, complex issues related to institutionalizing an aging parent surface. The need for assisted living and extended care has grown substantially. As a result, new possibilities for living arrangements and community involvement are being created (Aldwin & Igarashi, 2012).

To reduce family burdens, clinicians can help orient families to the greater range of options and community services that may obviate the need for nursing-home placement. Often families are unaware of home- and community-based services, such as supervised apartment programs with medical backup, assisted living options, adult day care, senior citizens programs, care from a visiting nurse, and respite care, all of which can help maintain aging parents in their homes and communities. It is valuable to distinguish among the need for professional assistance with cleaning, meals, and shopping, the need for routine caregiving that involves help with dressing, and bathing, and the need for skilled nursing care. Clarifying what is most appropriate is best achieved in collaboration with the aging member's primary physician or specialty care providers. Consideration of the course of chronic conditions over time facilitates a longitudinal and proactive planning strategy. Informing families about and promoting linkages to these various community supports can be empowering, instill a greater sense of hope, and counteract feelings of fear and helplessness. Access to services, any insurance coverage, and out-of-pocket financial costs are naturally of great concern to most families and must be taken into account.

Attunement to cultural values is paramount. For Asian Americans, caring for an aging member at home is an ethical responsibility, consistent with cultural values that emphasize the family unit, obedience to parents, respect for elders, privacy, and self-sufficiency. Placement in a facility can be seen as a failure to adhere to the value placed on filial obligation. An emphasis on privacy could hinder professional caregivers from coming to the home. Finding solutions that respect such values is crucial to family well-being and effective collaboration.

Exploring options and family expectations is particularly helpful to adult daughters, whose disproportionate responsibility for caregiving can leave them most vulnerable to blame and guilt when the specter of in-home caregiving services or placement arises. One woman with a demanding professional career and young children had to shuttle back and forth across the country to arrange simultaneously for her mother's nursing home placement and for her father's hospitalization and then funeral. Having a supportive spouse who could flexibly step in and assume greater childcare responsibilities and support his wife was essential to coping with the various family demands.

CHAPTER 13

Intimacy Issues for Couples

One of the most important marriage vows we make requires us to care for a partner "in sickness and in health," yet most of us celebrating a wedding have little idea what life together with an illness would mean. Chronic disorders can have devastating consequences for couples. To master the challenges, they must maintain a viable, balanced relationship while caring for an ill partner and coping with the uncertainties of planning and achieving normative lifecycle goals despite the threat of loss. A partner's serious condition powerfully challenges couples' relationship rules and boundaries. Studies have supported the use of couples and partner-focused treatments (Coyne, Rohrbaugh, Shoham, Sonnega, & Nicklas, 2001; Kuijer, Buunk, de Jong, Ybema, & Sanderman, 2004; Northouse, Kershaw, Mood, & Schafenacker, 2005; Northouse et al., 2007; Scott, Halford, & Ward, 2004; Shields et al., 2012). Further, research has shown that marital quality is associated with the health status and outcomes of both the ill person and the well partner across a wide spectrum of chronic disorders (Jaremka, Derry, & Kiecolt-Glaser, 2014; Kiecolt-Glaser & Newton, 2001; Martire et al., 2010; Traa, De Vries, Bodenmann, & Den Oudsten, 2015). There are, however, documented risks. For instance, elderly spousal caregivers with a history of chronic illness themselves, who are experiencing caregiver-related stress, have a 63% higher mortality rate than noncaregiving peers (Schulz & Beach, 1999). However, there is recent evidence that relational growth and physical well-being often occurs in the context of serious illness and caregiving (Kunzler, Nussbeck, Moser, Bodenmann, & Kayser, 2014; Roth et al., 2013).

In this chapter and in Chapter 14, the FSI model is used as a basis for a discussion of the typical issues couples have regarding intimacy, sexuality, communication, gender roles, coparenting, and relationship imbalances.

CONJOINT AND INDIVIDUAL SESSIONS

Intervention with affected couples benefits from a flexible integration of individual and conjoint sessions. Because patterns of secrecy and mutual protection are so common, as part of an initial assessment, I routinely meet with the couple separately and together. By doing this I can develop a better sense of the issues that can be openly shared and those that are closely guarded. Secret thoughts, feelings, and behaviors that are laden with shame, such as wishes to die or to leave the relationship or an ongoing clandestine affair, often need to be shared privately first with a neutral person. This needs to be done within a systemic framework.

Individual sessions allow thinking about which issues are best shared or kept private. A spouse may feel guilty about a brief affair; yet it may be unnecessary, even cruel, to divulge the affair to the partner. And if sharing it is warranted, a private consultation can help a partner do it sensitively. In one case a brief affair occurred when a woman was feeling overwhelmed and unappreciated as a caregiver for her husband, who suffered from heart disease. Her anger about his lack of nurturance was more significant than the affair. Several individual sessions helped reduce her guilt and her potential to be destructively angry with her self-absorbed husband. What was needed most was for her to express her needs and renegotiate the marital contract toward greater balance when conjoint sessions resumed.

In another situation, a woman experienced intense shame concerning her previously "perfect" husband's speech impediment that resulted from an accident. The husband's acceptance of his disability only heightened her sense of shame and prevented her from even mentioning her feelings, despite the fact that her ability to be close to her husband had been seriously affected. Individual sessions allowed her to express her feelings fully, to be assured that they were normal, and to then discuss them with her husband.

Combined individual and conjoint sessions are often useful when a couple enters a new illness phase. For instance, one couple dealing with the husband's terminal cancer needed conjoint sessions to bring closure on relationship issues and make plans for the funeral. At the same time, the husband required time alone to process personal feelings related to making peace with his own life, and his wife needed time to plan for a future without her husband (see Chapter 10). In terms of therapeutic process, it was important for the couple to be able to say to each other what they needed to discuss separately and why.

During medical crises or advanced stages of a disease, each partner may need to operate in different worlds. This need may impose severe limits on what a couple can realistically offer one another, particularly when the ill member is cognitively impaired or severely debilitated following major surgery, for instance. A conjoint meeting in which couples acknowledge these limits may be helpful. Also, individual consultation can offer support to the well partner.

INTIMACY IN ILLNESS AND DISABILITY

Couples' intimacy functions within a comfort zone that evolves over their life cycle. Their relationship processes determine whether this comfort zone allows intimacy to grow with the seasons of life or to become constricted and erode. Like other life challenges, illness and disability offer an opportunity for relationship growth and pose the risk of deterioration.

Illness onset forcefully challenges the emotional and physical boundaries of a couple's relationship. The condition is an "uninvited guest" that must be incorporated into the couple's lives. Its psychosocial type determines the nature and demands of this "intruder" and how it will develop and make its presence felt over time. A severe disability, such as a spinal cord injury, always has an effect on a relationship. A relapsing condition (e.g., disc disease) does so intermittently. Cancers in remission may not require daily caregiving, but the undercurrent of threatened loss can nonetheless permeate the couples' lives.

How Is Couples' Intimacy Defined?

Intimacy may have varied meanings for different couples and each partner, depending on factors such as gender, culture, race, social class, and phase of the individual and couple's life cycle. For instance, in middle-class U.S. culture, intimacy is often framed in terms of sharing feelings, interests, and a friendship. For a working-class couple, however, it may have more to do with helping each other survive economically, sharing responsibilities, and protecting each other. It is important to bear in mind that intimacy may be qualitatively distinct in different aspects of a relationship, such as the sexual, the spiritual, the intellectual, and the recreational.

Different attributes of intimacy help guide discussion. Each partner needs to be able to maintain some autonomy, with clear individual boundaries, while bringing "the self" into the relationship (Bowen, 1993). Wynne and Wynne (1986) emphasized both partners' ability to reveal themselves in verbal and nonverbal ways, trusting that the other person will be understanding and not betray that trust. Manne and Badr (2008) describe their relationship intimacy model as it relates to illness as involving *reciprocal self-disclosure* of concerns and feelings about the disorder intertwined with *partner responsiveness*, which is defined as feeling understood, cared for, and accepted by one's partner. Another useful concept is *relationship engagement*, which means viewing the disorder in relationship terms and engaging in behaviors intended to sustain or enhance the relationship (Manne & Badr, 2008). This includes an awareness of the challenges posed by an illness and a willingness to discuss these issues; a readiness to address aspects of the relationship that either have changed or need to change (e.g., relationship priorities or roles); and efforts to sustain the preexisting noncaregiving aspects of the relationship.

Weingarten (1991, 2013) describes how each partner needs access to areas of concern or interest of the other partner in order for them to participate in creating meaning together. With chronic conditions, "Moments of intimacy—that is, moments of shared understanding of each other's experience—are the goal, not sharing the same experience at the same time" (Weingarten, 2013, p. 97).

Intimacy When Facing Illness and Loss

"There is no love without loss" (Lifton, 1975, p. vii). All of us must grapple with the fact of our own mortality and the realization that intimacy occurs in the face of eventual loss. Serious conditions confront both partners with a powerful reminder of these existential challenges. When we are young and in good health, we tend to minimize this reality. Our cultural avoidance of these basic facts promotes patterns of intimacy based on a denial of illness and loss, relegating them to later life and hoping for a peaceful death (see Chapter 9; Becker, 1973).

Healthy coping with and adaptation to chronic disorders depend largely on a couple's willingness to address these basic issues of love, loss, and death. The diagnosis of a serious condition can heighten feelings of terror associated with loss, such that couples either draw away from or cling to each other. A prime reason for distancing is that the relationship can become a constant reminder of the universality of loss. Being a caregiver, receiving care, or observing the visible signs of illness or emotional strain can become powerful reminders of loss. Yet, it offers an opportunity to face the truth that all of us are mortal. Couples adapt best when they can harness consciousness of these facts of life in an empowering manner so as to live more fully in the present rather than impose constraints on their relationship. They can enjoy what they have now despite the imperfections, rather than postpone fulfillment based on an illusion of infinite time. Whenever I hear someone say, "I know I need to talk to him before he dies," I think, "If not now, when?"

Symptoms of chronic illness or pain fundamentally change the way in which individuals relate to themselves and those closest to them. Learning to live with limitations or a shortened life expectancy is humbling. Couples have an opportunity to reconsider what is really important versus what is trivial. For instance, when a condition may compromise sexual relations, couples generally adapt better if they can experience greater companionship. Couples in later life often make this change naturally. When younger couples can see that possibility not as a sign of old age but as the natural maturing of a good relationship, then they can explore new and deeper ways of sharing, not as a consolation prize, but as something most younger people do not learn to appreciate until later.

Competitive strivings between partners can diminish as a couple sees rivalries as wasted energy that detracts from enjoying each other. One 35-year-old man disabled by a construction accident felt a tremendous sense of relief when he really accepted his limitations. On one occasion he exclaimed, "For the first time in my life, I'm letting myself enjoy my wife and family without turning everything into pressured competition. I fought it like hell for a while, but I just couldn't make my body do what I wanted it to. When I finally could let go, I became a different person. I noticed possibilities I was blind to before. It may sound odd, but I feel healthier now than I did before my accident."

My Versus Our Shared Challenge

Seeing the challenge of illness or disability from a shared "we" perspective is fundamental (Badr & Acitelli, 2005; Kayser, Watson, & Andrade, 2007; Rohrbaugh, Shoham, Skoyen, Jensen, & Mehl, 2012; Rolland, 1994b; Skerrett, 2003). Couples who engage in conjoint coping, exemplified by the use of the word "we" or "our" to describe an illness and its challenges, experienced less psychological distress. Affirming a "we" perspective is perhaps the greatest preventive measure for all the other relationship imbalances described in Chapter 14.

When illness strikes, defining the problem as the exclusive domain of the patient will inevitably distort a couple's relationship. Focus on the highly technical and medical aspects of the patient's condition around the initial diagnosis and crisis phase promotes framing the problem as the ill partner's. Optimal couples' functioning depends largely on the willingness of both partners to challenge this fundamental assumption.

Facing and accepting loss should not be limited to the ill partner. It has never been limited to one partner and never will be. For any disability, the immediacy of loss may be heightened for the ill partner, but the well spouse faces many of the same dilemmas. There is no guarantee that the well spouse may not die first; no one can know or choose the moment of death. A health crisis provides an opportunity for couples to face this truth. Paradoxically, a serious illness in which one partner is more physically vulnerable challenges this basic assumption. If the illness-framing event is defined strictly as "my disorder and my problem," it places the illness within the patient, thereby skewing all the couple's interactions and promoting an unequal relationship. This enables the affected partner to exert power and control in the role of the sick person. Negotiating issues of power and control can become increasingly dysfunctional and lead to resentment, guilt, distancing, and a general erosion of intimacy.

One woman described how her relationship with her husband, who had had ALS, a serious, degenerative, neurological disorder, became more distant over the years. Finally, a marital crisis forced them to reconsider the basic beliefs that had been tacitly agreed upon in the initial crisis phase. She said, "We never really acknowledged the fact that Bill had a terminal illness. We never talked about the fact that I would die someday too, maybe before him. Because we never discussed these key issues, our relationship became hopelessly unbalanced. He felt entitled, and I felt it was my role to satisfy his needs. Only when our relationship came to the brink of collapse did we deal with these assumptions, which had guided our behavior for so many years. We needed to contemplate death together to reestablish our intimacy. Our last year together was our closest. So many problems could have been avoided if only someone had guided us early on." After their marital crisis, they asked her husband's neurologist why he had never urged them to talk about the life-threatening aspect of his condition. His forthright response was, "It was just too painful for me."

Couples are empowered when the condition is framed as a shared relationship issue. Then the psychosocial impact is defined in terms that acknowledge the physical and psychosocial burdens and include the illness-related roles of both partners—patient and caregiver. Reframing the issue also helps counteract the dangers of triangulation discussed later, where the disorder may be used as an "ally" by either spouse against the other regarding issues of control, entitlement, or sacrifice.

By introducing this concept of "our shared challenge" early on, clinicians provide an opportunity for couples to examine cultural and multigenerational beliefs about the rights and privileges of ill and well partners. In one situation, a well spouse grew up in a family in which she saw her mother care for her father, who suffered from emphysema, a progressive chronic respiratory disease, and never asked anything from him in return. She and her sisters were instructed not to bother their father with their needs. For this woman, powerful multigenerational beliefs and rules dictated extreme gender-based role relations in which the burden on a daughter of caring for an ill father or husband was never acknowledged. Chronic illness belonged to the husband or father, and female family members adjusted to that fact. The psychosocial experience of all family members was clearly subordinated to the biological condition of the father.

Communication

A long-term health condition and threatened loss present powerful challenges to a couple's communication skills. Research shows that supportive communication is correlated with positive health outcomes and negative communication with poorer outcomes in chronically ill persons (Fekete, Stephens, Mickelson, & Druley, 2007) and that problematic critical and controlling communications increased over time (Martire et al., 2010). Attempts to avoid a discussion of topics or concerns were associated with increased distress for both partners. Despite research that supports mutual sharing, couples coping with illness or disability often develop constrained communication in the mistaken desire to "protect" a loved one (Penn, 2001; Weingarten, 2013). This avoidance of issues that may cause the patient distress has been called "protective buffering."

Weingarten (2013) highlights asymmetric acknowledgement of loss by the ill and well partners as a problematic and significant source of conflict in couples. At the same time, she poignantly highlights the shared sorrow so common in couples coping with chronic disorders, whether acknowledged or not (Weingarten, 2012). While sorrow remains present to some degree, sharing it may reduce loneliness and isolation. Clinicians need to listen to and facilitate this shared experience of sorrow, while promoting what she describes as reasonable hope (Weingarten, 2010). Maintaining hope is essential. This may involve exploring ways to enjoy life despite the uncertainty about the course or outcome and to live and love well for as long as possible within the constraints of the condition.

Throughout this book, I have emphasized culturally sensitive, age-appropriate, open, and direct communication among family members living with chronic disorders. The couple's comfort zone and patterns regarding openness will affect the functioning of rest of the family system. Levels of personal disclosure that may have been functional before a disorder often become inadequate; discussions about living with threatened loss may represent new territory. My experience has been that couples and families with health care provider support are generally open to developing new patterns and areas of communicating.

Important issues that couples ought to discuss include the following:

- Understanding the illness and its psychosocial demands over time
- Beliefs about who or what caused the disorder and what can affect its course
- How to live with uncertainty and threatened loss
- Personal and relationship priorities
- The roles of patient and caregiver
- How to maintain a balanced, mutual relationship
- Living wills and advance directives concerning a possible terminal phase

One couple facing the husband's terminal cancer found the quality of their relationship enormously enhanced by early discussions about limiting life-saving efforts in the terminal phase. It gave the husband a sense of control over his death that reduced unbearable uncertainties and enabled him to focus his energies on living. It reduced his wife's fears about having to make life-and-death decisions without knowing his true feelings. To foster a balanced position, I always suggest that both partners discuss their desires, such as about treatment in the terminal phase, and draw up a living will. While acknowledging the immediacy of the ill partner's situation, I try to minimize differences between the two partners along with the illusion that loss is a concern of the patient alone.

As part of my consultative work with couples, I propose that each partner make two lists of illness-related topics: (1) a list of topics that he or she would like to discuss, but believes the partner would not, and (2) a list of topics he or she thinks should be off limits and why. In the second step, the partners share their lists with each other either alone or in a consultation session. Typically, to their pleasant surprise, they discover a significant overlap in what they want to discuss. This exercise facilitates the next step of choosing specific previously restricted areas to discuss. Common reasons for keeping to oneself include tentativeness about exploring new territory, concerns about hurting the partner or worsening the condition, and fears that the relationship will not survive being open with each other in certain areas. If certain topics are going to be restricted, couples should consider the consequences and reach a mutual decision (Imber-Black, 2014). Paradoxically, this process of defining taboo topics often helps dispel myths about acceptable limits. Multiple couple discussion groups, such as the MS Resilient Partners Program described in Chapter 4, provide a multiplier and normalizing effect. Couples hear that other couples struggle with the same challenges, some of who have problem-solved and overcome communication obstacles in healthful and relationship-enhancing ways. Support and encouragement from "fellow traveler" couples can't be overemphasized.

Couples need to appreciate that each partner may need to discuss important illness-related concerns at different times. This is often problematic because the partner who needs to talk may be intruding on the other's period of mental respite, when painful conversations are purposely avoided. Slipping into stereotypes of "worrier" and "spoiler" and cycles of the pursuer–distancer dynamic are minimized when both partners can share responsibility for initiating such discussions. Helping couples establish a planned time and structured process for talking about these serious matters often alleviates struggles for control about communication (see Chapter 14).

As is true for relationships in general, not all thoughts need to be communicated. A functional balance is necessary. However, many couples seek help at later stages with issues connected to areas of communication that have been completely stifled or avoided since the beginning of the disorder. Some of the most common include relationship imbalances, well-partner suffering, and discussions about death and dying.

Sometimes it may be functional for a well partner not to share a pessimistic belief concerning the anticipated outcome. In one situation, the husband, Paul, was fighting metastatic cancer. Although the physician had given the couple a 1-to-2-year prognosis, Paul maintained a belief that he could beat cancer. His wife, Betsy, believed he would likely die from it; but she confessed,

"I never wanted to interfere with Paul's goal, so I kept my feelings that he was going to die to myself or discussed them only with close friends. When Paul became terminally ill and needed to accept the inevitable, we talked more openly." In situations like these, I think couples can have initial "what if" discussions about the future that can prepare both partners for what may come, particularly the well spouse, while permitting different outlooks on the probabilities.

Expressing Anger

Anger is a nearly universal emotion experienced by both partners living with chronic disorders. The partner who has the condition will experience feelings of outrage at being victimized by the illness and fear losing control over his or her body or their future. Unfortunately, these feelings can easily be directed at the other partner. Couples function best when they are able to tolerate such strong emotions from either partner without applying shameful or pathological labels. Both partners ought to feel entitled to have and express their own intense emotions. At the same time, they may need help in not becoming reactive to a partner's outburst. Clinicians can help couples redirect their anger from the partner to the illness. Externalization of the disorder is helpful. Viewing the illness as the uninvited guest or intruder, as in *"The* (rather than my or your) asthma has been really difficult for us lately," is one way to externalize it.

Some people are extremely fearful about feeling or expressing anger. They may have a history of physical or verbal abuse or a family culture that values keeping feelings under control. A serious illness or disability can normally generate levels of distress well beyond anything experienced in the past, which can be terrifying. Clinicians can help such individuals differentiate normal outrage within the specific context of a chronic disorder from pathological anger or abuse.

The Gender Factor

The role of gender is a critical dimension in couples' experiences with chronic disorders. A meta-analytic research review suggests that in heterosexual couples coping with cancer, women experienced greater distress, regardless of whether they were the partner or patient (Hagedoorn, Sanderman, Bolks, Tuinstra, & Coyne, 2008). Also serious illness in the wife or mother can present the greatest overall risk to couple and family functioning because women generally fill so many of the practical and nurturing roles within families. Research confirms that women are more apt to assume the bulk of caregiving responsibilities with a disabled husband than is the case when the situation is reversed. Men, based on powerful cultural norms, often enlist other family members (e.g., adult daughters) or, when economically feasible, hire a part-time caregiver to take over a disabled spouse's role. Wives tend to try to assume their husbands' roles, despite the risks of overload (Zarit & Talley, 2013).

Initial Crisis Phase

In the initial crisis phase it is useful to inquire about what preconceived ideas couples have about who might become ill, dependent on the other, and die first, and how the other would survive. Often a spouse will fantasize about the kind of health problems a partner might develop based on family-related illnesses, such as heart disease, or risky health habits, such as poor dietary patterns, that may have been a source of conflict within a relationship. Typically, a couple's beliefs are gender based. Women are, on average, younger than their partners and have a greater life expectancy. For this reason women at midlife typically begin to rehearse the expectation that they may take care of or lose their partners some day. This gender-related difference in preparedness is reinforced by strong multigenerational patterns of caregiving by women. Men may need more guidance in adapting to a dependent partner, because illness or loss does not fit gendered social expectations. Psychoeducation can help reduce anxiety for men and help them to better take care emotionally of themselves, their partner, and their children. It is valuable to address any feelings of anger harbored by the male partner for being put in an unanticipated caregiver role and any feelings of guilt for the ill female partner for failing to stay healthy and becoming a burden.

Men, socialized to be tough and invulnerable, often feel that being nurtured and dependent is acceptable, if at all, only when they are ill or injured. For many men, their early memories of being nurtured are associated with mothering in periods of illness. The message from both their parents and the larger culture was that they should be strong. Often, illness and disability are experienced very ambivalently. On the one hand, powerful voices deride dependency and disability as a failure to fulfill the male role of self-reliant provider for one's family. This is most difficult in progressive and disabling illnesses, in which exerting control and remaining strong may have unavoidable limits. Conversely, a chronic condition may provide many men with a sanctioned reason to be nurtured. Clinician curiosity regarding such feelings can open a dialogue and allow a reevaluation of such deeply ingrained gendered beliefs.

Because of gender socialization, women and men often feel adept at different facets of coping. The psychosocial demands of a disorder can affect gender-based feelings of efficacy. Men tend to tackle the practical problem-solving aspects of coping, avoiding the emotional side of their partner and themselves. Managing home-based kidney dialysis may feel more in sync with a man's sense of competence. Women are typically expected to tend to the emotional demands of their husbands, children, and others, as well as to stifle their own needs. At the time of an initial illness crisis, couples tend to divide up coping tasks according to habitual patterns or stereotyped expectations. The risks are twofold. This division of psychosocial labor can become imbalanced and rigid, depending on who is ill and on gendered role expectations. Clinicians can help couples distinguish patterns that worked during the initial crisis from those that are more adaptive over the long haul. In this sense, a chronic disorder gives couples an opportunity to reexamine habitual gendered role constraints.

In one case, Marjorie had cancer that was in remission for a number of years, during a time of rearing her young children. Her husband, Alex, was very supportive, but uncomfortable in handling sadness and in being the nurturing parent. Throughout the illness, Marjorie had continued to monitor everyone's emotional needs, while minimizing her own. As her condition entered a terminal phase and she could no longer maintain her role as family nurturer, Alex felt ill prepared and overwhelmed by the emotional needs of his wife and children. An early intervention focused on renegotiating their gender-defined roles in a more balanced way, regardless of the outcome, is less crisis driven. It might have helped this couple to avert a double crisis in the final stages of the illness when they were facing impending loss and a need for role changes.

It is useful to ask couples how being male or female will affect their plans to organize around an illness. Are there any roles they feel particularly suited for and others for which they feel unprepared? Inviting each spouse to consider the positive aspects of untried gender roles is beneficial. For men, this may include allowing their softer side to emerge. For women, tackling the monthly account balances and insurance policies can enhance feelings of financial competency. Such inquiry facilitates bringing thoughts and feelings about gender into couples' discussions about coping strategies. It can promote some sense of mastery for couples dealing with a disorder wherein the medical course is largely beyond their control.

In many instances a couple's illness-related crisis can lead to positive realignments that change gender-based beliefs guiding the relationship, as in the following case.

Sam and Alice presented for treatment 8 months after Sam had suddenly developed a heart condition that left him disabled and unable to retain his job as a construction worker. Before this event, Alice had been at home full time, rearing their two young children, ages 4 and 6. Although Sam could no longer work at his job, he was physically able to assume the role of househusband. Initially, both Sam and Alice remained at home, his disability income enabling them to manage. When it became clear that Sam's disability was permanent, Alice expressed an interest in finding a job to relieve the financial pressures. Sam resisted at first, feeling that childcare and housework were appropriate only for a woman. He needed help in rethinking his gendered, rigid definition of family provider. With some encouragement, however, Sam agreed to try it. To his surprise, he enjoyed the time with his kids enormously, and the children loved it. Also, he became more fully aware of what he had missed with regard to his own father as he was growing up—a longing for closeness he had repressed since childhood. In spite of his disability, for the first time he felt a balance in his life he had never contemplated. "My job was important, but I'll only have one chance to spend time with my kids while they are still young."

Here, a systemic intervention would also need to explore the wife's feelings of having to forgo the satisfaction and bonding she had experienced in a primary parenting role. She is losing the chance to be at home with her children while they are young, and she may not have a satisfying job situation to compensate for it.

Challenging Role-Functioning Shifts

Dramatic role shifts can also present challenges for couples. In one situation, the husband, George, had sustained an injury that required a long period of rehabilitation at home before he could return to work. Until the injury, this couple had clearly defined traditional roles in which he supported the family financially and his wife reared the children. This arrangement had been satisfying for both. When George remained at home, he became involved with childcare and parenting functions that had been the province of his wife, Janice. His style of parenting was more authoritarian than hers. Intense conflict and struggles over control and turf emerged as previous differences in parenting surfaced more forcefully. Both acknowledged that these differences were nothing new, but had been less consequential because roles were only minimally shared. This case illustrates the need for couples to explore both the positive implications of and potential conflicts in shifting roles assigned primarily by gender.

Sexuality and Chronic Disorders

Chronic disorders can affect a couple's sexuality in a variety of ways (Agronin, 2015; Schover & Jensen, 1988; Sipski & Alexander, 1997; Verschuren, Enzlin, Dijkstra, Geertzen, & Dekker, 2010). Yet, a discussion of a condition's possible effects on sexuality and inquiry about any actual impact on a couple's sexual intimacy is often lacking (Hughes, Hertlein, & Hagey, 2011). Many times when I inquire, couples will state, "This is the first time we were asked." This is particularly true for older couples. When we providers don't ask, we reinforce the couple's hesitancy in bringing up any sexual difficulties. Unfortunately, this hesitancy fosters a barrier in communication between the provider and couple and inhibits healthy communication between partners.

Couples need clear information about how a particular disease or disability can be expected to affect sexuality physiologically and psychosocially.

Medical Treatments

The fatigue caused by debilitating conditions or certain treatments, such as radiation and chemotherapy for cancer, are typically associated with diminished desire. Neurological complications from diseases, such as diabetes, MS, spinal cord injury, or prostate cancer surgery, may interfere with erectile functioning. Medications for depression and hypertension may compromise libido and the ability to achieve orgasm (Seagraves & Balon, 2003).

Information about whether these limitations will likely resolve themselves or be permanent is very useful. In situations that require caution for a period of time, such as after a life-threatening health crisis, couples function best when explicit guidelines are given concerning any necessary limits on sexual activity and how long they should adhere to them. Charting this kind of information in a patient's electronic health record and, when appropriate, direct communication among his or her specialty and primary care providers is vital.

Many couples are unaware of technological advances and clinical interventions available to ameliorate many physical causes of sexual dysfunction. One young married man with MS had lost his ability to maintain an erection 5 years earlier. At the time his neurologist said, "What can you expect. You've got MS." Living in a semirural area, the couple and doctor were unaware of self-administered injections that were successful in temporarily restoring an erection for many afflicted patients, highlighting the need for clinicians to keep up-to-date on medical advances related to sexual functioning affected by chronic disorders. Learning how to give an injection is usually far less stressful than resignation to abstinence and a major long-term marital strain.

Psychosocial Impact on Sexuality

Almost any illness and disability can have secondary psychosocial effects on a couple's sexual life. Conditions with possibly fatal recurrences can easily convert sexual exertion into a dangerous activity fraught with anxiety. Disfiguring conditions such as facial burns, strokes, or a mastectomy can arouse anxiety about attractiveness and/or diminish sexual feelings for both partners.

Breast and ovarian cancer are intimately associated with reproduction and cultural symbols of female sexuality. In Western culture, women's breasts are emphasized as symbols of femininity and attractiveness. Loss or mutilation of a breast has significance for a woman's self-image and causes concern about her desirability to her spouse. She may not want to be seen or touched and may not believe her spouse's reassurances. Preventive psychoeducation and consultation are invaluable in such situations. Encouraging a sensitive dialogue between partners about the meaning of the loss for each of them should be a consultation priority.

Breast and reproductive disorders may require some men to address their sense of entitlement to an intact woman who will bear their children and assure continuation of the family lineage. Concerns about being judged failures by their male peers or fathers can heighten this attitude. One despondent young man, whose wife's ovarian cancer and radiation treatment precluded having children, stated, "I feel like I dropped the baton my father handed me." Unaddressed, such feelings represent a high risk to a couple's relationship.

Communication Challenges

Because illnesses easily disrupt a couple's sexual routines, those unaccustomed to communicating about their sexual life may need a crash course. Couples may need help in learning to discuss their feelings about limitations and preferences. A man suffering from chronic lung disease may find the customary missionary position too tiring. He needs to be able to tell this to his partner. In addition, if his disability has necessitated his wife's becoming the primary wage earner, he may associate her assuming a "superior" position during intercourse as symbolic of her new status in the relationship. This couple would need to discuss these issues to avert their sexual relations becoming tainted by unavoidable role changes that challenge the foundation of his definition of masculinity.

For someone who expresses intimate feelings mostly through sexuality, a partner's illness can create a serious crisis. This is more common among men than women. In one case, after a woman's operation for a bleeding ulcer, the husband continued to demand sex as a way to maintain a sense of contact at a time of uncertainty. The wife, not wanting to hurt her husband's feelings, passively complied. Because of physical pain and unexpressed resentment at his insensitivity, she responded in a distant, unimpassioned manner. This increased the husband's sense of desperation and redoubled his sexual demands, which only further angered his wife. In another situation, a wife felt in a double bind with her impotent husband: on the one hand, she thought that if she approached him in any way sexually, she would be labeled demanding or domineering, and if she did not, she would be seen as cold, passive, maternal, or treating him like a child.

A man who suffers a life-threatening health crisis, such as a heart attack, that limits his sexual performance and who feels less adequate in other areas of intimacy, may respond in two extreme ways. He may totally withdraw into a depression or, against medical advice, attempt to reestablish his intactness and manhood by pressing for sex. As discussed in Chapter 9, a wife who wishes to protect her vulnerable partner may decline, not from a lack of interest, but from a fear of precipitating a fatal recurrence.

Sometimes sexual activity cannot be sustained physically or is beyond the psychological limits of a couple. Openly discussing this is often extremely difficult for couples. Well partners may find the realities of caregiving or visible impairment of their mate an impediment to sexual intimacy. Often a well person's sexual withdrawal from a partner is fraught with feelings of shame and guilt, particularly if it is connected to general underlying feelings of not being nurtured or ambivalence or to escape fantasies. This is particularly important for female caregivers. Individual consultations may be needed with the well spouse to process such feelings before further conjoint meetings. Promoting open, sensitive discussion can help avert the risk of a spouse's general distancing from the relationship. Couples who can redefine intimacy and nurturance in terms broader than the purely sexual can successfully adapt to the loss of the sexual component.

It can be helpful to explore possibilities by asking questions such as, "If you were to view nonsexual nurturing as an acceptable compromise, how would that affect your feelings about the relationship?" Clinicians can help promote a mutually caring, companionable relationship in other areas, with shared interests and pleasurable activities.

Extramarital Relationships

How to deal with extramarital relationships in the context of chronic disorders is a particularly thorny question for clinicians. Our beliefs on the subject are enormously diverse, based on varied personal, cultural, and religious attitudes and mores. Personally, I subscribe to a nonjudgmental attitude, in which the context of each situation requires careful consideration. Standards that are applied to physically healthy couples may not fit the excruciating long-term strains of couples facing illness and disability.

I have seen many instances in which an affair was destructive and hastened the end of a marriage. I have also seen a number of occasions of protracted illness ordeals in which an extramarital relationship allowed a well partner to sustain his or her commitment to caring for a spouse, particularly when a long-term disabling condition strikes early in the life cycle. Couples confronted with advanced dementias, TBIs, or protracted terminal disease are prime examples. Also, it is worth noting that often the need for nurturance or for someone to share with emotionally is more important than physical intimacy. One woman, who took care of her severely disabled husband and reared three children over a 25-year period, stated, "I loved him, and I was committed to the marriage, taking care of him and raising the kids. But his ability to reciprocate was limited, and sex was physically impossible. I was 30 years old when he was diagnosed. I had a lover for many years, but I never considered leaving my husband. He and the kids always came first." I would consider this woman's experience adaptive in light of the primacy of her commitment to her marriage and family. This does not mean that I advocate affairs. But in certain situations of serious illness, an extramarital relationship can be one option to sustain a commitment. This is most relevant when a couple's relationship has, of necessity, become exclusively one of patient and caregiver.

Because a couple's relationship can become a constant reminder of illness and loss for both partners, an extramarital relationship can express a need to escape the ordeal and find respite or be nurtured. Both ill and well partners have described how an extramarital relationship helped them reaffirm a feeling of being normal. Closeness with someone outside the ordeal was not tainted with all the issues of patient and caregiver. Ill spouses, especially younger ones with terminal illnesses, can find it an escape and salve to the excruciating pain of facing a premature death. Sadly, often late in the chronic phase, couples have become so accustomed to these roles that they no longer find it possible to experience their relationship as separate from illness and adversity. For some, an affair may seem the only way to obtain a needed escape, to revitalize oneself, and be nurtured by an intimate.

These outcomes highlight the importance of early consultations with couples. These complicated issues are far less likely if, early on, couples can develop ways to discuss their needs for separateness and time together that is not governed by patient and caregiver roles (see Chapter 14). Sustaining a nonillness aspect to their relationship is essential (Navon, 1999).

When a long-term severe disability precludes sexual relations between partners, occasionally couples openly negotiate an understanding that the well partner may meet his or her sexual needs outside the marriage. This is an extremely delicate issue, one that requires a firm commitment to the primary relationship and sensitivity to discretion.

The advisability of disclosing an extramarital relationship needs to be assessed within the context of the total clinical picture. When it is suspected or discovered, and when relationship repair is the goal, a process of fuller disclosure and exploration of the couple's relationship is typically indicated. Also, when an affair is an expression of a deteriorating, dysfunctional relationship, disclosure may be necessary if the partner intends to continue the affair. On the other hand, disclosure of an affair may be counterproductive when it surfaces in situations, such as severe cognitive disability or the final stages of an illness when the patient may already feel overwhelmed and the original partnership may no longer exist or be possible. When clinicians agree that a well partner has realistically assessed an illness situation, the question of disclosure should be addressed in terms of "For what purpose?" The need to confess to an affair to assuage guilt needs to be considered separately from disclosure as a way to restore or repair intimacy. In instances in which the couple's relationship possibilities may be limited, disclosure and the resulting pain may only heighten guilt for the caregiver.

Regardless of a decision about disclosure, a clinician can play a critical role in helping normalize (not necessarily accept) an extramarital relationship that has occurred under unusual and stressful circumstances. Such understanding from a professional can help alleviate the suffering of a well partner and counteract survivor shame and guilt. In such cases, clinicians really need to examine their own ethical positions while maintaining a therapeutic role.

LGBTQ COUPLES

The 2015 U.S. Supreme Court ruling legalizing same-sex marriage nationwide eliminated many discriminatory legal barriers (e.g., family medical leave policies, survivor benefits, visitation with children of a deceased partner) for LGBTQ couples. Yet, LGBTQ couples facing chronic disorders still often deal with social stigma and homophobia in addition to all the same challenges as heterosexual couples. A major illness, with its attendant need for health care, can force a hidden or extremely private relationship to become public for the first time at a moment of great vulnerability. It typically brings same-sex couples into direct contact with health care systems and providers, not infrequently outside the LGBTQ community. Experiencing potentially cold or distant professional healers at a time of need can be a particularly poignant rejection. The intensity of this experience is magnified tremendously when gay couples face a stigmatized condition such as HIV, which a significant proportion of society still associates with a deviant lifestyle.

Clinicians, to be most helpful and "do no harm" to LGBTQ couples, need to be aware of and address their own personal prejudice and homophobia. Health care providers may experience discomfort in dealing with the couple together. Homophobia and antipathy are more containable if the health professional can define a health problem as limited to a biological issue or a part of the body rather than to the whole person and his or her intimate life. Yet, this kind of defense mechanism seriously compromises any provider–patient relationship.

Couples may need help when a health crisis brings their personal lives and families of origin together more intensively or even for the first time. Sometimes an embittered family may attempt to exclude the partner from caregiving or important rituals, such as a memorial service.

INCLUSION OF CLINICIANS IN THE COUPLE'S RELATIONSHIP

Chronic disorders often necessitate the intrusion of health professionals into the privacy of a couple's relationship. This is particularly true in cases of moderate or severe disability in which health care is delivered at home or when the ill member requires 24-hour care in a hospital or residential care facility. In essence, a second primary relationship can develop between the ill member and a health professional, for example, with a nurse or home health aide who tends to his or her physical needs. This new caregiver contact often coincides with decreased physical contact with one's partner. A nurse's emotional comfort through nurturing physical contact with a disabled or debilitated patient can contrast sharply with the emotional discomfort and distancing from physical contact that may have developed for a couple.

A professional who assumes caregiving functions that have become burdensome or anxiety ridden for the well partner can help a couple's relationship by handling certain tension-filled responsibilities. For one man, monitoring his wife's blood pressure following a stroke was a source of great anxiety. Although it was a simple procedure, he lived in fear that he would make a mistake and his wife would have a fatal recurrence. This led to hypervigilant monitoring of his wife that became a source of intense conflict and adversely affected their overall relationship. A regular visit by a nurse who assumed this responsibility solved the problem.

Although relief may be the predominant emotion for both partners in such a situation, divided emotions are not uncommon. When a health care professional provides intimate physical care (e.g., in bathing and dressing), jealousy can sometimes result. Also, the patient may experience intense anger that his or her partner is no longer providing all the care. This anger is connected to the inevitable separation process, described earlier, that may be especially terrifying for the patient. This underscores the importance of helping couples find alternative options for mutually satisfying interactions and activities.

When physical caregiving is required, the relationship implications of either the well spouse or professional assuming important caregiving functions should be explored in advance. This includes asking about any cultural or personal norms and meanings that may need to be acknowledged or, in some instances, modifications to accommodate strong values. Particularly in conditions that can have life-threatening crises, the possible effects on the couple need to be discussed. In one case, a husband who was a health care provider agreed to monitor his wife at home for life-threatening infections during a high-risk period when her immune system was depleted after each high-dose cancer chemotherapy treatment. Here, a missed infection could be lethal in 24 hours. His wife wanted desperately to rest at home rather than wait out the recovery phase in the hospital. The health care team complied with the patient's request to go home and encouraged the husband to agree to this cost-effective and expedient arrangement that his wife favored. The husband swallowed his fears, rather than appear weak to his colleagues. Eventually the strain of this arrangement and the couple's failure to discuss the husband's fears increased his feelings of anger and of being controlled by the situation.

CHAPTER 14

Rebalancing the Couple's Relationship

When a serious illness or disability becomes part of a relationship, a variety of imbalances are inevitable. This chapter addresses some of the most common ones and ways that clinicians can help couples compensate for structural and emotional changes.

ESTABLISHING HEALTHY BOUNDARIES

A key developmental task in the initial crisis phase is grieving the loss of life as it was normally led before the condition appeared. Part of this task involves couples acknowledging that their relationship will never be the same. Helping them see the possibilities for growth despite the loss helps counterbalance this painful process. A major risk for couples is that their relationship will become completely identified with a chronic condition. Couples' narratives can become burdened with metaphors of decline and loss, where living a normal life is outside the relationship and illness is within it. Although this process becomes more apparent in the chronic phase, the risk originates with framing assumptions about how a couple incorporates a condition, defines its boundaries, and begins to create illness-related meanings.

Naturally, setting boundaries becomes most difficult with disorders such as Alzheimer's disease or TBI, in which cognitive impairment is always present and directly affects all interactions (see Chapter 16). This also characterizes life-threatening conditions, such as after a heart attack, in which fear about further loss persists. It pertains to disorders that are permanently disabling, progressive, or require continuous care, such as chronic pain syndromes or a spinal cord injury. Here, the condition is ever present, demanding a couple's continual practical and emotional energies.

Creating limits is particularly important as couples emerge from an initial crisis phase that has been medically intensive and necessitated a period of immersion in learning about the condition. This is especially true when the initial crisis phase was marked by a life-threatening onset or a protracted period of disability requiring partner caregiving. Couples can benefit from advice about how and where appropriate boundaries can be established beyond these illness realities.

Crisis-Phase Life-Threatening Period(s)

Couples need explicit guidance in determining when an initial- or chronic-phase life-threatening crisis has passed. Misinformation about perceived risks heightens the power that the disorder and associated anxiety will wield over a couple. In a sudden-onset condition, such as a heart attack, a narrow escape from death requires an initial period of reduced emotional and physical stress for the patient that infuses the framing event with ambiguity and fear. In a situation in which this crisis can erupt suddenly, couples tend to cling, in a ritualistic way, to medical advice originally intended only for a limited period of time. Talking freely about emotional issues, expressing normal disagreements, or resuming sexual relations are often avoided to prevent another life-threatening recurrence.

Because conflict avoidance takes a heavy toll on a relationship over time (Gottman, 2011), providing clear guidelines about what is safe and what can exacerbate the illness is helpful. Are there any restrictions they need to continue 6 months from now, or even permanently? I routinely ask couples, "What activities do you think can make the illness worse?" Especially with potentially fatal conditions, couples can unnecessarily sacrifice healthy patterns of relating for fear that interacting normally might kill the affected partner. One Italian couple stopped having normal lively discussions about the wife's large extended family to avoid getting the wife, who had had a heart attack, too excited. Both the power of an initial life-threatening crisis and the insidious effects of slowly progressive or permanently disabling disorders can hinder couples' normal abilities to assess long-term risks to their relationships. Effective specialty and primary care collaboration regarding risks and precautions can help prevent unnecessary worry and discord.

Protected Time and Space

To counteract the tendency of the illness to subsume the relationship, clinicians can help couples learn how to circumscribe the time and space occupied by the disorder in their relationship interactions. Often, clinicians need to support couples in learning how to distinguish interactions that must explicitly include the condition from those in which it can become a dysfunctional form of currency. Adaptive minimization also needs to be distinguished from denial, which absorbs considerable psychic energy that compromises couples' relationships.

There are some simple strategies for keeping the condition in its place.

- Where possible, couples should arrange for times that are devoted to self-care and caregiving or discussing the illness and times that are preserved for other activities and discussions that do not become dominated by the condition.
- Specific areas of a home can be off limits to illness-related functions. For instance, not discussing the illness in the bedroom can help preserve romance.
- Couples often stop inviting friends to their home because it has become associated with illness. They should be encouraged to socialize with friends in their home and to try and preserve parts of their home life that have been pleasurable and keep them connected to their wider social network. Establishing clear caregiving boundaries within the home helps counteract the tendency for what is normal to become associated with what is outside the home and relationship.

Externalization

Putting a chronic disorder in proper perspective promotes functional boundaries. White and Epston's (1990) notion of externalizing the disorder or symptom is useful in this regard. A clinician might refer to a couple's struggle in coping with cancer in the following terms: "The cancer seems to be getting the upper hand lately, interfering with your experiencing the close times together you were accustomed to." Framing a serious disorder in this ways helps establish a boundary between the condition and the couple. This externalization unites the couple in relation to the disorder, which becomes a shared challenge; and it functions as a reminder that the person is not the illness, and that he or she and the relationship exist separately from the disorder.

Illnesses such as cancer can give rise to destructive metaphors that suggest a lack of control or a complete takeover of one's being. Such metaphors can become isomorphically extended, invading all aspects of a relationship. The lack of a boundary between the person and the cancer parallels the cancer's impact on a primary relationship. Externalization can help reduce feelings of being overwhelmed by establishing a functional boundary between the disorder and the couple, enhancing their sense of control, and reducing the need for denial as a defense.

Avoiding Triangulation

As discussed in Chapter 5, a chronic disorder can become a powerful third member in any dyadic relationship. In some relationships governed by unresolved struggles for control, a chronic condition can help the affected member gain the upper hand. For instance, for one couple with longstanding gender-related conflicts, the wife's chronic back pain legitimized her demands for her spouse to do more of the housework. The danger in allowing an illness or disability to serve as the rationale for change is that the change often remains dependent on continued symptoms or the threat of loss. For the woman in this relationship, this prevented her from getting well or reporting feeling better because the relationship shift had become possible only with her illness. Here, clinicians need to address the underlying issues related to power and control as a way of rectifying or preventing such a triangle. A preventively oriented psychosocial consultation in the initial crisis phase can anticipate any risks that the condition will become a third party in preexisting unresolved problems.

KEEPING THE ROLES OF PATIENT AND CAREGIVER WITHIN BOUNDS

The imbalances inherent in the long-term caregiving and dependency needs of an ill partner can foster challenges concerning hierarchy, power, and reciprocity (Scheinkman, 2008). A couple's expectations for shared, balanced role functions often become impossible to maintain when one partner has a significant disability. A new version of balance needs to be negotiated; otherwise, old relationship understandings become a "hollow shell" creating role strain and confusion for the couple.

Sustaining intimacy depends largely on establishing viable caregiving boundaries. Even the strongest relationships are strained by the discrepancies in shifts between two forms of relating: patient–caregiver and equal partners. Couples function best when they can discuss such challenges openly.

Psychosocial Typology and Time-Phase Guidance

Early education about the physical and psychosocial demands of a condition over the long haul gives couples a sense of the degree and timing of caregiving demands and helps them take greater control of their lives. Some progressive disorders require a greater amount of caregiving that will eventually require 24-hour care. Clinicians can help couples create a workable boundary between a future time, when they will relate more as patient and caregiver, and the present, when they can more fully relate as equal partners. Other conditions, such as arthritis, may necessitate intermittent care when flare-ups occur, but have clearer boundaries. Disorders with an uncertain course and outcome (e.g., MS) make planning more challenging. Some conditions (e.g., chronic fatigue syndrome or dementia) fluctuate daily, with better functioning earlier in the day. The psychosocial typology and time-phases framework can inform couples about periods when imbalances will be inevitable (e.g., in mornings versus evenings, during flare-ups, and in the later stages of progressive disorders). The type of disability predicts which aspects of a relationship are likely to become skewed and which will be preserved. Although a physically disabled man may no longer be able to share physical household tasks or provide income equitably, his potential for helpful communication about practical issues and for emotional support may be unaffected. Making these distinctions and clear thinking about aspects of functioning that will be unaffected can help couples negotiate role changes, while trying to preserve some balance.

Caregiving by Patient versus Family Member versus Health Care Provider

Couples need clear professional guidance concerning which aspects of caregiving can be realistically carried out by the patient, which require another person, such as a spouse, and which need professional assistance. Also, they need to know under what circumstances care warrants including another person or a health care professional or requires transfer to a skilled-care facility. This basic information helps spouses establish healthy boundaries so that the ill partner's dependency needs and fears and the well partner's sympathy do not take over. Having this knowledge helps address questions pertaining to the timing and meaning of potential caregiving changes.

- What would it mean to their relationship to have professional help with caregiving?
- What would it mean to each partner?
- What would this mean from a couple's cultural perspective?

Santiago and Luciana are coping with her severe, advanced Parkinson's disease and increasing dementia. Both partners were raised in families that have powerful multigenerational legacies involving feelings of shame. Luciana's father had died in a state hospital, with a dementia resulting from years of chronic alcoholism. Her father's condition had been a source of intense family conflict and embarrassment within their extended family and local community. Santiago's mother had had a progressive illness, and he had left caregiving to his sisters, which resulted in unresolved guilt feelings after his mother's death. These histories severely restricted this couple's perceived options, as Luciana's illness worsened. Santiago felt that it was essential to remain the primary caregiver until his wife died to avoid repeating his behavior during his mother's illness. For Luciana, becoming institutionalized because her symptoms could not be adequately controlled would represent a humiliating repetition of her father's inability to control his alcoholism. When Luciana's motor and cognitive disabilities became overwhelming in the terminal phase, the couple's unwillingness to consider other options caused an impossible situation in the home and for the adult children who understood their parents' histories. After seeking family behavioral health consultations that included their primary care doctor, Luciana was finally admitted to a nursing home. It's important at the outset to assess constraining multigenerational legacies and the willingness to engage extended kin or adult children in giving respite to the well partner.

Clinicians should also consider how the well partner feels about caregiving. Are there certain aspects that are too frightening or repelling? Frequently well partners, usually women, believe that they should handle everything.

One woman found that tending to her husband's advanced psoriasis interfered with her continuing to feel attracted to him. She had provided his physical care without questioning whether he could manage it himself, and the husband had assumed that his wife would want to do so. He was unaware of her feelings, and there had been no discussion about the possible adverse impact on their relationship. In fact, he was capable of applying the medicinal ointment himself and readily agreed to the change once the issue was raised. Although not intended as part of the consultation, a discussion of the issue led to a broader dialogue regarding caregiving and role functions in the couple's relationship more generally.

Couples need to negotiate understandings about the caregiver–patient role that fits the condition's realities. Does the couple have a sense of limits? Or are they driven by multigenerational legacies and belief systems that promote unrealistic and ultimately dysfunctional roles? Couples with preexisting issues concerning control, attentiveness, or nurturance are most vulnerable to unhealthy caregiving bargains based on who is indebted to whom.

When caregiving is extensive, both partners need a transition from a patient–caregiver mode to other ways of relating. Sometimes spending time alone is needed first. Sharing moments about lighter or humorous topics can help. When this kind of transition is bypassed, one or both partners can feel emotionally blocked or violated. An avoidable cycle of anger, hurt, and rejection can ensue at a time when a couple may desperately need to reconnect in old, comfortable ways. A disabled husband who wants sex may easily offend a tired spouse, who may need close, quiet time together with or without sex.

Transition from Crisis to Chronic Phase

Couples often do not have a good sense of the stamina required in the chronic phase or when it may be advisable to renegotiate a typically intensive crisis-phase caregiving arrangement for the foreseeable future. This renegotiation process influences whether a key chronic-phase task will be successful: maximizing autonomy for all family members, given the constraints of the condition. During the transition to the chronic phase, when issues of permanency need attention, clinicians can encourage couples to talk frankly about how they can best handle the emotional and practical demands of the disorder while protecting their relationship. As previously mentioned, a clinician's silence on the subject can inadvertently be interpreted by couples as encouragement to retain crisis-phase relationship guidelines indefinitely.

Negotiating Reasonable Caregiving Limits

Depending on the type of disorder, couples commonly tilt into a number of skewed patterns, including ill versus healthy, disabled versus able, in pain versus pain free, dependent versus independent, and confined versus out in the world. These asymmetries can easily foster feelings of resentment and guilt when well partners develop a long-term pattern of concealing personal needs and goals so as to not offend their ill or disabled partners. Patients can resent their illnesses and their partners' health. They can feel guilty about being a burden and preventing partners from living normal lives. Sometimes, to alleviate such emotions, the patient behaves in provocative ways to drive the well partner away. Especially in young couples, the well partner often feels both resentful about his or her constricted life-cycle options and shameful about having such feelings. Because of gender-based socialization, women as well spouses are much more likely to accept limits on their own needs and development stoically and without question.

Normalizing these emotions is a good starting point. Then couples need help devising ways to make flexible autonomy possible. Any relationship inequalities should be acknowledged. It cannot be stressed enough that *the long-term viability of the relationship may depend on openly discussing and legitimizing both partners' needs.* I have seen countless relationships deteriorate or end when these issues are not addressed.

Open communication about caregiving limits may be very painful, but for clinicians to collude in avoiding this subject is a prescription for disaster. The well partner, in particular, may need permission to voice concerns and reasonable limits, which can be very difficult when the ill spouse is acutely symptomatic. A profound health imbalance between two partners typically can make the well partner's claim of entitlement to any semblance of equality seem shameful. Yet, defining limits is a critical point in solidifying long-term relationship bargains around a chronic condition. Facilitating this process at the outset promotes resilience and helps to reduce the ambivalence, escape fantasies, and survivor guilt that so often surface in dysfunctional ways later on.

Rachel was facing the slowly progressive, very disabling, fatal illness of her husband, Frank. She said that her decision, made openly, not to be her husband's sole primary caregiver allowed her to commit to the long haul. On one level,

Frank rationally accepted Rachel's choice; it lessened his anxiety that he would burden her. On another level, it generated intense anger and a sense of abandonment, which, unfortunately, did not surface until much later, during a marital crisis. Sadly, Frank's natural reaction was not openly discussed at the time of Rachel's caregiving decision.

TOGETHERNESS AND SEPARATENESS

With serious illness, couples adapt best when they can acknowledge different needs for separateness and togetherness. The ill partner's increased need for dependency typically fosters a desire for greater closeness. Simultaneously, the well partner may need respite time and space apart from the demands of the illness and to prepare for a future possibly without the ill partner. This process can be very painful and threatening to the ill person, who may feel abandoned, and often expresses this fear as intense anger. As in the previous case vignette, if Rachel had not decided to limit her caregiving, she might have felt powerless and totally controlled by Frank's condition. Eventually this could lead to strong resentment, wishes for his demise, or a decision to leave him when life became intolerable. Frank, in turn, had to face a boundary between Rachel's needs and his own. The immediate physical imbalance and the tragedy of Frank's life-shortening illness had to be acknowledged. At the same time, the basic fact that two committed, equal individuals are entitled to make personal decisions needed to be affirmed. Couples adapt best to chronic disorders when they can transform their understanding of "we-ness" to include a new version of separateness that acknowledges different needs and realities.

Couples, and especially the well partner, need reassurance that emotional distancing that occurs out of fears of loss is a natural initial reaction and not a profound statement about loyalty to the relationship. Such reassurances help counteract feelings of shame that contribute later to survivor guilt or unresolved grief.

It is important to distinguish between each partner's need for separateness within healthy intimacy and situations in which distancing occurs because of fear. Exploring couples' worst fears, such as concerns about inadequate pain control, in a normalizing and educational manner can diffuse them. Often, both partners have fears, and hesitating to talk about them prevents the couple from giving each other support. Openly sharing their concerns and clarifying limits and expectations often facilitate mutual comforting. One man distanced himself from his wife because he feared that he would need to take complete charge of the dying process for her, including actively helping her to die. When they discussed the subject, his wife specified what she would want and when she heard about his fears, agreed to take a more active role by talking with her doctor about assisted dying options, rather than make her husband primarily responsible for helping her.

RECOVERY AND ADAPTATION IMBALANCES

Often partners differ in the pace at which they adapt to an illness diagnosis or crisis. Such discrepancies can be a major source of misunderstanding and conflict. Clinicians need to distinguish between arrested or blocked adaptation, characterized by denial, and normative differences based on personality style or different roles assumed during the initial crisis phase. Examples of conditions wherein adaptation is likely to occur at different rates in couples include major mental illness, TBI, and conditions with very arduous initial treatments, such as intensive and prolonged chemotherapy. The following case illustrates the skewed timing of adaptation for each partner.

> Jerry had suffered a serious head injury in a near-fatal car accident. After months in a coma, he regained consciousness and began a 2-year recovery that, by all accounts, was miraculous. During this time, he had cognitive and speech deficits that slowly resolved. Late in his recovery, he and his wife, Marge, sought treatment for an accumulation of strains in their relationship. He complained that Marge seemed depressed and unable to celebrate his return to almost normal health. She protested that Jerry was unavailable to talk about and attend to her need to discuss what had happened. While he was regaining his former state of health, Marge had become more irritable and vocal about how hard life was. Both spouses felt invalidated.
>
> Jerry, who had an iron will and was fiercely independent, had come to terms with his injury and its meaning for him alone over the weeks and months of recovery. While he was incapacitated, Marge had been totally absorbed in tending to him and their three children as the bulwark for the family unit. Her all-encompassing caregiving and parenting responsibilities had, until recently, not allowed her time to process the events. As is often true for the primary caregiver, processing what had happened became possible only near the end of Jerry's recovery, when he was no longer so vulnerable and could handle her feelings of distress. This couple was completely out of sync with each other for two reasons. Jerry's personal style was geared toward working out emotional issues alone, while Marge needed a collaborative process. Also, he was more focused on personal recovery and less aware than she was of the need for the relationship to recover. The pace of adaptation for each partner needed to be validated and normalized.

> In a similar situation, one woman had recurrent depressions over a 2-year period that required repeated electroconvulsive treatments resulting in amnesia for that time period. She was perplexed by her husband's anger once she recovered. As though awakening from a dream, she was unprepared for the aftermath and could not comprehend the anger directed at her.
>
> Both cases demonstrate that when there is an extended period of cognitive impairment, the affected partner, because of problems with recollecting the event and the different perceptions of time, may have difficulty understanding a partner's needs. Also, after intense suffering, often the ill partner

may have difficulty with reliving the experience. He or she can be considered to have a form of posttraumatic stress reaction in which processing events with one's partner resembles a flashback experience. Clinicians can help the healing process by facilitating a gradual sharing of two equally valid realities.

BELIEF SYSTEM IMBALANCES

In times of adversity, differences between partners' beliefs can precipitate a relationship crisis. Especially after an initial health crisis, couples have an opportunity to shift constraining beliefs in more healthful directions. Some couples choose to work on altering basic beliefs, as the following case illustrates.

> Jack, age 33, and Katherine, a 32-year-old nurse, presented in a marital crisis. Jack was very depressed and despondent. Diagnosed with a mild case of MS 1 year ago, he expected to be wheelchair bound, mentally impaired, and seriously compromised in the fathering of his two small children. Katherine was intolerant of his attitude and thought he could lead a good life, even with a chronic illness like MS, believing that "disabilities become handicaps if you let them take over."
> Jack's family background was significant in that, as he put it, "Everyone has a cross to bear. Everything is a catastrophe. Suffering brings status." When Jack was growing up, his father had a chronic anxiety disorder that had controlled family life. Since the diagnosis of MS, whenever Jack and Katherine visited Jack's family, his relatives granted his every wish: at the age of 33, he clearly had the biggest cross to bear.
> Katherine's basic beliefs were "When you get hurt, you get hugs and kisses, and then you get out there and fight, like my grandmother who escaped from the Nazis after being shot in the leg." Her parents had divorced when she was 10, and her mother had successfully obtained a job and reared the kids.

Their different fundamental beliefs about health issues and how to manage adversity were the focus of treatment. Each partner had very different legacies and family scripts concerning control, the meaning of illness, and the rights and privileges of being sick. These came into full play during the initial crisis phase of an illness with an uncertain course. In Katherine, Jack could see values that would align with his own and others that would challenge him. Katherine, as a nurse, had a great capacity for caregiving, which his helpless side found attractive. In her belief in mastering adversity, Jack saw something foreign to his experience, but something that he admired and wanted to emulate. Their underlying different beliefs now expressed themselves fully during a health crisis. Changing his values, which he gradually did, meant not only relinquishing the status attained in his family of origin and his desire for the kind of attention his father had received, but also exchanging values that granted status at the price of shame for more empowering beliefs that strengthened their marriage.

In some Hispanic and Asian cultures, for example, it is expected that the family should protect the patient (Tse, Chong, & Fok, 2003); in other words, the spouse, not the patient, should be informed of the diagnosis, prognosis, and disease course. This cultural expectation can powerfully influence a couple's ability to cope and adapt. Such prescribed cultural norms regarding how medical information is communicated should be acknowledged between partners and with the health care team.

LIFE-CYCLE IMBALANCES

Life-cycle imbalances are typically experienced most acutely at transition periods in both individual and couple life cycles. The disorder, of necessity, needs to be brought into bold relief at these times, often revealing stark differences in each partner's capacities to envision and fulfill life-cycle goals. Previously manageable gaps can now be experienced as unbridgeable chasms that threaten the core of the relationship. Open dialogue is essential at these times.

The type of disorder can clarify the degree to which an illness (1) currently interferes with life-cycle planning and (2) how the future progression, disability, and shortened life expectancy may affect each partner's and the couple's development. These factors can help focus the discussion of each partner's and the couple's developmental goals. The psychosocial demands of the illness over time and individual and couples' development each need consideration separately and as an interwoven whole.

Because of skewed abilities, attention to balancing both a partner's and couple's goals is most valuable. As discussed in Chapter 7, for couples living with a serious illness, a well partner's ability to pursue individual goals can facilitate commitment to a relationship and strengthen the couple's bond. Especially with disabling conditions, where well partners may have a tendency to defer (or deny) individual needs, clinicians' explicit inquiry about and support for these needs legitimizes them and promotes effective dialogue between each partner. Madsen's (2011) useful concept of collaborative helping maps facilitates viable planning by offering a clear vision of individual partner and couple goals and the constraints and the resources available to achieving those goals. Couples who best master challenges are those who have the broadest and most flexible definitions of acceptable roles and have alternative means of satisfying developmental needs.

Younger Couples

Life-cycle imbalances are most evident in younger couples at early stages of their relationship, when chronic disorders are most untimely. Research suggests that young adults experiencing chronic illness for the first time may experience greater distress and difficulty with collaborative dyadic coping (Berg & Upchurch, 2007). Most individual and collective dreams have yet to be achieved, and so the sense of loss and of being robbed is more acute. The distinctions between the couple and their age peers are often exquisitely apparent. Redefining personal and relationship goals in the context of imposed limitations can strain both partners. The ill partner often becomes more aware of the pragmatic difficulty of achieving normative goals, such as beginning a family or pursuing career goals. The ill person may not want to burden or disappoint the partner, and therefore may minimize her or his actual limits. The well partner often realizes that the price of commitment to the relationship may mean forgoing key personal or relationship dreams, such as having children, or that achieving such goals will require unusual persistence and possible hardship.

Clinicians can help couples anticipate life-cycle points at which issues of imbalance, autonomy, limitations, and complexity become heightened. At these key junctures, couples can be helped to negotiate issues of pursuing individual and collective goals in a balanced and mutually respectful manner. As the next two cases illustrate, it is often at these transitions that couples have an excellent opportunity to grow as a couple and redefine the constraining aspects of a relationship.

For Carlos and Maria, the decision to start a family meant that each of them had to accept compromise. Maria had continual chronic pain from a severe accident. Because of her disability, Carlos needed to acknowledge that there would be an inherent imbalance in the practical tasks of parenting, and he would have to scale back his personal goals for career advancement. Maria needed to face her limits more directly, as she poignantly stated in the first few months after their daughter was born, "Although I tried to prepare myself, it was a painful time for me. I had to accept my limitations in a way I never had to before."

Some couples may decide not to or be unable to have children.

Stan and Alice, in similar circumstances, decided to forgo raising a family. As a result, Alice planned to expand her career aspirations. Although this was a healthy way for her to ensure that the relationship would not stifle all areas of her individual development, it heightened a sense of loss for her disabled husband, who suffered the double blow of not having children and not being able to work. Stan became depressed. Alice assured Stan that, even though he was disabled and could not work, her freedom to pursue some of her personal dreams strengthened her commitment to the relationship. Out of this process, Stan decided, for the first time, to become involved in community activities and volunteer work within his physical limits. Alice's pursuit of her own dreams had triggered a developmental crisis for Stan, in which he finally had to choose between expanding his personal options or remaining despondent. This couple's process was helped by the fact that remaining childless has become a more common, active choice, and that couples can express their need for generativity in diverse ways.

With untimely conditions, couples often have trouble finding age peers with whom to share relationship and life-cycle concerns related to living with illness and disability. In this regard, younger couples tend to become more isolated. Generally, support groups are disease specific; less commonly are they geared explicitly for couples; rarely are they organized according to age groupings. For instance, a cancer support group, although it addresses many concerns common to couples at different ages, may not meet the life-cycle dilemmas of a younger couple. When feasible, clinicians can be extremely helpful by promoting networking among couples coping with chronic disorders at similar phases of development. Time-limited multicouple discussion groups or 1-day workshops as described in the MS Resilient Partners Program in Chapter 18 are particularly useful to younger couples. Often such groups address sensitive subjects, such as sexual intimacy, more rapidly than might otherwise be achieved in standard conjoint sessions. Inclusion of sensitive topics, such as sexual relations, into the group psychoeducational component facilitates couples initiating discussion. One couple who opens up about such challenges can draw other couples into conversations that have been previously avoided. When useful, group dialogue can be combined with an individual couple's consultation for a more in-depth, private discussion.

Just as healthy couples may avoid friends who are coping with serious illness, couples coping with a chronic condition may also become avoidant of and tentative about reaching out to friends, furthering their own isolation. They can become extremely self-conscious and insecure, feeling that their peers cannot understand their situation. Often they are dealing with issues that are more normative in later life-cycle phases and experience being out of sync with their friends. Sometimes tentativeness and fears by both well couples and those dealing with illness can lead to an escalating cycle of distancing that results in a breakdown in relationships. Couples who prevent the disorder from becoming their total identity and can accept any unavoidable imbalances with peers can best counteract the tendency to isolate themselves.

Midlife and Later-Life Couples

For couples in middle or later life, the transitions of launching children and retirement involve the end of major commitments that have lasted for many years. Release from these commitments typically creates time for each partner to reevaluate his or her personal goals and their relationship as a couple. Fantasies about and plans for the use of leisure time come to the fore. The compromises necessitated by a chronic condition may heighten feelings of being robbed. Plans for traveling more or moving to a new place that needed to be deferred and have kept spirits up during arduous times now may need to be confronted as unrealistic and require revisioning. In our work-ethic-driven culture, all of us need to be reminded that life offers no guarantees, and that, when feasible, we need to set aside time for pleasures, even small ones, at all life phases.

Especially at midlife, ending a relationship burdened by a longstanding illness may feel more attainable when parenting obligations no longer exist. Generally, for both partners, the risks of ending the marriage, starting an affair, and experiencing depression are highest at these times. When faced with more serious and debilitating illnesses, long, unmet relationship needs may interact powerfully with an awareness of one's mortality and the realization that there is still enough time to establish another life. As one woman put it, "I raised three kids by myself for the past 20 years while my husband was disabled. I want a chance to live while there is still time." This woman's feelings of anger and entitlement were counterbalanced by a sense of guilt that she would be abandoning her disabled husband to living alone or to be cared for by her daughter, who would then unfairly inherit her burden. To navigate this family's complex transition required sessions with the couple, the adult children together and individually, and the family unit.

To work effectively with such couples, clinicians need to be aware of their own biases that might align them with the particular values of one partner or preconceived ideas about older couples' being unchangeable or about illness as just a part of old age. Loss of a satisfying sexual relationship can be just as painful for older couples as for younger ones. The realities of a couple entering late adulthood after years of stress and weariness from living with a chronic condition are very different from those of a healthy couple worrying about future infirmity. An older couple who knows all too well about living with chronic illness may be acutely aware of what their relationship could withstand if the well partner were to become ill or disabled. These couples may benefit from help in addressing realistic concerns about the need for enlisting greater support from adult children or extended kin or hiring a part- or full-time caregiver. In cases of more severe disability, they may need to consider a move to an assisted living or a skilled-nursing facility and possibly being separated in the process. Fostering open patterns of communication and joint decisions about future eventualities are the best preparation for these critical life-cycle junctures.

CHAPTER 15

Individual and Family Challenges in the New Era of Genetics

The study of genomics is changing the way illnesses are conceptualized, diagnosed, treated, and potentially prevented (Collins, Green, Guttmacher, & Guyer, 2003; Nussbaum, McInnes, & Willard, 2015). There is an increasing recognition of a genetic component in most serious physical and mental disorders. The burgeoning field of epigenetics studies how genes get switched on and off and how the expression of heritable traits can be modified by environmental influences, including individual and family lifestyles and processes (Reiss, Neiderhiser, & Hetherington, 2009; Schermerhorn et al., 2011; Spotts, 2012; Tienari et al., 2004).

New genetic technologies enable physicians to test for a heightened risk of developing a serious illness before it actually occurs. Testing for a genetic risk for common health conditions is increasingly entering mainstream medicine in primary care settings. The boundary between health and chronic illness has become blurred by the designation of "genetically at-risk." Individuals and families may live with illness-risk information long before loved ones, including future offspring, have developed symptoms of those conditions (Miller et al., 2006). The knowledge of future disease risk through genetic testing must be managed within a context of family relationships, cultural beliefs, outside resources, and the wider health care and societal systems.

These scientific advances confront families and clinicians with unprecedented and complex clinical and ethical challenges. Some fundamental questions include:

- Under what circumstances would individuals and families benefit from genetic risk screening and knowledge about their health risks or possible fate?
- How can we best help family members reach decisions about whether to pursue predictive testing?

- Who are the relevant family members to include in these decisions? Spouses or partners? Siblings? Extended family?
- How will testing affect families' lives if they are found to be at a genetic risk for a disorder?
- How will a couple's relationship (in terms of their commitment or decisions about having children) and their relationship with their extended family be affected?
- How, and at what age, should children be told they are at risk for a genetic disease or carrier status and that genetic testing is available?

Building on the FSI model, this chapter describes the Family Systems Genetic Illness (FSGI) model as a framework for organizing the expanding and complex array of genomic conditions (Rolland & Williams, 2005) and discusses key clinical issues, especially those related to living with uncertainty and using a developmental perspective (Rolland, 2006a). Myriad ethical challenges and issues related to cultural diversity are woven throughout.

Because most health and mental health conditions have a genetic component, clinicians need to assess families' assumptions and knowledge about how genetics and illness are linked. Even for those illnesses that don't have a known genetic aspect, there may be misperceptions or beliefs about a genetic component that need clarification.

With the advent of genomic medicine, attention to the *dimension of time* is more critical than ever. The FSGI model expands the definition of disease to include the nonsymptomatic period of living with genetic risk information prior to a clinical diagnosis. Family members will experience throughout their lives increasing amounts of available information about risks for traits (e.g., hearing loss), specific illnesses (e.g., Parkinson's disease), or a constellation of conditions (e.g., cardiovascular or autoimmune diseases or schizophrenic disorders). Genetic testing is utilized for multiple purposes, including preconception and prenatal screening and diagnosis, newborn screening, carrier testing, diagnosis and prognosis of a genetic disorder, and presymptomatic and predictive testing.*

The availability of these genetic tests offers the *possibility* of learning more about the degree of risk. The possibility of incurring future illness affects the individual psyche, specific relationships, family identity, and meaning-making.

---

*A presymptomatic test is used to identify the high likelihood that a healthy person will develop an inherited disease (e.g., Huntington's disease). For some disorders, predictive testing of genetic susceptibility identifies genetic factors that increase the likelihood that the person with a family history of the disorder will develop the disease (e.g., hereditary breast and ovarian cancer (HBOC)). Carrier testing is used to identify if a person has a mutation in one copy of a gene for a recessive condition (e.g., cystic fibrosis and Duchenne muscular dystrophy). In most cases, carriers do not have symptoms of the disease, but have a 50% chance of passing the gene with the mutation on to their children. Newborn screening seeks to diagnose children with medical conditions for which early treatment can reduce morbidity and mortality.

Responses can influence affected members' health from conception to death, including life-course decisions and developmental paths, such as forming a committed relationship, starting a family, and career and retirement plans (Rolland, 1999).

THE FSGI MODEL: PSYCHOSOCIAL TYPOLOGY AND TIME PHASES OF GENOMIC DISORDERS

The FSGI model is intended for conditions with a genetic component for which testing is, or may become, available. This schema is flexible enough to be adapted to ongoing genomic scientific advances and potential reclassification of diseases. It groups disorders that have similar patterns of psychosocial demands during the nonsymptomatic phases before and after genetic testing.

The typology of genomic illness highlights four variables.

1. Likelihood of developing a condition based on genetic mutations
2. Overall clinical severity (regarding symptoms, disability, and outcome)
3. Timing of the clinical onset in the life cycle
4. Whether effective treatment interventions that can alter the clinical onset and/or progression exist

These variables are hypothesized to be the most psychosocially significant for a wide range of genomic disorders and, as with the typology of chronic disorders, provide a vital bridge between the biological and psychosocial worlds. Testing is intended to clarify whether or not a person has a specific genetic mutation. Test results may show the existence of a mutation, but uncertainty about the likelihood, timing, and severity of the condition still remains. The typology includes disorders in which individuals can be *carriers of a genetic mutation* related to a specific disease, such as cystic fibrosis (CF). Individuals who have carrier status may have no risk of the disease themselves. But, from a broader multigenerational family system perspective, the risk of CF exists for offspring. Carriers or potential carriers of the CF mutation bear a psychosocial burden—not for their own personal risk of symptomatic disease, but for their children, particularly when considering a committed relationship and family planning. The next section of this chapter looks at each of the components of the typology in more detail.

Psychosocial Typology of Genomic Illness: Components

Likelihood of Developing a Condition Based on Genetic Mutations

This variable addresses the likelihood of clinical onset, including the degree of risk that can be clarified for a condition through current testing. Genomic conditions can be grouped in terms of (1) a high likelihood, that is, a high level of penetrance of a genetic mutation (see Table 15.1); (2) a variable likelihood, or (3) a lower likelihood, reflecting complex multiple gene and gene–environment interactions. Traditional autosomal-dominant inherited conditions, such as Huntington's disease, are at one end of the continuum, with a very high likelihood. If the person chooses testing and is positive, the individual and family members must absorb the near certainty that the disease will develop.

Many recent genomic discoveries are currently in the variable range. They consist of multifactorial disorders, such as many forms of cancer that are determined by the interaction of single or multiple genes and environmental factors. For instance, individuals with a mutation in a gene for breast and ovarian cancer have a heightened risk, but they may or may not develop these diseases. An example of a "lower-likelihood" mutation involves a common variant of the gene for apolipoprotein E, which is present in over 25% of the U.S. population and increases the 3% baseline risk for Alzheimer's disease in later life only modestly (Nussbaum et al., 2015).

A highly penetrant genetic mutation presents a qualitatively different form of stressor to family members than one with a lower penetrance. Because of the increased odds of disease onset with highly penetrant mutations, families may be more likely to prepare for what lies ahead. Yet, it can interfere

TABLE 15.1. Useful Genetic Terms

Autosomal dominant inheritance: a pattern of inheritance in which every child of a patient, regardless of gender, has a 50% chance of inheriting the gene that causes the disease.

Epigenetics: the study of the way in which the expression of heritable traits is modified by environmental influences or other mechanisms without changes in DNA sequence.

Genetic mutations: alterations in a DNA sequence.

Genetics: the study of single genes and their effects.

Genome: an organism's DNA.

Genomics: the study of the function and interaction of all the genes in the human genome, including their interactions with environmental factors.

Multifactorial: denotes conditions or diseases in which multiple genetic and environmental factors contribute to the presence of the condition or disease.

Penetrance: the likelihood that, in a given population, persons with a specific gene mutation will manifest signs of a disorder.

Recessive inheritance: a pattern of inheritance in which a variant of a gene causes clinical symptoms only when two copies are present on a pair of autosomal (not sex) chromosomes.

with life-cycle planning and a sense of hopefulness about the future (Brouwer-Dudokdewit, Savenije, Zoeteweij, Maat-Kievit, & Tibben, 2002). With lower-penetrance mutations, a salient adaptational challenge for families involves living with more ongoing uncertainty.

Overall Clinical Severity

This variable involves the expected degree of disease burden. When considered with the "likelihood of development" variable, it entails practical and emotional meanings for those contending with whether or when a disease will occur. For instance, Huntington's disease onset is inevitable; it is also progressive, highly disabling (including dementia), and fatal. In contrast, an increased genetic risk for hereditary breast and ovarian cancer (HBOC) is much more uncertain in terms of whether cancer will occur and, given the available treatment options, the trajectory or disease burden if it does. Living with such ambiguities can be extremely taxing psychosocially (see Chapter 9).

Timing of the Clinical Onset in the Life Cycle

The timing of onset of a genomic disorder in individual and family life cycles has major implications. Three broad time periods of typical onset are *childhood and adolescence, 0–20 years old* (e.g., most cases of cystic fibrosis and asthma); *early-to-middle adulthood and the child-rearing years, 20–60 years old* (e.g., Huntington's disease, HBOC); *and later life, over 60 years old* (e.g., most forms of Alzheimer's disease).

Considering the timing of clinical onset in relation to life-cycle development clarifies both the immediate and long-term challenges. For instance, disorders that strike a parent during the early-to-middle child-rearing phase are most disruptive to parenting and overall family stability (Werner-Lin, 2008). They affect key family developmental tasks, challenging a couple's relationship, child rearing, financial and household demands, and prompting a realignment of relationships with extended family and of grandparenting roles (Rolland, 2016).

Prevention and Treatment

Conditions can be categorized as to *the availability of effective treatment interventions that can alter the clinical onset and/or progression*. For instance, with Huntington's disease, no treatment currently exists to prevent clinical onset or halt progression. Individuals with the gene mutation will get the disease, and it is fatal. By contrast, individuals who carry an HBOC mutation have access to early detection methods, such as increased mammographic surveillance, which may improve prognosis; to options like preventive chemotherapy or a bilateral mastectomy that decreases the risk of clinical onset; and to a variety of treatment strategies if cancer is later diagnosed. Some conditions, like HBOC, may involve more than one illness type: those that are more highly responsive to preventive treatment and those that are less responsive. Advances in pharmacogenetics are beginning to alter treatment strategies for many health conditions.

A Psychosocial Typology Matrix

A useful typology can be generated by combining the above variables: the likelihood of developing a condition based on genetic mutations (high, variable, or lower), the overall clinical severity (high or low), the timing of clinical onset in the life cycle, and the availability of effective treatments to alter clinical onset or progression. Each type of condition has a distinct pattern of psychosocial demands based on its biological and environmental responsive features. Analogous to the psychosocial typology described in Chapter 2, thinking about the independent and combined effects of these variables can facilitate discussions with patients and their families. For instance, most forms of Alzheimer's disease have a lower likelihood of development, occur in later life, have a high severity, and lack effective prevention or treatment options.

Expanding the Concept of Illness Time Phases

Genetic testing allows us to expand our thinking about the time phases of chronic disorders to include the time before clinical onset. The nonsymptomatic phases include (1) awareness, (2) crisis I pretesting, (3) crisis II test–posttesting, and (4) long-term adaptation (see Figure 15.1). Each nonsymptomatic phase poses distinct developmental challenges (see Table 15.2). The phases are distinguished by concerns about living with uncertainty (Rolland, 2006a) related to the potential amount of genetic knowledge medically available, decisions about how much of that information various family members choose to access, and living with the psychosocial impact of those choices. They can guide periodic family consultations, or "psychosocial checkups."

Awareness Phase

The nonsymptomatic awareness phase begins with some recognition of possible genetic risk, regardless of whether genetic testing is available, and before actively considering actual testing. Key goals include (1) establishing initial communication in the family about the illness and genetics; (2) seeking information about the genetics of the specific illness from one's primary care provider or a genetic specialist; (3) considering whether individual family members could pursue genetic testing (based on family rules regarding need for consensus); and (4) coping with and adapting to concerns about genetic conditions appearing in the media, but for which no genetic test yet exists.

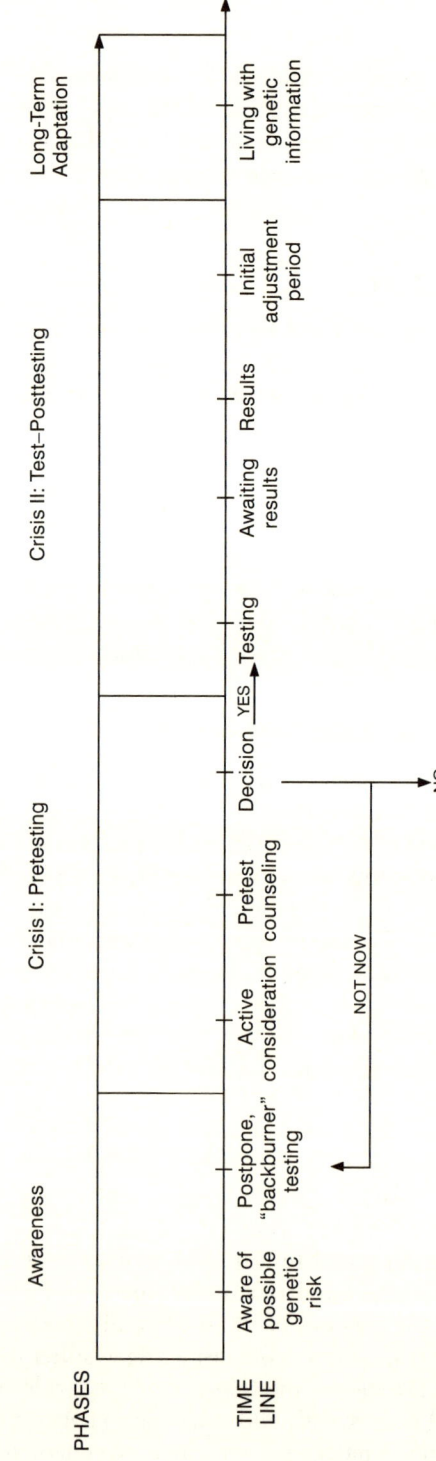

FIGURE 15.1. Nonsymptomatic time phases of genetically linked disorders. Excerpted from Rolland and Williams (2005).

TABLE 15.2. Nonsymptomatic Time Phases of Genomic Disorders: Developmental Challenges

Awareness Phase (Begins with awareness of possible genetic risk)
1. Establish initial communication in family regarding genetics of illness.
2. Seek basic information regarding the genetics of specific illness from primary care provider.
3. Consider whether individual family members could pursue genetic testing (e.g., rules on the need for family consensus or individual autonomy).
4. Cope with and adapt to concerns about conditions where no genetic testing yet exists.

Crisis Phase I: Pretesting
1. Consider how a decision might affect different nuclear and extended family members.
2. Gain an understanding of the genetics of illness.
3. Gain a psychosocial understanding of the illness in practical, emotional, longitudinal, and developmental terms.
4. Gain an appreciation of the developmental perspective (individual, family, and illness).
5. View the challenge of genetic knowledge as a shared one in "we" terms.
6. Consider who in the family may be at risk and who to inform.
7. Consider whom to include in decision making (e.g., spouse, other family member) about whether to test.
8. Explore family beliefs about the meaning of genetics (e.g., blame, stigma, special).
9. Reach a decision about whether to test now or to defer until later.

Crisis Phase II: Testing and Posttesting
1. Crisis coping and adaptation to new genetic knowledge.
2. Accept the permanence of genetic-testing knowledge.
3. Maximize the preservation of family identity before obtaining genetic knowledge.
4. Create meaning that promotes personal and family mastery.
5. Acknowledge possibilities of loss related to genetic risk, while sustaining hope.
6. Develop flexibility in the face of uncertainty.
7. Consider implications of testing results for family members who test normal and at-risk members who have not been tested.
8. Establish functional collaborative relationships with health care providers.
9. Adapt to any preventive treatments and health care settings.

Long-Term Adaptation Phase (if results are positive)
1. Maximize autonomy and connectedness for all family members within scope of genetic knowledge.
2. Minimize relationship imbalances.
3. Mindfulness about the possible impact on current and future phases of family and individual life cycles.
4. Live with anticipatory loss and uncertainty.
5. Balance open communication (vs. avoidance and denial) and proactive planning with the need to live a "normal" life, keeping threatened illness in perspective.
6. Maintain up-to-date genetic and medically relevant information.

Adapted from Rolland and Williams (2005).

In a family with a multigenerational history of a genomic disorder, such as heart disease, there may be an undercurrent of concern about vulnerability. With known genomic conditions, such as hemophilia, the perpetuation of an illness in the family system may be expected, despite uncertainty about which members will develop it. When a family's multigenerational experience seems genetically unremarkable, members are usually not concerned about lurking genomic conditions. They may be unaware of genetic risks or illness patterns or attribute diseases in the family to other causes. Those who have not been sensitized to life with genetic-risk information may have the sharpest emotional transition as new genetic tests become available for a range of common conditions.

In many families, multigenerational stories have evolved about a condition that "runs in the family." With genetic testing, these family stories collide with information attainable from high-technology medicine, often clarifying both a diagnosis and its inheritance pattern. In one family, a history of "increasing incoordination" now has a name, spinocerebellar ataxia. If you have the genetic mutation, you will not only get the disease, but you will also have a good idea of the age at which it will likely strike and, based on advances in DNA analysis, a good prediction of its severity. With this new technology, living with uncertainty is transformed to include the process of deciding whether and when one may want to clarify individual risk.

For inevitable, fatal disorders like Huntington's disease, the issue becomes deciding between different ways of living with anticipatory loss—either informed by genetic testing or not. While illness and death are universal experiences, knowing that one will very likely develop the disease at midlife clarifies the likely timing and form of a fatal illness. For some, acquiring this knowledge is emotionally debilitating; for others, it can focus their priorities and life planning, enhancing a sense of control. For disorders, such as genetically-influenced heart disease, in which the likelihood of development is highly variable and effective prevention and treatment are available, the trajectory is very uncertain, both in terms of disease onset and outcome. For these kinds of conditions, the experience of uncertainty is quite different. For some people, the idea of identifying any mutation can be crushing; for others, preventive steps, when available, may help foster a sense of mastery in meeting a biological challenge.

DISEASE WITH KNOWN MANIFESTATIONS AND A MULTIGENERATIONAL HISTORY

Stories concerning a specific condition, such as hemophilia, are often passed down through the generations. They commonly provide basic family scripts for the affected and unaffected family members (Byng-Hall, 2004). Emotional intensity often is greatest for at-risk members who have directly known and witnessed another family member's experience of living with a particular disease. Some may have been caregivers for a family member with the same condition they are vulnerable to. It is valuable to inquire about such prior sensitization and its role in creating meaning about the genetic condition in the context of family identity (see Chapter 6). Witnessing forms of suffering or disability may result in quite different attitudes. In one family, 10 years of grueling caregiving for a family member who was reduced to a helpless state and who did not recognize loved ones, left a legacy of dread of dementia. One son stated, "If I'm ever disabled like my dad, I'd rather be dead." Yet in another family, the son said, "Even when my father had Alzheimer's, he still was loving and seemed to enjoy being with our family. It's inspiring and helps me appreciate that even if I get Alzheimer's, I will have something to live for."

ACCESS AND AFFORDABILITY

Families that lack adequate health care are particularly disadvantaged, heightening health disparities for underserved populations, including low income, immigrant, and persons of color. They may be unaware of predictive testing for hereditary forms of illness, such as colorectal cancer, and lack access to early and regular screening to diagnose and successfully treat precancerous polyps and the early stages of the disease. The costs of genetic tests or preventive interventions may be prohibitive.

Crisis Phase I: Pretesting

This phase involves the active consideration of testing, an understanding of relevant genetic knowledge, and the psychosocial ramifications of testing for oneself and the family. It continues through the period of decision making about whether to get tested. One key task for the individual is to consider the effect that genetic testing might have on the rest of the family and on family dynamics. Individuals must think carefully about what other family members may be at risk, what members to inform about testing, and with whom to communicate the results. Who does the person want to include in making a decision about whether to undergo testing? In some cases, this would be the spouse or partner and in other cases, the parents, children, and siblings.

Clinicians can help an individual to understand (1) which relatives are at risk, (2) the correct, essential information about the genetic risk, and (3) strategies for sharing the information with different family members of varied ages. To promote accurate communication, it is useful to provide other family members with informational aids, such as a copy of the family ancestry diagram, basic information about genetics, and a copy of personal risk information. The individual can ask the provider to review an "informational" letter that he or she plans to send to other family members. Data support the belief that family members' accurate knowledge about a genomic condition is associated with less decisional conflict about genetic testing (Cameron & Muller, 2009).

The decision to proceed with genetic testing is associated more with a perceived risk rather than with scientific data about the risk (Lerman, Croyle, Tercyak, & Hamann, 2002). As such, inquiring about the meaning of risk information as filtered through cultural and multigenerational perspectives will help clarify the key factors in the decision-making process. This process is more intense if the mutation is highly penetrant and causes a severe, life-shortening disease, such as Duchenne muscular dystrophy, for which prevention and treatment options are limited.

Families need the latest information on advances in preventive medical surveillance and lifestyle options that can affect disease onset or outcome. Outdated information might contribute to misinformed testing decisions and concerns, especially in families with a multigenerational history of diseases, such as breast or colon cancer. Relatives in the past may have had a relentless course with a fatal outcome, leaving a legacy of hopelessness (Reibstein, 2004).

INDIVIDUAL RIGHTS VERSUS COLLECTIVE FAMILY RESPONSIBILITY

A right to privacy is a basic tenet of health care and the physician–patient relationship. Genetic testing challenges this idea because it has the potential to affect many more lives and the future of the entire family system. Yet concerns about stigma and discrimination breeds secrecy. In my work with the breast cancer service at the University of Chicago, I reviewed the histories of families that were potentially at a high genetic risk according to the genograms of biological relatives. I was most struck by the large number of family members affected by genetic risk both vertically across generations and horizontally within each generation. Because one family member exploring his or her genetic risk can affect so many others, we need to consider carefully, in each case, our ethical positions about privacy, responsible communication, and the advisability of scheduling pretesting family consultations. I strongly encourage individuals in committed couple relationships to share their decision making with their spouse since the results affect both the partner and the relationship. Developmentally, partners need to consider how the outcome might influence future hopes and dreams, family planning, potential caregiving, and spousal loss.

Distinguishing family member privacy from potentially destructive secrecy is crucial. If the decision is made to keep genetic testing hidden from the extended family, there are real risks for future blame, shame, and guilt. Secrecy may come back to haunt the individual if an uninformed relative develops a serious condition and would have benefited from knowing about it earlier, especially if preventive steps are available. One useful way to be collectively responsible and still maintain some privacy is to inform the extended family that testing is being done for a particular genetic mutation, how it is inherited, who is at potential risk, and where other family members can get professional genetic counseling. Families that have estranged relationships are of particular concern. Offering pre- and posttesting consultations can help individuals explore the implications of maintaining ruptures and secrecy in the face of genetic knowledge, which may have life and death implications. Optimally, those considering testing can view the issue of genetic knowledge as a shared challenge with loved ones.

TIMING OF CONSIDERATION OF TESTING

The nonsymptomatic crisis phase often begins when a genetic test becomes available, or a physician suggests possible testing. For others who are aware of an existing genetic test, an active desire to consider testing may occur as they reach a milestone or major transition in the individual or family life cycle (e.g., a relationship commitment). For instance, some women decide to test for HBOC genes when they reach the same age as that of a blood relative who was diagnosed with breast or ovarian cancer. They believe they are entering a heightened "danger period." Some consider testing when they contemplate starting a family and worry about passing on a genetic vulnerability to their children; others do so when another family member pursues testing and learns of a genomic condition in the family.

The decision-making process may not be a one-time event; some individuals consider and postpone testing more than once. One woman with a strong family history of early breast cancer had a sister who tested positive for a HBOC gene, BRCA1. She considered predictive testing at age 20, and again at 24 before getting married. Although she was anxious about her future risk, she deferred testing until her and her husband's discussion about starting a family tipped the balance at age 26.

When a family member is the first to seriously consider testing, a larger question arises: Is this disease hereditary and therefore part of the family's identity and destiny? If so, how would this information affect how family members see themselves, and how others see them as a family (e.g., flawed, stigmatized, special, doomed, or resilient) in the face of adversity?

PRESELECTION

Often, family members will informally identify those members who they believe are more likely to inherit a genetic disorder and those they think are likely to be spared. Typically, this decision is based on gender or resemblance to an affected member. But this approach can be risky if others decide not to be tested, neglect regular preventive care, and the disease is then detected at an advanced stage. Preselection beliefs often help to define life choices and future planning, yet are not openly discussed among family members. Clinicians can inquire about preselection from a life-cycle perspective: "Are there ways you and your family have already organized your lives in relation to beliefs about your genetic risk?" And "What might be the implications for all of you if you get expected or unexpected test results?"

Crisis Phase II: Testing and Posttesting

Whether family members test positive or negative for an illness, either outcome can precipitate an immediate crisis. As with the crisis phase of an illness onset, families face specific developmental challenges. These include (1) accepting the current genetic information, with the knowledge that new scientific developments are rapidly expanding, (2) preserving valued aspects of personal or family identity, (3) creating meaning about the genetic information in a way that preserves a family's sense of mastery, and (4) developing family flexibility in the face of future uncertainty and loss to maximize preservation of key life-cycle goals (Rolland, 2006a).

In one family, the ailing father was diagnosed with spinocerebellar ataxia, an inherited progressive neurological disorder with severe muscle incoordination and speech and swallowing difficulties. The five young adult offspring then pursued testing; two learned that they were highly likely to develop the disease; three tested normal. Family consultations encouraged all members to discuss the significance of the test results and their relationships and to begin to anticipate future caregiving needs, role changes, and financial support. These discussions deepened sibling bonds and laid the groundwork for facing future challenges collaboratively.

UNEXPECTED TEST RESULTS

A person who expected to have a specific genetic mutation, but postponed testing, may experience grief for the opportunities not taken when later learning of normal test results.

In one case, a man, who assumed he would develop his father's progressive degenerative neurological disease at midlife, tailored his life choices in early adulthood to accommodate this expectation. He married a woman whom he felt would be a good caregiver when he eventually became ill and disabled. Further, he had a vasectomy to ensure that this genetic disease would not be passed on and because he thought he would be a burden to his wife and an inadequate parent if, as expected, he did not survive the child-rearing years without disease onset, disability, or even death. Finally, he abandoned his ambition to pursue a career in medicine because of the lengthy training period, and instead, chose a more modest career path as a computer technician. When specific testing became available, he tested normal at age 35 for the specific mutation. Afterward, he became despondent, feeling that he had needlessly sacrificed having children and becoming a physician. His depression and a serious marital crisis led to referral to a family therapist. A combination of individual and couple's sessions helped him and his wife realize that they made good life decisions based on his reasonable expectations and the uncertainties at the time. Then they explored new reproductive options to having children, including adoption.

Clinicians can ask adolescents or young adults about their future dreams and how fears regarding any familial illnesses may influence their life planning. This inquiry can stimulate a discussion of the pros and cons of formulating life goals in relation to a perceived or actual risk.

Sometimes a family member's informal attribution of high or low risk turns out opposite to expectations, as in the following case.

Mary, age 27 and married for 2 years, was referred a month after testing positive for BRCA1. Her family history was significant: A maternal aunt had recently died at age 49 of breast cancer, and Mary's mother had been diagnosed with in-situ breast cancer a year earlier, electing a bilateral mastectomy. Her 25-year-old sister, Jane, strongly resembles their mother, while Mary is strikingly similar to her hardy father, physically and in personality. Also, Mary had always been "the protector" of her younger, somewhat physically frail sister. Mary and her husband had discussed testing before marrying, but they decided to defer testing for what they saw as "low risk." When her sister, Jane, became engaged, she and her fiancé decided to pursue testing. Mary then decided to be tested at the same time to be supportive of her sister, whom she assumed would be BRCA1 positive. The testing results revealed that Mary was positive and Jane negative. Mary was shocked and devastated, completely unprepared to find that she carried the BRCA1 mutation, and not her sister. For the first time she was in the unfamiliar position of needing support from Jane, who was unaccustomed to being the supportive sibling. This unexpected news started a process of reshaping their relational dynamics and rebalancing their relationship to be more mutually supportive. In doing so, they redefined competence more flexibly to include life challenges and areas of strength as well as vulnerability. Both became more resilient individuals as they strengthened their bond.

This case highlights the value of brief family psychoeducation before and after genetic testing to minimize the possibility that individuals and their families will be shocked by unexpected test results.

ALTERED RELATIONSHIPS BETWEEN THOSE WHO TEST NORMAL AND THE AT-RISK GROUP

Genetic testing creates three distinct subgroups: (1) those who test positive for the specific mutation, (2) those who test negative, and (3) those who have yet to be tested and remain potentially at risk. Relationship realignments can occur among these subgroups. Those that test positive often remain psychologically linked to those who remain potentially at risk and who still live with a heightened awareness of risk. Both groups live with anticipatory loss, albeit with different degrees of knowledge. Their common threat may strengthen their relationship bonds. Other bonds between those anticipating future illness and those without genetic risk may fray. A family member with normal test results may fear the premature loss of a close member who tested positive. Optimal prevention includes pretesting consultations that educate family members about these challenges and promote ongoing open dialogue and periodic follow-up consultations.

SURVIVOR GUILT AND ALTRUISTIC INTENTIONS

Family members not at risk might say, "How can I enjoy life and my own good health, when she will likely get breast cancer and maybe die from it." Survivor guilt may lead them to conduct their lives in self-defeating ways or take risks that undermine their own health. Psychoeducational family consultation can explore and normalize these complex emotions.

For those who test normal, compassion for those less fortunate, as well as survivor guilt, can be channeled in positive ways through altruistic actions (Perry & Rolland, 2009; Williams, Schutte, Evers, & Holkup, 2000). After her two sisters tested positive for BRCA1, a third sister, who tested normal, became involved as a volunteer for the National Breast Cancer Foundation, which provides public education, advocacy, and peer counseling for those affected or at high risk. This gave her a sense of purpose that offset her feelings of being the "lucky one."

ONGOING RELATIONSHIP TO HEALTH CARE PROVIDERS

Posttesting contact with the health care system, unlike that needed for those with active disease, may be minimal or periodic (e.g., more frequent mammograms or colonoscopies). Yet the psychosocial impact may be enormous, and individuals and families may benefit from periodic emotional support that is timed with difficult transitions. This situation is at odds with the current design of our health care system; psychosocial care, when provided, tends to occur around symptomatic health crises.

Long-Term Adaptation Phase

This phase is the time span between positive genetic testing results and the manifestation of the condition. It may vary from a short time to decades or even one's entire life if the illness never emerges. Major adaptational challenges in this phase involve minimizing relationship imbalances between the genetically affected and unaffected family members and their ability to live as fully as possible, given their heightened genetic risk. Several other keys to family mastery include (1) remaining mindful about the possible effect of genetic knowledge on current and future phases of family and individual development and (2) keeping up to date with new information about genetic risk and advances in preventive or symptomatic treatment (see Table 15.2).

Families are strongly affected by the concerns of "if" and "when" a condition might strike. As discussed earlier, some genomic conditions can be expected to occur within a certain period of the life cycle. If so, increased anxieties about threatened loss might surface as individuals and families approach that specific life-cycle phase. It might occur as the person approaches the age at which another family member developed the specific condition. Note the age of illness onset for affected family members. Prevention-oriented individual and family consultations are valuable at these junctures.

VIGILANCE IN LOOKING FOR "FIRST SIGNS"

Looking for the first sign of a genomic disorder is similar to remaining vigilant about a recurrence of cancer. With conditions of variable likelihood, the first signs can crush any hope of not getting the disorder at all. For nearly certain inherited conditions like Huntington's disease, looking for the first sign is not a question of if but when. Experiencing the first signs means transitioning from anxious waiting to entering the world of living with an active disease with high severity, major caregiving needs, and a fatal outcome. Anticipatory loss can be especially intense for highly penetrant disorders with high severity (see Chapter 9).

For individuals who test positive, fears about genetic susceptibility can continue throughout life. Every ambiguous symptom and medical appointment induce apprehension. One woman, age 55, who had a strong family history of colon cancer and who had tested positive for the specific high-risk mutation, got regular screening colonoscopies over many years that revealed benign polyps but no cancer. Despite the number of years in which she was cancer-free, she revealed, "Whenever I get a pain in my body, not just my abdomen, my first thought is that I finally got cancer and it will now kill me." Anxieties may be triggered, not only by annual checkups, but also by a diagnosis of another serious illness in an immediate or extended family member or friend or genetic testing by another family member. Since this is a typical experience, psychoeducation focused on these adaptational challenges in the early posttesting period can be very helpful.

Vigilance for the first signs of a genomic condition is particularly difficult when the common normative experiences of aging, such as memory lapses, occur. Clinicians can help families maintain a functional awareness without resorting to disabling hypervigilance for the onset of conditions like

Alzheimer's disease. Individuals with a blunting style of coping, in which symptoms are minimized, tend to be less vigilant with perceived risk in an emotionally adaptive way (Hurley, Miller, Rubin, & Weinberg, 2006). A higher-monitoring style of coping that involves an extensive focus on health threats and detailed health-related information is more useful in situations wherein early detection and treatment intervention might affect the course and outcome. Often different family members or spouses take these positions in a complementary manner. These normative differences in style and role functions can become polarized and conflictual in the context of uncertainty, where the stakes are very high at significant medical or life-cycle junctures, as in the following case.

Joan and Bill sought a couple's consultation with a family therapist for increasing marital discord. Joan had tested positive for BRCA1 several years earlier. Her blunting style led her to minimize any symptoms, such as lumpiness in her breasts, while her husband, Bill, with a more monitoring style, became very anxious about her minimizing concern over possibly significant symptoms. At times when she was due for her annual mammogram, her laissez-faire style of scheduling the exam conflicted sharply with his insistence on prompt and timely appointments. He felt that she was being insensitive toward him and irresponsible. She felt that he was both morbidly obsessed with disease and death and overinvolved in trying to be in control of her body. This led to escalating conflict in a vicious cycle. The more she told him to leave her alone, the more his hypervigilant anxious behavior escalated, and in turn, the more she "dug in her heels." This relational impasse was complicated by the fact that, when Bill was a teenager, his own mother had died of colon cancer that was discovered in an advanced inoperable stage.

Here interventions that help family members respect and balance both monitoring and blunting positions can diminish stylistic differences that become skewed and polarized. Also, useful information can guide the family in distinguishing significant warning signs from insignificant ones. Exploring prior sensitization to loss in either spouse's multigenerational history can facilitate an empathic understanding rather than reactive anger.

The existence of a genetic mutation in a family casts a shadow on future generations. In essence, learning about a genetic risk can involve loss of a common dream or the universal hope that one's children will have a better life (Sobel, Cowan, & Brookes, 2003). This is especially true with mutations that can cause severe illness with currently limited preventive options, such as Huntington's disease. As an antidote, clinicians can encourage families to sustain hope for future medical advances that may prevent a clinical onset or progression. It is also vital to stress that a family's process of deriving some meaning from genetic knowledge preserves their sense of value and competence.

CULTURAL MEANINGS AND BELIEFS

Ethnocultural values and attributions of meaning can strongly influence the personal and family experience of genetic testing and living with risk information (Paniagua & Taylor, 2008; Rolland, 2006b). Providers need an appreciation of the cultural norms and traditions of patients, families, and communities and anticipate how they will influence the way in which families interpret and act on genomic information (see Chapter 8). They need to understand the strong convictions about genetic testing or attributions about ancestors' genetic legacies held by highly religious groups, indigenous peoples, and non-European immigrant families, as well as the differences in beliefs across generations.

Because of culturally ingrained meanings, families might equate the word "genetics" with fate or stigma. With the advent of genomic medicine, in which multiples genes and environmental factors interact with genetic risk to cause disease, health practitioners need to help families deconstruct outdated deterministic meanings. It is particularly important to explore beliefs about the significance of genetic information, about the cause or inherited risk of an illness, and about mastery over and acceptance of a future risk that may be beyond their control.

Communication

Cultural norms vary in the kind and degree of open communication about genetic risk, including (1) between health care practitioners and the individual and family, (2) within the immediate family, (3) with extended family members, and (4) with the wider community.

For instance, in many Asian, Middle Eastern, and Muslim cultures, sharing a family history with outsiders is traditionally not considered appropriate behavior (Daneshpour, 1998). Seeking a complete family and medical history could be interpreted as an unwarranted intrusion and as an attempt to make the family responsible for an illness. A genetic condition brings shame and could seriously affect the ability of any offspring to marry. In these circumstances, a family's reluctance to convey crucial medical information can easily be misinterpreted by the clinician as noncompliance. Simultaneously, a highly valued cultural norm is to revere health care providers, such as physicians or genetic counselors, as experts who should be obeyed. The family may be in a significant bind. Here, collaborative conversations and decision making are culturally dissonant, and sharing a family illness history may conflict directly with a fear of shaming one's ancestors.

Tremendous cultural variation exists as to who among family members or friends should or should not be included in reaching decisions about genetic testing. Sometimes, seeking help outside the family, including from health care practitioners, may be seen as publicly shameful. Such beliefs can place serious constraints on utilizing genetic services (Sue & Sue, 2012; Wang, 2001). We can understand such beliefs as intended to protect the family from making detrimental decisions or taking actions that might bring shame on the entire family and its ancestors.

Diagnostic and Intervention Options

Cultural or religious beliefs can influence diagnostic and intervention options. For instance, some Asian-Pacific Islanders believe that blood and other body fluids carry the essence of life and must be conserved. This belief can foster a resistance to amniocentesis and diagnostic tests that require blood samples. Many Latino cultures value having an optimistic outlook about future health outcomes and use folk beliefs and religious faith for reassurance. This optimism can result in reducing the significance of genetic risk information in reproductive decision making (Penchaszadeh, 2001).

Ethnic and Racial Disparities and Differences

Increasingly, genomic research is discovering links between major health conditions and specific ethnic groups. Type 2 diabetes, heart disease, hypertension, obesity, and some cancers are more common among Hispanic populations; Tay-Sachs and HBOC in Jewish groups; sickle cell anemia in African Americans; and CF and phenylketonuria in U.S. whites (Nussbaum et al., 2015). As such, some diseases can become associated with specific groups due to increased prevalence, heightening their risk of stigma and discrimination.

Racial and ethnic differences in the use of genetic testing have been documented in a number of areas, including BRCA1/2 (Sherman, Miller, Shaw, Cavanagh, & Gorin, 2014) and amniocentesis testing (Saucier et al., 2005). Such usage disparities are due, in part, to factors such as socioeconomic status, objective risk, risk perceptions and attitudes, physician recommendations, and a lack of awareness of genomic services (Hall & Olopade, 2006). African Americans are less likely to endorse the health benefits of testing and to believe that testing could provide reassurance, and more likely to believe that genetic tests for cancer would be anxiety provoking and to express concern about the government's use of genetic testing information (Peters, Rose, & Armstrong, 2004). Historically, the African American community has rejected sickle-cell carrier screening because of concerns that it would increase discrimination or support claims of genetic inferiority. They also feared that such community-wide screening would result in government involvement in family life and reproductive choice and attempts to limit the African American population (Wailoo, 2001). There are many similar distrust issues in Native American communities. For Latinos, the influences that affect decisions about prenatal screening include language barriers and miscommunication, a lower degree of acculturation, traditional beliefs, and religious affiliation.

Basic Clinical Questions

Some useful questions to ask regarding socioeconomic, cultural, or religious influences include the following.

- What does the word "genetics" mean to you and your family?
- Are there any aspects of your culture that influence your beliefs about genetics?
- Does your culture make it difficult for you to tell me about health conditions that may run in your family? What should I (we) be aware of in your culture that makes this difficult?
- Are there specific cultural or religious rules regarding pursuing any diagnostic or predictive genetic tests or treatments?
- In your culture, are there rules about who in your family or community would be included in or excluded from communicating and making decisions about genetic testing?
- Do you have any concerns about how genetic information may get used or misused?

ADDITIONAL LIFE-CYCLE ISSUES

Increasingly, predictive testing may occur at earlier life-cycle phases, many years before a disease would likely occur. Early testing means that future disease challenges may feel remote to individuals, their family, and health care providers. Without any signs of overt disease, it can be challenging to connect a genetic risk with a later presentation with anxiety, depression, or psychosomatic complaints or a relational crisis in a primary care setting.

Life-Cycle Transition Points

Clinicians should inquire about life-cycle transitions that are expected over the next 3 to 5 years to explore how specific genetic knowledge might affect major upcoming decisions. Prevention-oriented consultations that encourage flexibility in life-cycle planning are often useful at these later transitions.

Courtship and Early Marriage

Communication about genetic risk can be complex for a young couple or family at early life-cycle transitions. Often, these challenges are experienced as occuring "off-time" when compared with most age peers. During courtship and early marriage, the partner at potential genetic risk may feel vulnerable to being rejected as defective. He or she might overemphasize the risk in order to test the commitment of the other partner or may minimize the risk and its potential impact on their lives. The unaffected partner may minimize concerns out of a lack of real-life exposure to the specific disease (e.g., Parkinson's disease) or a desire to provide reassurance and preserve a positive vision of the couple's future.

Childbearing Decisions

Another common transition point occurs with making decisions about having biological children (see Chapters 7 and 9). Some important considerations include (1) whether to explore various reproductive strategies or adoption, (2) whether to pursue prenatal testing, (3) beliefs about terminating a pregnancy of a genetically affected fetus, and (4) possible onset and progression of a disease during child rearing and potential role changes that would occur with functional losses or early death (Brouwer-Dudokdewit et al., 2002). As discussed in Chapter 9, when thinking about starting a family, couples need to realize that they will be making a 20-year commitment. The experience of future risk complicates long-range planning, especially with a disorder that typically begins during the child-rearing period, such as HBOC, early-onset Alzheimer's disease, or Huntington's disease. The latter diseases would be particularly stressful, posing an intense caregiving burden on top of child-rearing demands.

Genetic risk must be considered for both parents and their children. Basic concerns include:

- The anticipation of illness onset in the at-risk parent and complications that interfere with effective parenting.
- Genetic transmission to children, affecting their lives and possibly those in the following generation.
- The threat to their hopes and dreams for children who may develop the disorder at some point in life.

Child and Adolescent Adaptation

Research (Rowland & Metcalfe, 2012) demonstrates that children adapt best to their genetic conditions when parents treat developmentally appropriate communication as an ongoing process through childhood. Children also benefit from talking with health care providers about risk and its implications. Early discussions also reduce parental anxieties that disclosure will come from an unwitting source.

Witnessing parental illness can affect any phase of child and adolescent development, and a youngster's anxiety can be magnified if genetics is involved. In one family, when the father, in his forties, had a serious heart attack linked to a familial form of cardiovascular disease, it raised concerns for his teenage children about their own genetic risk. Some will respond by actively considering predictive testing, while others may avoid it out of intense fear and sometimes withdraw from the family. Withdrawal can lead to substance abuse, depression, anxiety, oppositional behavior, or intense conflict with the parents. The following case highlights a few of the complex themes at play when at-risk children witness a parent's genetic disorder.

In the Ruiz family, Carla, the mother, has polycystic kidney disease (PKD), inherited as an autosomal dominant disorder, that usually affects 50% of the children. It is a progressive condition characterized, most commonly, by ever-enlarging cysts on the kidney, ultimately leading to renal failure and the need for dialysis or a kidney transplant. Hypertension, heart valve abnormalities, and cerebral aneurysms are additional risks. Often PKD remains clinically "silent" until an advanced stage. Carla learned of her disease at age 32, when her two sons were ages 5 and 7. Because she knew her sons were at risk, she always tried to shield them from her disease complications, which began when the sons were in their early teens. The complications included dialysis and later a kidney transplant. Carla and her husband, José, have had a good marriage in spite of the challenges.

Because lifestyle adjustments can alter the course of PKD, both sons were offered presymptomatic testing when they reached 16. Juan, the older son, chose to proceed with testing, and learned that he was indeed positive for the mutation. Arturo adamantly refused testing and distanced himself from the family. Arturo, now 25, has suffered from depression, lives alone, and moves from job to job. Despite family members' concern, he continues to deny that the risk of PKD matters to him. Juan is now married. Because of the risk to offspring, he and his wife decided to adopt two children. Like his mother, he is optimistic and enjoys his career, his marriage, and raising children in spite of the challenges. He believes that his mother and his parents' relationship inspired him in the "art of the possible," which meant accepting what he could not control and seizing opportunities to make the most of possible options.

Individual counseling for Arturo combined with family consultations gradually addressed the meaning of his potential disease risk, his fears, and how his life became stuck in the wake of his refusal to be tested.

At the time testing was initially suggested, a family-centered biopsychosocial consultation might have averted Arturo's difficulties. It could have included education about the disease and its psychosocial implications for the future, particularly concerns about loss and the specific issues for adolescents transitioning to early adulthood. In this scenario, if Arturo had still declined testing, the clinician could have suggested future reconsideration.

COMBINING THE FSGI AND FSI MODELS

The FSGI model is intended for use sequentially with the FSI model (see Figure 15.2). The latter model is designed for conceptualizing illnesses after they

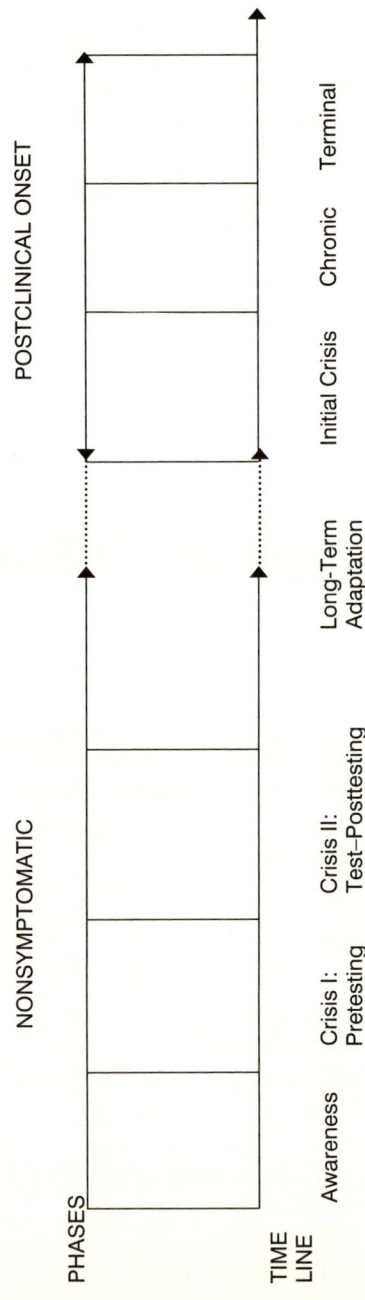

FIGURE 15.2. Time phases of genetically linked disorders. From Rolland and Williams (2005).

become clinically apparent. At the time of clinical onset, the overall clinical-severity variable in the genomic disorders typology can then be separated into its key components: type of onset, course, outcome, disability, and level of uncertainty. Together the FSGI and FSI models conceptualize a genomic condition through the nonsymptomatic and symptomatic phases and in relation to individual and family development.

As an example, consider one family. The father, Jim, age 50, was the first family member diagnosed with Huntington's disease, with onset at age 40. At that time, his son, Sam, and daughter, Sarah, were in their early teens in the *awareness phase*. This condition can be categorized, according to the FSGI model, as high likelihood of development, high severity, onset in early-to-middle adulthood, and no effective treatment to prevent onset or alter progression. When Sam decided to go ahead with testing, he went through the *crisis I and II pretesting and posttest phases*, learning that he carries the mutation. He then entered a *nonsymptomatic long-term adaptation phase*, until his clinical symptoms emerged. Then, the course of his illness can be tracked by the FSI model.

In this case, HD can be categorized as *gradual clinical onset, progressive course, fatal outcome,* and *highly disabling*. This reality will influence the nature of challenges facing Sam, his partner, and any children they have as they go through the *crisis, chronic, and terminal phases postclinical onset*. Sarah (who deferred testing), may assume caregiving responsibilities for her father and, possibly, for her brother, Sam, while living with her own uncertainty of developing the disease. How all these stressors will affect her life-cycle planning will need to be carefully considered.

INTEGRATED COLLABORATIVE PRACTICE

The FSGI framework guides both assessment and clinical intervention. In the awareness or pretesting phases, clinicians can help family members acquire a shared understanding of the practical and emotional demands of living with a potential or actual genomic condition over time. Clinicians can assess a family's strengths and vulnerabilities in relation to both present and future phases. A time line can help to reveal a clustering of stressors or the concurrence of nonsymptomatic time-phase transitions with other symptoms in the family, such as a child's behavior problems. These symptoms may reflect an expression of concern about an at-risk member, as in the following case.

Phong, age 8, from a traditional Vietnamese immigrant family, was suffering anxiety and declining school grades. Her maternal grandmother had recently died of breast cancer, and her maternal aunt currently had breast cancer. She revealed to her pediatrician her secret fears that her mother would get breast cancer and die. Family communication was constrained by the cultural belief that discussing genetic risks could harm at-risk family members. Further, they believed that genetic risk meant incurring an inevitable disease and preferred to leave matters up to fate. A culturally sensitive and collaborative intervention included the pediatrician, a genetic counselor, and a medical family therapist. Sessions with the genetic counselor provided accurate information about the BRCA1/2 mutations, early detection, and preventive steps that could alter the course of HBOC. Genetic testing was recommended for the mother. In this crisis-pretesting phase, the family therapist explored the parents' concerns and clarified that living with increased genetic risk would not inevitably lead to cancer. The mother decided to have genetic testing, and learned that she was BRCA1 positive. Posttesting consultations with the family therapist facilitated more open discussions among family members, which included Phong and her siblings, about the threatened loss of both the aunt and the mother and the recent loss of the grandmother. With the mother's positive results, they also faced dealing with a possible genetic risk for Phong, and with the help of the genetic counselor decided to defer making a decision about her testing until late adolescence. The family faced both posttesting crisis-phase challenges for the mother and awareness-phase issues for Phong.

The time phases and transition points can inform the timing of psychosocial consultations.

In one family the most common form of hereditary colorectal cancer, hereditary nonpolyposis colorectal cancer, was carried on the father's side. The father, age 40, had been receiving screening colonoscopies for over 10 years. The family physician suggested a consultation with the parents regarding the usefulness and timing of genetic testing for their 16- and 17-year-old sons. They were approaching early adulthood when screening colonoscopies should begin for those carrying the mutation. Follow-up consultations with a medical family therapist, family physician, and genetic specialist working collaboratively facilitated family communication, while they respected each son's autonomy concerning whether and when to seek genetic testing.

The FSGI framework can facilitate the development of prevention-oriented psychoeducational or support groups (see Chapter 4). New models of family involvement are especially needed for individuals in the nonsymptomatic long-term adaptation phase.

ETHICAL AND LEGAL CONSIDERATIONS

The expanding landscape of genetics research and testing has raised profound ethical and legal issues. For example, genetic risk information has implications for the health care issues of multiple family members, including reproductive issues. Misuse of genetic information is another major concern. A few key family issues are discussed in the next sections. (See McEwan, 2006; Ormond & Ross, 2006; Ross & Fost, 2006 for more in-depth discussion.)

Legal Parameters

Clinicians in the United States need to be aware of several important landmark legal documents. In 2008, the U.S. Congress enacted the Genetic Information Nondiscrimination Act (GINA). At its core, it prohibits discrimination based on genetic information in determining health insurance eligibility or rates and employment suitability, yet it has some exemptions (e.g., obtaining life insurance). The Affordable Care Act prohibits discrimination against persons with genetic diseases by refusing to cover them for preexisting conditions.

A number of legal cases involve issues of patient confidentiality and circumstances in which a health care provider would have a duty to disclose information to at-risk family members. This applies when the provider has made reasonable attempts to guide patient disclosure to relevant family members. According to HIPAA regulations, overriding patient confidentiality is ethically justifiable when failure to do so has a high probability of resulting in imminent, serious, and irreversible harm to the relative, and when communication of the information will enable the relative to avert harm. Because most testing results are indeterminate and probabilistic (e.g., 60% lifetime risk), ad hoc decisions to breach confidentiality are currently very murky.

As predictive testing becomes a part of routine health care, questions will increasingly arise regarding legal rights of, access to, and use of genetic information by third parties outside the family. Major areas of risk include (1) insurance; (2) employment; (3) education (e.g., discrimination against children with genetically linked psychiatric disorders); (4) child custody litigation; and (5) adoption. The potential risks for discrimination and stigma are enormous. For instance, in divorce and custody battles, parental rights have been linked to testing a spouse who is at a potential risk for Huntington's disease to determine his or her fitness as a custodial parent. A particularly complex disclosure issue is how to manage an unexpected finding, such as misattributed paternity. Various viewpoints on appropriate management exist, often hinging on the ethical position of the health care provider. Clearly, these situations require a family therapy consultant.

Ethical Issues

Reproductive genetics involves counseling individuals and couples about potential preconception and prenatal testing through methods such as ultrasound and amniocentesis to assess the risk of having a child with a genetic condition. Genetic risk counseling occurs during the course of genetic screening and/or testing. Typically performed by a genetic counselor, geneticist, or a genetic nurse, the goals of counseling are to impart knowledge, address uncertainty, weigh the pros and cons of different options, and maximize adjustment. Family systems-based consultations are a valuable way to examine the interplay between the genetic information, a couple's functioning, and each partner's values as they may affect embryo selection and pregnancy termination. The following case vignette illustrates.

Leah and Rich came in for a consultation when Leah was 11 weeks pregnant. Rich had recently learned that his mother, age 63, who was diagnosed with breast cancer at age 35, had a recent recurrence and tested positive for BRCA1 mutation. This meant that he had a 50% chance of carrying the mutation, and if so, his offspring would have a 50% risk of inheriting the condition. Leah, who lost a close friend to breast cancer, was eager to test the fetus and consider terminating the pregnancy if the fetus was affected. She felt that breast cancer would be a horrible disease for the entire family. Rich believes that his mother did well living with the disease. The genetic counselor informed them that not everyone with the mutation develops the disease and that screening and preventive treatment are usually not recommended until after age 18. Also, Rich's deep religious convictions made ending the pregnancy unethical, except in extreme circumstances. A consultation with a medical family therapist helped the couple explore their respective values about how prenatal testing would influence decision making about possible pregnancy termination, their perception of this child, and potential effect on their marriage. After three consultations, the couple decided that pursuing testing at this time was not in the best interests of either their relationship or the family.

States vary tremendously on the requirements and range of tests offered for newborn screening. With the rapidly declining cost of genome sequencing, it is economically arguable that it is more cost-effective to sequence the entire genome than carry out individual genetic tests. This economic imperative collides with profound ethical questions. The increased availability and use of prenatal testing presents moral issues on where to draw the line between invaluable medical advances that may save lives and prevent disease and suffering and a societal fixation on "the perfect, healthy body." How we define a "quality life" will affect the discourse about these highly complex issues. As the disabilities community has noted, a risky by-product of more genetic screening will be an increasing tendency to devalue the lives of many human beings with disabilities, heightening their sense of otherness, marginalization, and isolation. Dr. Adrienne Asch, former Director of the Center for Ethics at Yeshiva University and blind since birth, once remarked how her blindness was not the major problem in her life; it was others' relationship to her blindness that was the most difficult.

The basic policy for adult-onset conditions is that genetic testing of children and adolescents is reasonable only if medical intervention exists that would help prevent or mitigate the condition's severity. The advantages of reduced uncertainty and pragmatic planning need to be weighed against possible stigmatization and discrimination, the potential of altered parental expectations, and the disruption of family relationships.

Use of Assisted Reproductive Technologies for Genetic Reasons

Couples may decide to prevent transmission of a genetic risk to their children, and adopt a child, which continues to be the prime alternative. Additionally, medical advances now offer individuals and couples a stunning array of reproductive technologies that facilitate the road to parenthood. A few of the most common methods are embryo selection; in vitro fertilization combined with preimplantation genetic screening of embryos for genetic risk; and, when pregnancy termination is acceptable, prenatal screening through amniocentesis. If a woman has a genetic risk for a specific condition, the husband's sperm can be used with an anonymous egg donation or a donation by another relative, such as an unaffected sister. Couples might consider surrogacy (use of the surrogate's uterus and eggs) as one way to avert transmission of a mother's genetic condition. For a man, sperm donation is common. Such choices allow for varying degrees of the spouses' genetics to be part of their child.

With any of these options, consultations with couples, potential donors, and surrogates are essential. Exploring ethical concerns and the potential impact on family relationships is particularly vital when the donor or surrogate is a family member, as shown in the following case.

Mary and Tom want to have kids, but Mary is a carrier of the Duchenne muscular dystrophy mutation: a progressive, incurable, fatal, sex-linked disease (50% of sons will get the disease and 50% of daughters will be carriers). Mary witnessed her own brother's suffering and death from the disease. Mary and Tom do not want to have a child with the illness, but are religiously opposed to pregnancy (or fertilized egg) termination. Her sister, Julie, who already had two children and does not carry the mutation, offered to be an egg donor as a gift of life to Mary and Tom. Julie provided the egg, which was fertilized in vitro with Tom's sperm and then implanted in Mary's uterus, resulting in a healthy baby girl.

Before proceeding with this plan, there were separate family consultations with Mary and Tom, with Julie alone, with Julie and her husband, and with both couples together. In the course of the consultations the quality of existing relationships and their views regarding the potential impact on couple and family relationships were assessed, and psychoeducation regarding potential benefits and challenges over time was offered. Additional psychosocial check-up consultations that continued for the first 2 years were valuable in addressing any anticipated or unanticipated feelings or relationship issues (e.g., attachment between Julie and her niece).

CONCLUSION

In this burgeoning era of genomics, we have expanding opportunities to learn about future disease risk through genetic testing. Gene-editing possibilities will increase. To meet this challenge, biopsychosocial models of health care will need to shift from focusing on intervention after disease onset to more predictive and preventive approaches. Individuals and families will increasingly be challenged to make decisions about acquiring and using information about the genomic aspects of disease risk. The FSGI model, anchored in a developmental systems framework, offers a way to help address the major psychosocial challenges.

CHAPTER 16

Neurocognitive Impairment
Mastering Challenges over Time

Conditions involving neurocognitive impairment, such as Alzheimer's disease and TBI, present heart-wrenching challenges for individuals and their loved ones. Because these conditions alter the capacities for relational connection in varied ways, they can profoundly affect couple bonds and family life (Ablitt, Jones, & Muers, 2009). Health care of dementias is among the costliest chronic disorders (Alzheimer's Association, 2015; Hurd, Martorell, Delavande, Mullen, & Langa, 2013). The greater health and mental health morbidity for dementia caregiving relative to other chronic conditions is well documented (Alzheimer's Association, 2015), especially for elderly caregivers with a chronic illness themselves (Schulz & Beach, 1999). The higher intensity and statistically longer caregiving duration are major factors (Kasper, Freedmen, & Spillman, 2014).

An extensive literature on dementia caregiving and effective multicomponent interventions focuses on the primary caregivers (Belle et al., 2006; Mittelman, 2013; Zarit & Talley, 2013) and on reducing caregiver depression and anxiety (Joling, van Marwijk, Smit, van der Horst, & Scheltens, 2012; Mittelman, Brodaty, Wallen, & Burns, 2008). However, these approaches tend to focus narrowly on individual caregivers and their dyadic relationship with the neurocognitively affected member. The broader relational impact for couples and families is considerable and is well documented (Fisher & Lieberman, 1994). While there has been a greater use of family therapy with dementia (Benbow & Sharman, 2014; Boss, 2005, 2011), a broad family systems approach that takes into account family processes over time is underutilized.

This chapter is a revised and expanded version of Rolland (2017).

Using the FSI model as a guiding framework, this chapter addresses some key family and couple challenges, such as communication issues, ambiguous loss, loss of decision-making capacity, placement decisions, and life-cycle issues, that are involved in caring for a member with mild to severe cognitive impairment and progressive dementias. Core concerns, such as intimacy, sexual relations, and revising hopes and dreams, are highlighted for couples. Guidelines that help couples and families master these complex challenges, deepen bonds, and forge positive pathways ahead are provided.

NEUROCOGNITIVE CONDITIONS: SYMPTOMS, PREVALENCE, AND ETIOLOGY

The traditional terms *dementia* and *mild cognitive impairment* are being phased out in favor of newer scientific terms, *major* and *minor neurocognitive impairment*. Major neurocognitive conditions can affect executive functioning (that is, difficulty with planning, rate of processing, judgment, mental flexibility, abstract thinking, and problem solving), as well as memory, attention, learning, ability to use language, perception, and social cognition. These conditions can affect mood, causing depression and other myriad behavior changes. For example, behavior can become inappropriate (exaggerated or apathetic) or agitated, and can entail wandering and personality changes, such as paranoia and delusions. They interfere significantly with a person's everyday independence and functional abilities, such as dressing, eating, managing medications, or paying bills. The conditions typically require caregiving assistance. Minor cognitive impairments are of lesser severity and everyday independence is preserved.

The most common neurocognitive conditions are dementias, which increase in prevalence with aging and affect around 10% of those over 65 and nearly 50% for those beyond 85 years. Alzheimer's disease accounts for about 60–80% of cases, with vascular causes (e.g., stroke, atherosclerosis/ischemia) making up about another 20–25%, and Lewy body disease about 5–10% of cases (Alzheimer's Association, 2015). Other significant causes of neurocognitive impairment include frontotemporal dementia (FTD); seizure disorders, TBI, and chronic traumatic encephalopathy (CTE); infections (e.g., HIV, meningitis); degenerative diseases (e.g., Parkinson's disease, MS); chronic alcohol-related syndromes; advanced kidney, liver, and heart disease; autoimmune disorders (e.g., systemic lupus); genetic conditions (e.g., Huntington's disease); and serious, persistent mental illness (e.g., schizophrenia, depression). Complications from treatments (e.g., brain surgery, radiation, chemotherapy) or antihypertensive or psychopharmacologic medications can also impair cognitive functioning. Many chronic conditions, like Parkinson's or heart disease, can include a neurocognitive component alongside their other major disease symptoms or as a future manifestation or complication (as in advanced hepatitis and metastatic lung and breast cancer). For other individuals, cognitive impairment looms as a potential disease. Thus, cognitive impairment is implicated in a wide range of disorders with varying trajectories and associated challenges.

PSYCHOSOCIAL TYPOLOGY ISSUES

Because a variety of conditions can affect neurocognitive functioning, the psychosocial typology and time-phases framework can help organize clinical practice. The most common symptom with dementia is apathy, which tends to occur early on and remains stable through the course of the illness. Agitation, irritable mood, and emotional lability are more prevalent as the disease progresses. Disinhibition occurs in about a third of dementia cases and is characterized by a lack of restraint manifested in a disregard for social conventions, impulsivity, and poor risk assessment.

Type of Onset

Gradual Onset

With gradual-onset conditions, such as Alzheimer's disease, their timing and course may vary considerably. The impact is experienced and understood slowly over time. Although providers may inform family members about the common symptoms of dementia, families often need to revisit and reprocess initial information in the context of their actual lived experience.

Acute Onset

As discussed in Chapter 2, strokes and major TBI are different in that the patient and family experience an acute onset of neurological deficits, typically with an extended period of improvement and uncertainty about residual long-term deficits. With acute-onset conditions, a crisis often occurs when a plateau of recovery is reached. At this point, hopes for a more complete resolution of cognitive deficits are relinquished, and adjustments to permanent disability must be addressed. Family members may psychologically reach this juncture at different times, complicating the process of transition. Clinicians need to walk a fine line, preparing family members so that they might begin to adapt to a realistic chronic phase, while keeping hope for a fuller recovery alive as long as possible. When caregiving, financial, or health care coverage resources are limited, earlier problem solving and implementation of an alternative plan may be necessary. In both acute- and gradual-onset illnesses, periodic family consultation timed with points of progression or recovery is very beneficial.

Traumatic Brain Injury (TBI) is most often due to an acute event, such as concussion from an auto accident, fall, or a gunshot wound. In the United States, over 5 million people live with disabilities caused by a TBI (Centers for Disease Control and Prevention, 2014). Children 0–4 years of age, adolescents 15–19 years of age, and older adults over 75 have the highest rates of significant TBIs. Increased attention is being given to TBI in returning war veterans (Lindquist, Love, & Elbogen, 2017) and to CTE from contact sport head injuries, such as repeated concussions. Symptoms of TBI can resolve eventually or leave the affected person with a continuum of mild to severe permanent neurocognitive impairment. Additionally, mounting evidence suggests that this type of trauma may incur the added risk for progressive dementia years or decades later, saddling families with further concerns about anticipatory loss.

A proactive life-cycle-oriented family systems approach is essential with this population. In pediatric cases, some chronic effects of TBI often are delayed, manifesting later in such areas as behavioral difficulties or academic performance (Gerrard-Morris et al., 2010). Clinicians need to assess whether abuse is a cause and yet be aware that such difficulties often have been mistakenly attributed to parenting problems or the child's "laziness" (Wade et al., 2006). Delayed effects are also becoming more evident with other types of TBIs in young adults and veterans. For many veterans, the presence or extent of injury is not apparent until they return to civilian life with their families (CDC and NIH, 2013).

TBIs in adolescents and young adults often necessitate continual caregiving and prolonged or permanent dependency on the young person's family, sometimes blocking natural transitions in the family life cycle. The impact on younger couples, who are in the early years of marriage or child rearing, is well established and can be profound. However, systemic research that examines the relationship between marital quality and stability from the perspectives of both the caregiver and TBI-affected spouse is lacking (Godwin, Kreutzer, Arango-Lasprilla, & Lehan, 2012). Mood swings, emotional outbursts, and fatigue have the highest correlation with marital dissatisfaction. A specific Brain Injury Family Intervention model, which includes psychoeducation, skills building, and psychological-support components, has been effective with this specific population (Kreutzer, Stejskal, Godwin, Powell, & Arango-Lasprilla, 2010).

Course

Understanding the expected pattern of cognitive impairment over time can help families organize patterns of daily living and anticipate future challenges. For instance, seizures are likely to recur; they have a relapsing course. The residual deficits of TBIs and stroke are relatively stable and have a constant course. Family members may be heartbroken because their loved one will remain unchanged cognitively day after day, stretching into the foreseeable future.

Conditions, such as Alzheimer's disease and multi-infarct (repetitive small strokes) dementia, are progressive. For Alzheimer's disease the expected course is 5 to 15 years from symptom onset to death. Because progression implies a progressive loss of cognitive and relational abilities, the importance of family communication from the outset cannot be overemphasized (and is discussed in a later section). With progressive loss of cognitive functioning and the high stress of caregiving, family members are at a high risk for losing work time and opportunities for social and leisure activities. Findings suggest that particular difficulties, such as agitation and incontinence, tend to accelerate nursing home placement (Smith, Williamson, Miller, & Schultz, 2011). Clinicians need to be aware that early symptoms, such as memory loss, do not prevent family members from generally experiencing the affected member as still the same person. Personality and behavioral changes begin to emerge with increasing disability. Families can benefit from psychoeducation explaining that dementia symptoms, such as agitation or frightening temper outbursts, are generally part of the condition rather than displays of intentional hostility toward caregivers.

Threat of Future Cognitive Impairment

The threat of future cognitive impairment, such as with Huntington's disease (see Chapter 15 on genetic conditions), MS, or REM sleep behavior disorder, can tax couple and family relationships (see Chapter 9). This uncertainty can interact with multigenerational illness legacies involving dementia, as the following case demonstrates.

When Sandra and Ken were both in their 50s, Ken was diagnosed with REM sleep behavior disorder, which causes affected individuals to physically act out their dreams. The acting out included kicking, punching, and flailing his arms in response to the content of action-filled dreams, in which he was being chased or defending himself. Once while dreaming he hit his wife while serving a tennis ball! The physician informed them that he was at higher risk for other serious illnesses, including dementia with Lewy bodies, a progressive condition like Alzheimer's disease. Sandra's family history was noteworthy for her father's over 20-year struggle with Parkinson's disease, including cognitive impairment that was behaviorally very difficult to manage in the later stages. Despite her generally positive outlook, her greatest fear was to reexperience this kind of ordeal and suffering with her husband. Ken, a teacher, lived well with the uncertainty. His attitude, consistent with his overall beliefs, was that he would continue to teach and enjoy life as long as possible. He made financial preparations for Sandra and his adult children for the worst-case scenario, and then went about living fully, not knowing whether the dementia would ever occur.

However, Sandra closely monitored her husband for occasional lapses in memory that in her mind signaled early dementia and an anticipated excruciating ordeal as she endured with her father. Despite baseline and repeated neurocognitive psychological testing that revealed normal age-related functioning, Sandra was not convinced. The couple's relationship suffered and became conflicted.

Ken's beliefs and positive approach to living with uncertainty and threatened loss collided with Sandra's catastrophic fear of a repeated "dementia" ordeal with her husband. The following therapeutic steps in this case proved to be helpful.

- Coaching Sandra to be more assertive in asking questions of the neurologist (and informing him about her sensitizing experience with her father). This enabled Ken's neurologist to be both more reassuring and pragmatic regarding what types of "lapses" or symptoms would be of concern.
- Helping Sandra and Ken to keep her prior experience "in its place," to be mutually supportive regarding her history and his neurological risk, and to minimize the impact of both factors on their relationship.
- Facilitating more thorough conversations with their adult children regarding future caregiving options, including expectations of them. This entailed a more detailed discussion of Ken's condition and future neurocognitive risks. This process, for the first time, drew their children into the "inner circle" of communication and made them part of a future caregiving team.
- Encouraging Sandra to discuss her wishes should she develop a serious health condition. Part of her previously unexpressed fear was getting dementia like her father. Some of her worry regarding Ken represented projected fears about her own future health.
- Encouraging the couple to explore alternative living options, such as assisted living and moving closer to their children and grandchildren.
- Facilitating a discussion of life plans and relationship priorities, and positive ways that Ken and Sandra could harness their future health uncertainty to enhance their marriage. This involved rebalancing future goals to include a greater proportion of short- and medium-range versus longer-term plans.

Disability and Severity

The kind of neurocognitive impairment (cognitive or behavioral), the expected disease course (progressive or constant), the timing of disability (during the crisis or chronic phase), and the degree of severity are crucial to family psychosocial understanding and proactive planning.

Fluctuating Severity

Often cognitive deficits fluctuate in severity and are very susceptible to fatigue, especially later in the day, such as "sundowning" with dementia. These uncertain fluctuations can intensify frustration and confusion. As with other invisible symptoms, such as pain, family members can become exasperated. Similarly, proneness to sensory overload is a common feature of cognitive impairment. Coaching patients and families to avoid overstimulation and to plan visits or certain conversations for earlier in the day can be very helpful. Informing families that they can expect that a person with advanced Alzheimer's disease may have brief periods of lucidity can help offset the inevitable emotional pain of re-experiencing the former person and then losing him or her again in an instant.

TIME PHASE-RELATED ISSUES

Neurocognitive impairment often persists or worsens over many years. The FSI time-phases framework provides a pragmatic guide to the ongoing, evolving caregiving process for such disorders.

Initial Crisis Phase

Diagnosis

Scientific views about the boundaries between normal aging and early diagnosis of dementia are evolving rapidly and becoming more blurred. Increasingly sophisticated neuroimaging techniques are able to show brain alterations well in advance of the clinical signs of dementia. Mild cognitive impairment is increasingly diagnosed as a separate condition, with additional risk for dementia. Concurrently, an increasing array of genetic mutations for susceptibility is being identified, some of which confer a modest increased risk in later life. Other rare mutations (e.g., Presenilin 1) predict the almost certain onset of Alzheimer's disease closer to midlife (see Chapter 15). Like genetic conditions, current advances in technology and diagnosis for neurocognitive conditions far outpace effective clinical interventions. The lack of diagnostic clarity and the relative lack of treatment options present patients and their families with complex dilemmas.

On average, there is a 2- to 3-year interval between symptom onset and medical evaluation. One major reason for the lag is the confusion about normal versus abnormal memory decline. Another is denial and fear of a dire prognosis. With an unclear medical diagnosis, clinicians or families may attribute negative psychological or relational motivations to the affected member's behavior. Yet earlier detection can enhance planning for the impaired member and his or her loved ones (Smith & Lunde, 2013).

Communication of a Diagnosis

Despite general agreement among health providers that patients have the right to know their diagnosis, dementia presents a more fraught situation. Although the provider disclosure rate for diagnosis of patients with the most common cancers or cardiovascular diseases is over 90%, it is below 50% with Alzheimer's disease and even lower with other dementias (Alzheimer's Association, 2015; Werner, Karnieli-Miller, & Eidelman, 2013). Providers are significantly more likely to disclose a dementia diagnosis to caregivers than to patients, yet the disclosure rate to caregivers is still below 60% with dementias. Provider hesitancy may also be due to their uncertainty regarding the diagnosis, the lack of effective treatment, and a fear of upsetting family members. The severity of the patient's cognitive impairment by the time a diagnosis is reached also can also constrain a frank discussion by providers. These concerns lead clinicians to avoid conversations that could be crucial for patient and family adaptation.

Because the patient may already have significant cognitive deficits at the time of diagnosis, it is especially important for a primary caregiver to be included in any initial provider communication about the condition. Despite evidence that supports the disclosure of a dementia diagnosis to both patient and caregiver (Alzheimer's Association, 2015), caregivers are often reticent about disclosing the diagnosis to an affected family member owing principally to their fears of upsetting the affected person and/or other family members.

A fear of stigma is one powerful factor that inhibits communicating a diagnosis of dementia. Just as individuals experiencing memory lapses and other early signs of dementia often hide their symptoms from other family members, health care practitioners may try to spare the person from a stigmatizing diagnosis (Batsch & Mittelman, 2012). Cognitive impairment, and particularly dementia, continues to carry a stigma for affected individuals and their families akin to the stigma attached to psychiatric diagnoses. However, a frank, but sensitive, explanation of the diagnosis and its neurological base promotes better decision making, especially early on, when the patient is capable of understanding and giving informed consent to current and future options. This includes medical and caregiving choices and getting financial and legal affairs in order. For the family, knowing the diagnosis facilitates expressing grief and fears and developing effective caregiver coping strategies. Often the diagnosis provides relief from the uncertainty of ambiguous cognitive symptoms, allowing families to move forward in developing an action plan.

Providers should be attuned to the effect that the word "dementia" has on patients and their families, connoting inevitable deterioration, burdensome caregiving, and anguish for loved ones, even when it remains "only" a possibility. In one person's case involving a full battery of medical tests, the neuropsychological testing report alone mentioned "consistent with Alzheimer's type dementia." The primary care physician discussed the relationship of the patient's memory difficulties to preexisting heart disease and did not mention Alzheimer's disease. Unknown to the provider, the family became preoccupied with dread and despair by the mere mention of "Alzheimer's" in this one report. In this case, with the patient's permission, I conferred with the primary care physician and neurologist, and then coached the family to raise their concerns at their next scheduled appointment. Timely clinician inquiry about such meanings can help avert unnecessary suffering.

Important Communication

Early proactive family communication about progressive neurocognitive conditions that includes the affected member as much as possible promotes optimal adaptation. Advance directives, written wills, funeral and memorial service preferences greatly reduce the potential for later family conflict, when the affected member can no longer communicate effectively. Addressing old conflicts and relational wounds early in the disease process can prevent disappointment and complicated grief and can maximize quality time. If cognitive functioning can worsen suddenly and dramatically (as with stroke), the urgency is even greater. When the patient and family have discussed dementia-related wishes and planning at an early stage, it provides information about the patient's wishes that can inform discussion among family members who might later disagree about looming decisions, such as placing the affected member in a nursing home and proxy decision making (Rolland et al., 2017).

Community-Based Services and Educational Resources

Providing information about supplemental home and skilled-facility services is especially important with neurocognitive conditions. Because the sheer demands of protracted hands-on caregiving with cognitive impairment and associated behavioral issues (e.g. wandering and emotional lability) are especially burdensome, asking families about their own caregiving resources (e.g., family members, community), access to health care provider caregiving services, and cultural preferences is vital. Psychosocial information about the specific neurocognitive condition, combined with guidelines for stress reduction, sustaining care, and resolving disagreements, are key elements of the consultation process. Such consultations support a family's physical and emotional caregiving needs in the chronic phase.

Linking families to educational and internet resources is vital. The Alzheimer's Association, the National Institute on Aging, and AARP are examples of large national organizations that provide an array of information and links to dementia-specific services. Memory Club is an example of a community-based program that provides group psychoeducation to persons with dementia and their care partners (Gaugler et al., 2011). There are a plethora of books (e.g., *The 36-Hour Day*); personal and informational websites, DVDs, interactive Web-based programs, films, and documentaries (e.g., *Away From Her* [2007], *Still Alice* [2014], *The Forgetting* [2008]); and personal accounts of spouses (e.g., *A Curious Kind of Widow: Loving a Man with Alzheimer's Disease* [2006]), of adult children caregivers (e.g., *The Alzheimer's Action Plan* [2009]), and of younger children (e.g., *What's Happening to Grandpa?* [2004]). Such educational resources can be integrated into family consultations and contextualized to fit diverse family situations and cultural orientations.

Beyond these very useful resources, there is a dire need for family systems-based psychoeducational programs, such as time-phase-oriented multifamily group formats. Those geared to the initial crisis phase, when the affected member can often still participate, are the most beneficial.

Pharmacological and Integrative Health Strategies

In the initial crisis phase, it is important to alert families to pharmacological treatments (e.g., donepezil or low-dose antipsychotics) that may benefit memory or ameliorate disruptive behavior. Because persistent depressed mood, anxiety, or sleep disturbances can worsen cognitive impairment, a willingness to consider possible psychopharmacological treatment is beneficial. Mindfulness meditation and cognitive behavioral techniques can help the affected member improve focus and concentration, thereby offsetting some of the memory and other cognitive challenges.

Chronic Phase

Mild Cognitive Impairment

With milder cognitive impairment, such as mild TBI, ongoing efforts to cope with the losses are a constant issue in family relationships (Landau & Hissett, 2008). Poor communication can heighten the affected person's own loss of identity and the experience of loss for family members. Often a person with milder deficits can appear relatively normal to outsiders but seem like a different person to a spouse, children, or other family caregivers. Family efforts to appear unchanged to the outside world foster isolation and secrecy that hinder effective adaptation.

The impaired person is often painfully self-conscious about such deficits as forgetfulness, difficulties comprehending previously manageable tasks, and an inability to keep up with a partner or children. Family members, especially spouses, may report that certain conversations are no longer possible. Errors of judgment, such as in financial matters, may occur in an erratic, unpredictable fashion, reducing a sense of trust and risking mismanagement. Also, concerns about embarrassment and being stigmatized can contribute to family isolation. For conditions involving milder, often nonprogressive, impairment, health care providers need to be particularly attuned to the development of these common issues, along with psychological fatigue, since they often emerge independently of any changes in medical status.

Problems are compounded when the disabled person denies or minimizes his or her deficits. An impaired member with milder deficits may vacillate between two extremes: "I'm fine," in an attempt to deny or minimize difficulties, and "I can't do anything right," reflecting an underlying sense of devastation and helplessness. Both extremes can leave family members feeling frustrated and isolated and impede adaptation. Yet, confrontation can be very difficult, because family members tend to want to protect the impaired person's self-esteem by acting as a buffer between him or her and the world. Often this protective pattern escalates until a needed confrontation does take place. One man had been left with cognitive deficits from a postoperative encephalitis. He could handle one task or interact with one person at a time, but not hold conversations involving more than one person or multiple trains of thought. For a long time, his wife protected his self-esteem by saying nothing. Finally, in one therapy session, she turned to him and exclaimed, "You can still play each instrument well, but the mixer is broken!" The husband burst into tears. Yet, this overdue confrontation was unavoidable and was a first step in openly adjusting relationship patterns for the long term. This involved the husband achieving greater acceptance of his disability; his making others aware of his challenges at times; and both partners communicating more openly when he struggled or she perceived him doing so.

Progressive Moderate to Severe Impairment

With progressive neurocognitive impairment, families are strained pragmatically and emotionally by the continual recalibration and renegotiation of family relationships. The affected member's participation in family dialogue and in reaching decisions becomes increasingly tenuous.

Coping with Ambiguous Loss

The experience of ambiguous loss underlies neurocognitive impairment (Boss, 2005, 2011). With progressive dementia, family relationships can become more parentlike and limited to caregiving. A family may perceive the affected member as increasingly psychologically absent, yet physically present. Boss describes end-stage situations where an ill member becomes "psychologically dead," but remains physically alive, as in Alzheimer's disease. Uncertainties about the illness trajectory combined with the unending strain of boundary ambiguity can push families to extremes. Is the impaired member in or out of the functional family system? Does the family reorganize without the affected member, or do they minimize the demands of the illness and unrealistically expect the ill member to maintain his or her usual family responsibilities? Both strategies are attempts by the family to gain a sense of control over the excruciating uncertainties of progressive losses and caregiving strains.

Clinicians can note communication patterns that bypass the ill member. Often, when asking the affected member a question, another family member will automatically answer it. Or family discussions will not include the cognitively impaired member, as if he or she were not in the room or part of the family circle.

Coping and adaptation are especially difficult, because the ambiguity is continually experienced in the present. A key therapeutic goal for family members is "learning to hold a paradox—that someone we love can be both absent and present at the same time" (Boss, 2010, p. 141). This both–and mindset helps members regain a sense of control and more equanimity regarding the unavoidable ambiguity. Just as caregivers struggle with ambiguous loss, those with the impairment struggle with their loss of self, and in nonprogressive illnesses also struggle with learning to live within the limits of their current abilities, while continuing to have hope and try to improve. This fosters resilience. As part of this both–and approach, an adult child often needs support in adjusting to the dual experience of being a son or daughter, who also provides caregiving for a parent (Walsh, 2016a).

Grieving Losses

In progressive, fatal conditions, such as Alzheimer's, grieving the significant loss of "the person" and their accustomed relationship occur incrementally over time and before he or she actually dies. In the later stages, this loss includes that of having eye contact, of hearing the impaired member's voice, or most painfully, of being recognized. Combined with the ambiguity of the losses, the grieving process is distinct from that of the finality of death. There are no normative rituals, like a funeral or memorial service, to commemorate the loss. All this can complicate the grief process. Offering consultation can enable family members to acknowledge and grieve these incremental losses as they unfold.

Health care providers who do not acknowledge progressive deficits and the patient's attempts to minimize them may block a caregiver's bereavement process. Clinicians can help avert unnecessary suffering by affirming caregivers' experience and the need to mourn the loss of a cherished relationship as normal long before medical intervention has reached its limits.

A spouse (or a caregiving adult child) can feel lonely and isolated in grieving, even with other family members. Mutual support is facilitated when a spouse, other caregivers, and close family members can acknowledge this change with one another. This "inner circle" may need to appreciate that extended family and friends may have not arrived at the same emotional transition. Providers can help normalize these common discrepancies in the bereavement process.

Concurrent with these losses is the process of revising family members' relationships (including attachment) with the affected member. Enjoying the aspects that are still available blends with grieving the parts of the relationship that are no longer present. As Boss (2010) poignantly notes, "The goal is not to disconnect, but rather to balance new human connections and social activities with the attachment to someone who is fading away" (p.144).

Family Rituals

It is useful to inquire about the ill member's continued participation in family rituals (Imber-Black et al., 2003; Imber-Black, 2012). Often family celebrations are skipped, or a member's participation eliminated to avoid both the pain of loss and embarrassment or awkward interactions. A more adaptive approach is for the family to acknowledge the losses and arrange participation to the extent possible, with other members fulfilling former role functions.

Major Memory Loss and Communication

A hallmark of most dementias is memory loss, particularly that of short-term memory. Long-term memory is often intact until late stages of the disease. Accurate recall of the details of family gatherings years earlier may be juxtaposed with no recollection of what was had for breakfast. Reminiscing about good times long ago and sharing old photos can be a source of pleasure for all. Although recalling past events and having conversations with an affected member may be limited and frustrating, often other senses are intact. Since sustaining physical touch is often possible even with advanced dementia, coaching families in this regard can be very emotionally beneficial. Also, listening to music or singing familiar songs together can be a shared source of enjoyment and connection.

Stamina

In the chronic phase, clinicians should be alert to the exhaustion experienced by family caregivers. Especially in cases of neurocognitive impairment, they can experience a growing, profound weariness that isn't directly related to the degree of impairment. Commonly, this weariness is intertwined with the experience of ambiguous loss and ambivalence about the patient's continued survival. Our health care system's tendency to designate one primary caregiver, most often a wife or daughter, overburdens that individual, leaving other family members unsure about how to help. Useful strategies include offering family systems-oriented consultations to maximize flexible division of responsibilities among the caregiving team, and including additional family or professional caregivers when needed. Family members, even those living at a distance, can collaborate as a caregiving team and offer ongoing help and respite to the primary caregivers.

In these cases, families tend to underestimate the amount of stamina needed and the effect that intensive caregiving has on their relationships with the affected person. These predispositions, coupled with the fact that many neurocognitive conditions are not life threatening and often have a protracted and unpredictable course, can lead to enormous family strain and weariness over the long haul. With dementias, "beating the odds" in terms of rate of progression and life expectancy is often fraught with complex, ambivalent family emotions and increasing burnout. One case of FTD, which typically has a progressive, fatal 5- to 7-year disease course, highlights these issues.

Tom, age 54, has had a very slow progression of FTD for the past 7 years, leaving him disabled and unable to work (with mounting financial strain) and is experienced as "not the same person" by his wife, Mary Lou, and their adult children. At his next annual medical appointment, the neurologist reached the conclusion that Tom had a "phenotypic" variant of FTD and an uncertain future course. This prognostic "good news" created a crisis. Mary Lou, who for some time had felt the loss of her life partner in terms of their close and caring bond and his attentiveness to her needs, became significantly depressed in the following weeks. The couple had barely managed financially on his disability income and her salary as an administrative assistant. She lived with his slowly deteriorating executive functioning and erratic behavior, which included periodic temper outbursts, behaving inappropriately, and making comments that led to embarrassing situations and a gradual distancing of friends.

Their former excellent marriage and the time-limited aspect of Tom's prognosis had helped Mary Lou withstand an emotionally wrenching and exhausting situation. Now, she envisioned only a gradually worsening ordeal with no end in sight. Intervention at this juncture resulted in the following changes.

- Mary Lou's need for more separate time alone was discussed and acknowledged. Tom's mental capacities were sufficient for the couple to broach this delicate issue. Aware of his own deficits and the impact on his marriage, he fully supported Mary Lou's needs. She decided to pursue some independent interests, and began taking photography workshops and volunteering at their church.
- Tom agreed to a psychiatric consultation to discuss the possible use of medication to decrease his FTD-related irritability and reactivity.
- The couple discussed communication strategies to help improve their awareness and management of times when Tom's potential cognitive overload and increased risk of his illness-related reactivity might occur.
- Family meetings with their adult children facilitated more balanced teamwork and a division of labor more consistent with a longer illness trajectory.

Transition to Major Cognitive Impairment

A nodal point in family caregiving occurs when the affected member needs help with basic activities of daily living, such as bathing, eating, and toileting. Because of the inherent strain, timely consultations can help family members reevaluate shared caregiving responsibilities and the need to hire direct-care workers, such as nurses' aides, home health aides, and personal and home care aides. A decision to hire outside help may be difficult for families who are financially pressed or constrained by cultural beliefs that all caregiving should be done by family members. Also, at this point family members may need help in adapting to a time when the affected person no longer recognizes them.

Long-Term-Care Facility Placement

A decision to place a family member in long-term care may also arise at this juncture. The exorbitant cost of skilled nursing facilities, coupled with a lack of or limited long-term care insurance coverage in the United States, presents major financial challenges to affected families. Even if obtaining Medicaid benefits is a viable option, the process of qualifying for them can be lengthy and can overwhelm families. Cultural values that place great importance on continued family and home-based care can generate serious family disagreements, similar to those related to terminal illness (see Chapter 10).

Family consultations are vital in addressing different perspectives and facilitating family decision making and expressions of grief and loss. Often, the viewpoints and support of key health care providers can facilitate adaptive family processes and decision making. Clinician support can help alleviate any feelings of blame, shame, or guilt and normalize the experience of family caregivers, who may have reached their limits, and sensitively address cultural beliefs about caring for the ill member until death.

Available options range from standard custodial care that can often be dehumanizing to innovative person-centered care models that emphasize retaining a person's remaining abilities, preserving autonomy and dignity, and building on strengths. The recent growth of special care units for dementia facilitates these goals. The architectural design and daily programs can be tailored to meet safety needs, while preserving privacy and group interaction. Emphasizing familiar activities, such as food preparation or gardening, is helpful. The Green House is one innovative U.S. model that provides person-centered, small-group home care based in neighborhood settings. Emerging evidence shows the positive effect that person-centered care can have on family involvement and well-being (Lum, Kane, Cutler, & Yu, 2008). Often family caregivers are eager to continue to provide aspects of care, such as dressing and feeding (Gaugler, Anderson, Zarit, & Pearlin, 2004), and their ongoing participation as partners is crucial.

Once away from familiar surroundings, a cognitively impaired family member may have greater difficulty recognizing their spouse or children during visits. The impaired person may also form an intimate bond with another resident who has dementia, and clinicians should forewarn loved ones about these normative possibilities. Sometimes, the resident is able to go home for weekend visits. This can be a mixed experience for families, as shown in the following situation.

Lydia, age 55, had had extensive treatments for a brain tumor that left her with a profound executive function disability, including a severe memory deficit about her past, as well as the ability to create new memories. After several attempts to care for her at home, it became clear that she required near-24-hour care and she moved to a nearby nursing facility, where her family could visit regularly. On weekends, Michael, her husband of 30 years, would take her home and, with the help of their two adult children, they managed for several days. For him it provided some glimpse of their former life together, but it was exhausting. Lydia could joyfully reconnect with her home and family, but on Sunday night, when it was time to return to the nursing facility, she would become very confused and upset, not understanding why she had to leave her home again. This was heartbreaking for Michael and their kids. It heightened their experience of chronic sorrow (Weingarten, 2012).

LIFE-CYCLE-RELATED ISSUES

Any transitions in illness, individual, and family development are nodal points in adaptation (see Chapter 7). Family strain can be heightened when cognitive impairment exists or looms as a future threat. The following case highlights key challenges.

Fiona, a bright, vivacious woman, age 38, had a progressive form of MS for 10 years. It required her to relinquish her career, to go on permanent disability, and to move back in with her parents 3 years ago, after the breakup of a long-term relationship. Besides coping with daily fatigue, she dealt with slowly increasing cognitive impairment, involving difficulties with memory and executive functioning. She has one married brother, Robert, who lives nearby with three small children. Her parents, Maggie and Sal, are in their mid-60s. Maggie has been Fiona's primary caregiver since she moved back home. Sal recently retired from his factory job after a mild heart attack and worsening osteoarthritis in both knees and hips. They sought a family consultation because Maggie is experiencing more caregiver burden, and she and Sal feel constrained about caring for their daughter at a time when they see their own window of opportunity for independent living narrowing.

Developmentally, Sal and Maggie are transitioning into later life. Sal is contending with heart disease and slowly increasing pain and disability from arthritis. Robert and his wife both work and are immersed in raising small children. Fiona has a progressive disease with increasing cognitive impairment at midlife. She faces the emerging painful realizations that she is permanently disabled from working and supporting herself and that her dreams of having a long-term relationship and raising her own family are becoming unrealistic. Fiona's losses and the prospect of further disability interact with the life-phase challenges of the rest of her family. My consultations were organized around an awareness of these developmental issues and Fiona's physical challenges.

They involved family meetings with (1) Fiona, her brother, Robert, and her parents, Maggie, and Sal; (2) with Fiona and Robert as siblings; (3) with Robert and Jackie, his wife; and (4) with Maggie and Sal as parents. Meetings with each of them individually clarified their own priorities in relation to the caregiving needs of Fiona.

A central theme involved having the family see themselves as an evolving caregiving team in relation to each member's caregiving limits. I focused on improved collaborative teamwork, sharing responsibilities, and having reasonable expectations for each member. For instance, Sal took over handling medical- and disability-related paperwork. To provide respite for his parents, Robert would invite Fiona to dinner once a week. Within her limitations, Fiona agreed to help with specific housekeeping chores and to pursue some community volunteer work several mornings a week through their church.

Looking toward the future, Robert felt a daunting sense of responsibility in terms of potentially adding caring for his sister to his responsibilities as a spouse and parent. Since his aging parents' ability to manage Fiona's care was precariously time limited, he was concerned that he might need to assume responsibility for their needs as well as hers. As the "fortunate" well sibling, he needed affirmation for his own concerns. Culturally, the parents did not want Robert to assume caregiving responsibility for everyone. They also felt strongly that it was essential to protect and provide for the needs of their grandchildren. This meant acknowledging their limits and making difficult choices regarding future caregiving resources. Fiona expressed an understanding of and appreciation for her family's loving support and their own needs. It was important to meet once with Robert and his wife, Jackie, to better understand their relationship and her perspective. Since Jackie also had normative issues of caring for aging parents, she and Robert needed to reach their own agreement regarding joint and individual responsibilities to both their families of origin. Fortunately, they had a strong marriage and shared common values.

Overall, the family developed a life-cycle-sensitive plan. It took account of these various developmental needs, it could be adapted to possible changing circumstances (including health status), and it would be reviewed periodically. Anticipating Fiona's as well as Maggie's and Sal's future prospects, the family had preliminary exploratory meetings with several group homes (for Fiona) and assisted living facilities in the region. Because of the very real potential that Fiona's cognitive limitations would become more severe, it was vital to have these conversations when she was still able to actively participate.

Younger Couples with an Affected Partner

Cognitive impairment in a younger adult is an enormous challenge for younger couples who are also parents. More often, the impairment results from a TBI due to trauma, stroke, or a spontaneous hemorrhage. The following case demonstrates some key issues.

James and Hannah, a couple in their early thirties, were raising three small children, ages 4, 7, and 8, when Hannah suffered a stroke that left her with both physical and cognitive deficits. Although she could, with difficulty, manage activities of daily living, she required a cane and could no longer drive. Her stroke caused her to have daily chronic fatigue. Due to neurological damage, her personality became much more apathetic, irritable, and erratic; her speech was labored and difficult to understand; and she had cognitive and emotional difficulty with most complex activities, such as cooking, helping her children with homework, or consistently nurturing them. Various psychotropic medications were tried with limited success. James, who worked full time as a bookkeeper, assumed most of the responsibilities for raising their children and tending to Hannah's needs. Hannah's parents provided some help a few mornings each week.

Over the first few years, couple and family sessions helped them through the initial crisis and early chronic phase, but as time passed both the couple's and Hannah's relationship with her children gradually became more limited and distant. Sadly, even with persistent efforts by James to revitalize their marriage, her cognitive and emotional impairments interfered, and his bond with Hannah became much more limited to caregiving. The deterioration of both the couple's relationship and that between Hannah and her children represented a profound loss for all. James committed fully to raising his kids and staying with Hannah until they reached adulthood. He had a wonderful relationship with all three children. For years, he took the entire family on summer vacations, despite the intense demands on him. Their kids all transitioned well into early adulthood, went to college, and are now beginning their careers, with two of them getting married in the past year. This process included family sessions, in which both parents made it clear that they wanted their children to have an independent life of their own, pursuing their dreams.

James, now in his early fifties, feeling that he had met his commitment to raising his kids and providing for Hannah's needs, including her future security, decided to better address his own needs. It was a wrenching decision, fraught with potential shame and guilt, but one that I felt that I could support, given the whole illness narrative and his life-cycle phase. We openly explored these issues in couple and family sessions. His adult children longed for their father to enjoy his life and understood all too well the profound limits of the relationship with their mother. After helping her move into a smaller apartment with professional caregiving support, he separated from Hannah, and moved into his own apartment. Initially, Hannah was furious and felt abandoned by James. However, in collaboration with her individual therapist, their children, and the extended family, everyone supported the decision, as well as affirmed ongoing support for Hannah. This included James having dinner once a week with Hannah, regularly calling her, and committing to provide continued financial support.

GENERAL FAMILY CHALLENGES

Different Perspectives on Neurocognitive Abilities

Clinicians need to appreciate that patients and their family members will have different perspectives about the kind and degree of cognitive impairment, which often involves safety risks that can have immediate consequences. For instance, erratic behavior or compromised judgment may be most evident to a primary caregiver, while the patient and other family members may not recognize it or minimize the risk, as the following case illustrates.

Enrique and Gloria, both in their early sixties, were dealing with Enrique's early mild cognitive impairment from Parkinson's disease. With Enrique disabled from work, Gloria worked full time, which meant that Enrique was at home all day. On several occasions, he had absentmindedly left the kitchen while cooking, almost setting the house on fire. He also had some difficulties with balance and had used poor judgment by climbing a ladder to change light bulbs and fell, barely averting a serious head injury. Further, he had become easily distracted while driving, resulting in some near accidents. Enrique minimized these issues, while Gloria became increasingly anxious and exasperated. She insisted that he agree to some ground rules, such as not using ladders or leaving the kitchen while cooking, as well as getting his driving evaluated. Their daughter, Isabella, who was very close with Enrique, felt conflicted about taking her Mom's side and restricting her father. Entering the caregiving arena was new territory for her. The following interventions over the course of four consultations encouraged a more collaborative approach.

- Enrique, who had gone to his neurology appointments alone in the past few years, agreed to go together with Gloria and Isabella to the next one.
- I collaborated with the neurologist, who was apprised of the family situation. We decided that she would see the couple and daughter together at Enrique's next appointment. Also, she would recommend neuropsychiatric testing and a driving assessment at the medical center's specialized testing facility.
- I suggested that Enrique and Gloria develop lists of reasonable risk-reduction behavioral limits for discussion at the next family therapy session. Enrique, who prided himself on thoroughness, surprisingly thought of several items that hadn't occurred to his wife. This resulted in some moments of shared humor and greatly eased tensions, facilitating mutual agreement and compromise. For instance, they agreed that Enrique could use a ladder, but not go higher than the second step.
- Isabella was included in some of the discussions pertaining to disease progression and caregiving, with present and future life-cycle considerations framing the conversation.
- Sensitive discussion of Enrique's painful losses of autonomy and control sparked an awareness of needs to affirm his abilities, value his contributions to the family, and respect his pride and dignity.

Confronting the Affected Person with Reality versus "Let It Be"

Families coping with dementia can be continually barraged with the affected member's distortions, confabulations, outright confusion, and delusional thoughts. At an early phase, they may repeatedly attempt to correct the affected member. This can become very tedious. When safety is a concern, intervening may be necessary. But often it is not.

After my father developed dementia at age 97 and moved into assisted living, he had several weeks of feeling down. One late afternoon, when I called him from Chicago, he was very upbeat, the best I had heard him sound in a while. When I inquired about his day, he related that he had had lunch with my mother at their favorite restaurant. However, my mother had passed away 15 years earlier! My first thought was to correct him by saying, "You know, she died years ago." Fortunately, I caught myself and said, "That's great Dad. How is she?" He said, "Wonderful! In fact, she is meeting me soon and we are going to dinner." My response was, "That's great. Please give her my love." For me, it was poignant. I was sad about his confused state and the sadness triggered my own thoughts of missing my mother. But he was happy and, in my mind, there was nothing to be gained by correcting him. In fact, I would have needlessly burst his brief bubble of joy.

Letting such delusions be does not mean to *just* relax and accept all the difficulties with neurocognitive impairment; it also means to "let" a new personal and relational reality develop consistent with the current level of cognitive abilities.

Working with a Self-Awareness of a Loss of Function

At the heart of the experience with neurocognitive impairment is the experience of the affected person's sense of loss of oneself, along with the losses in family members' relationships with the impaired member (Landau & Hissett, 2008).

Todd, retired and in his seventies, struggled with a slowly progressive dementia. He experienced increasing difficulty with remembering words, retaining focus, and keeping track of a conversation. As a result, he withdrew from socializing with friends and from talking with his adult children's families. He often uncharacteristically retreated into silence. Growing up in poverty, he was a highly competitive person, who had become very successful and rarely had to compromise his standards. Having prided himself on his intellect and ability to express himself, he experienced deep shame over the loss of cognitive functioning.

In couple sessions, his wife, Sandy, and their adult children, shared her view that, although his difficulties were apparent, he was exaggerating them. She observed that friends valued his participation in conversation, even if he no longer was the lead person. When I inquired about how it affected their relationship, Sandy said that it was a bit challenging at times, but that they could still talk at a deep level. She noted that it became more apparent when socializing with friends or in groups. Sandy felt that his withdrawal and distancing from their children and friends was a great loss to their marriage.

The consultations focused on the following key interventions.

- Individual meetings with Todd to help him work through his feelings of shame and revise his standards of "excellence," while preserving his sense of dignity. He needed to expand his beliefs about mastery. This included

striving to accept and find joy within his current (and future) level of neurocognitive functioning and attaching greater value to his emotional connections (which were intact) rather than to his intellectual prowess.
- Coaching the family to have more one-on-one socializing and smaller gatherings (e.g. with each adult child and their families) to help offset his difficulty focusing on and tracking conversations in larger groups.
- Given Todd's greater ability to focus on and recall the past, coaching family members to engage him more about his life experiences and what they meant to him.

CHALLENGES FOR COUPLES

Conditions involving cognitive impairment are among the most difficult for couples (Borden, 1991; Daniels, Lamson, & Hodgson, 2007). Unlike other forms of disability in which the potential for intimate connection is preserved, cognitive disability often necessitates losing aspects of intimate bonds and certain coparenting roles that cannot be salvaged.

Transformation of Intimate Bonds

For many couples, a major attraction in the choice of a life partner involves a suitable fit at both intellectual and emotional levels. A loss of cognitive abilities that were once a vital part of deep connection can be devastating. As one woman described the impact of her husband's stroke, "The most painful part is that he's not the same person anymore." To the degree that this occurs, the old relationship must be transformed, posing a profound crisis. An altered relationship has to be forged, often with very different and limited possibilities for intimate sharing. Yet, these situations also provide a new opening for forming a more loving relationship. A gruff or domineering spouse may soften with dementia and become more cuddly and affectionate.

Some couples get mired in thinking that either the relationship must be restored or all is lost. It is useful to highlight unaffected areas and strengths of a relationship and to emphasize the development of new, shared interests, such as less cognitively oriented activities (e.g., taking walks or listening to music together). Also, with advancing dementia, the affected spouse increasingly becomes incapable of meeting the needs of the caregiving partner, affecting couples overall coping strategies as well (Schulz & Martire, 2004). When important parts of a relationship are no longer possible, the well partner needs help deciding how those important needs can be met in different ways or with others, without threatening the relationship. Both partners may underestimate a relationship's resilience and flexibility, and affirming the possibility of positive changes is vital.

Revising Intimacy and Sexuality: Reaching Limits

Especially with progressive cognitive impairment, a well partner can increasingly struggle with ambivalent feelings about how—or whether—to continue to invest in a revised version of intimacy or redefine the relationship in basically caregiving terms. The well partner can become exhausted and demoralized by the ongoing process of revising their intimate bond in a downward spiral. When a couple's relationship becomes primarily that of a caregiver and patient, well partners often experience relief, once this ambiguity is clarified. They may reach this "wall" sooner than other family members (e.g. adult children, geographically distant members). Prevention-oriented family psychoeducation with the spouse alone, or together with adult children or key extended kin can sensitize everyone to this spousal experience.

SEXUAL RELATIONSHIP

A couple may become painfully out of sync in terms of their sexual relationship. Sexual desire often remains completely intact despite the loss of many cognitive abilities. Unfortunately, once there has been a fundamental change in the capacity for intimate connections, the well partner may lose sexual interest in the affected mate. In my experience, this commonly occurs for women, who are less likely to separate sexuality from other relational aspects. An impaired male partner may be sexually unaffected and value performing sexually to bolster his feelings of self-worth and enjoy one of his remaining pleasures. Clinicians should be alert to concerns of abuse if a spouse insists on sexual relations with a cognitively impaired partner. As discussed in Chapter 13, with long-term cognitive impairment, complexities of extramarital relationships may arise.

When possible and with knowledge of the illness trajectory, promoting sensitive couples dialogue at an earlier stage before cognitive impairment constrains effective communication can help prevent some of the potential suffering related to couples' sexual relationships. Also, where appropriate and culturally congruent, it is valuable for clinicians to affirm and support the well partner's legitimacy to set limits and boundaries on sexuality. Because of cultural norms, this is particularly important for female caregivers (see Chapter 14).

PART IV
THE CLINICIAN'S EXPERIENCE AND COLLABORATIVE PRACTICE

CHAPTER 17

Personal Themes for Clinicians
The Shared Experience of Illness

Working with serious health conditions stimulates concerns related to our own physical vulnerability and mortality. To optimize our clinical effectiveness, we need to address our own personal issues; the ability to work successfully with illness and loss is tied to how comfortable we are in dealing with the existential realities of our own lives and those of our loved ones. Having an awareness of and being able to process our personal experiences are key to becoming more clinically effective. It is vital to take stock of our belief systems, current life-cycle phase, and multigenerational issues concerning illness and loss.

This chapter addresses the challenges of facing loss and of our limits in the context of work demands, while maintaining a satisfying personal and family life. In the last section I provide an in-depth case example involving a personal illness story and its intersection with a couple coping with cancer.

FACING LOSS AND PERSONAL LIMITS

Working with illness and loss heightens awareness of our own mortality. A "we–they" attitude toward the patients and families we encounter is not realistic or helpful. We are helping them with issues that are inevitable in our own lives and families. For many practitioners, this is different from working with patients who have serious mental disorders that we and our own families may have been spared; our own fears and vulnerabilities concerning mental disorders can feel more remote, fostering a "we–they" mindset.

We need to be cognizant of our prior experiences with illness and loss that have made us more resilient, as well as any unresolved or painful issues that may complicate our clinical effectiveness. Naturally, any personal situation of recent or threatened loss is likely to affect our attitudes working with families in similar circumstances. This is not inherently good or bad; rather, it requires an ability to be mindful of the impact of such situations. Clinicians commonly feel torn between their subjective feelings of overload and a professional credo to remain objective and persevere with any case no matter what the circumstances. To behave otherwise could be experienced as a shameful failure.

I am reminded of an experience during my training, when I was presenting a difficult case to a supervisor. I had recently made a home visit to a family in which the mother had been diagnosed with metastatic cancer. The supervisor interrupted my case presentation and said, "You're radiating ambivalence about this case all over the room. What is going on?" Only at that point did I tell her that my own mother had died 4 months earlier of a heart attack. In medical school I had been taught that you wall off personal experiences and just keep going. By devoting more attention to medical details one could more easily be distracted from personal emotional issues. Here, where my explicit purpose was psychosocial, I could not defend myself the same way. The supervisor, who must have sensed my feelings of professional inadequacy and personal sadness, told me that after her own mother died she felt unable to work effectively with certain cases and transferred several of them to another colleague and, for more than a year after, declined others involving major loss. She did not tell me to transfer this case, but she was giving me permission to be human and acknowledge my limits.

This vignette highlights the importance in professional training of self-understanding about illness and loss and accepting personal limits that are consistent with a positive, professional self-image. When we neglect this self-analysis, we can become isomorphic with some family caregivers who have unrealistic expectations of competent caregiving and who see respites as shameful signs of weakness. Our inability to share our limits with colleagues can lead to covertly communicating the same unwavering "tough-it-out" mentality with patients and their families. One of the most difficult tasks for well family members is to feel entitled to their own nurturance. Often the very thought generates intense shame because the caregiver burden is deemed a light one compared to the fight-for-survival burden shouldered by their loved one.

When we model the same behavior in our professional roles, we can generate feelings of shame about our clinical performance, which risks limiting our effectiveness. The unacknowledged expectation that colleagues might judge us negatively is a major impediment to sharing personal feelings about working with illness and loss. Generally, this fear represents a projection of our own feelings about not living up to idealized, unachievable professional standards. This can contribute to a hidden, shame-based, and impaired professional self-concept. If we are reticent about sharing these issues with family and friends, we can become truly isolated and alone with our suffering. Such isolation can have far-reaching negative implications for long-term professional survival and general quality of life. It may be connected to the high rate of depression and suicide among physicians (Gold, Sen, & Schwenck, 2013). Nevertheless, most health professional training still advocates maintaining a stoic attitude, in which revealing feelings or vulnerabilities is discouraged.

When undergoing professional training, clinicians commonly experience a period of intense awareness of personal themes related to illness and loss. If there is no opportunity to acknowledge or discuss them, then these issues are, of necessity, repressed and driven underground—otherwise, it would be impossible to continue. This process of "psychic numbing" (Lifton, 1982) adversely affects our ability to remain sensitive and open to the emotional processes of families facing serious illness and is a major contributor to symptoms of professional burnout. Typically, clinicians who work with repeated loss in hospice or oncology units, for example, encounter a psychological wall (compassion fatigue) that represents a combination of immersion in patients' and families' experiences with suffering and death, unsustainable personal standards of professional competence, and a reawakening of personal themes related to loss. At this critical juncture, clinicians may change careers (usually with a sense of personal failure); develop a rigid, self-protective, hardened, clinical style; or more adaptively, reexamine basic issues related to illness, death, and past losses.

In one hospice, the director of social services instituted a preventive group program for all new clinicians that was based on a developmental model of the typical psychosocial experience over the first year. In many respects the developmental tasks for the clinician mirrored those experienced by families in the crisis and chronic phases of adaptation to illness. On a cost-effectiveness basis, this program significantly reduced staff turnover and the use of sick and personal days and generally improved clinician morale and productivity.

It is useful to have opportunities to discuss our multigenerational experiences with illness and loss and how they influence our work with different patients or disorders. A conscious decision to incorporate personal experiences into case discussions or peer-supervision groups has enormous payoffs. Difficulties with particular cases, overall job satisfaction, and issues of burnout can be intimately connected to unexpressed emotional reactions and beliefs. This is isomorphic with the kinds of complications that occur in families in which core beliefs have not been articulated among family members or with health care providers.

Discussing relevant beliefs and feelings within one's professional family (e.g., in a clinic, unit, or department) is the most fruitful. However, institutional constraints can make this difficult, unless a commitment is made to establishing a structured, ongoing process with ground rules that deal with concerns about clinician vulnerability. Clinicians often feel uncomfortable sharing personal feelings about loss with coworkers they will have to continue working with. A consciousness of hierarchy can inhibit airing vulnerabilities with a supervisor who is responsible for performance reviews. A candid discussion about such fears, perhaps with a consultant, can help a professional group decide on the best approach. Sometimes, because of institutional constraints, clinicians need to find alternatives, such as organizing a monthly peer group to talk about issues of joint concern in working with illness and disability. In one city, oncology social workers formed such a group and hired a consultant, who met with them on a monthly basis.

In my experience teaching in medical schools and psychiatry departments, I have found that status and gender tend to prevent physicians from sharing personal vulnerabilities with nonphysicians, such as nurses, psychologists, and social workers. The image of the (male) doctor as the technological expert in control further constrains physician self-disclosure. Many female physicians feel that to be accepted as equals in a traditionally male profession requires being psychologically tough. More generally, issues of hierarchy severely restrict sharing among disciplines (e.g., between psychologists and social workers). Physicians usually do not want to let down their guard and risk potentially tarnishing their professional image publicly in the eyes of other professionals, who are traditionally trained to look up to them. Unfortunately, most health care systems minimize or disregard the need to invest time in preventively addressing personal concerns that emerge for clinicians at all levels of health care delivery.

Emotional Burnout and Compassion Fatigue

Just as the ultimate cost to families is much higher when respite from caregiving and processing of feelings are deferred, such deferment is also harmful to clinicians (Paris & Hogue, 2010; Rosenberg & Pace, 2006). Health and mental health professionals often adopt a "we haven't got time to talk about those issues" stance that parallels that of families. Burnout and overload become apparent only after the underlying signs have become overt.

Sadly, clinicians often know that they are heading for emotional burnout, but feel there is no space for attending to their emotional needs, and they are right. Our culture's avoidance of issues related to loss combined with our current health care system's laserlike focus on productivity conspire to create rigid institutional structures that bypass the emotional needs of clinicians. Only when we more openly admit that the stresses and strains on families coping with illness and disability apply also to clinicians involved in their care can we truly implement a model of care that tends to providers' needs.

Most institutional philosophies and structures do not account for the psychosocial demands of disorders over time, and this failure is dysfunctional for families and clinicians alike. Families in a health crisis tend to model their illness system after that of the health care team, which, as described in Chapter 3, becomes part of their initial crisis phase "framing event." This dynamic can be overtly or covertly transmitted to families if clinicians have no forum in which to discuss their own concerns related to working with actual or threatened loss. Such dynamics can foster distant or overinvolved clinician interactions with patients and their families. Distancing may occur because a clinician feels that it is dangerous to listen to family issues that are the same as those he or she is repressing or neglecting. This may take the form of avoiding a particular patient, family, or painful topic. Overinvolvement or inappropriate personal sharing may occur with a family when there is no other outlet for burdensome feelings that would naturally arise in the process of working with serious conditions.

Clinicians need to be particularly aware of situations in which their own fears about infirmity and loss collide with professional beliefs about competency. Neglecting to do so can often lead to counterphobic behaviors. A clinician may express fears about a loss of control triggered by a particular case by admonishing the patient or family that if they tried harder the patient would recover. Such a cavalier attitude about an illness such as Alzheimer's disease, that may have a relentless course, conveys insensitivity in the face of an excruciating family ordeal. Vulnerable families are readily shamed by such behaviors, although they may reflect a clinician's own difficulties. Popular cultural beliefs that promote taking personal responsibility for an illness as a vital step toward regaining health can heighten this experience.

We need to give ourselves permission to step back from a case to reflect and consult with colleagues. Otherwise, we replicate dysfunctional family dynamics. The strain inherent in working with illness and disability often gets expressed dysfunctionally among colleagues. Far too often in high-stress work settings characterized by frequent loss, conflicts develop between clinicians who feel overwhelmed in caring for their patients and families. Or difficult patients and families are scapegoated. Both patterns resemble the patterns typically seen in families coping with these problems over an extended period.

Once, I was invited to consult with a hospice program because of intense staff infighting that had developed in recent months. A previous consultation had been unsuccessful because the consultant attempted to encourage the expression of negative feelings among the staff, which only left the clinicians feeling more frustrated and helpless. First, I met with the administrative and clinical directors. This discussion revealed that the program under new leadership had been enormously successful, but the increased service demands had overloaded the staff. Having no vehicle for mutual support and reluctant to take their problems home, the clinicians began to fight with one another. Affirmation and normalization, like that provided for burdened families, laid the foundation for a supportive environment for further discussion. Labeling the conflicts as a sign of the program's overall success fostered a new, positive narrative that facilitated better ways of solving problems in the context of the program's normative developmental challenges.

CLINICIANS' MULTIGENERATIONAL LEGACIES WITH ILLNESS AND LOSS

The FSI model, coupled with a personal family genogram, can be an extremely valuable educational tool in furthering clinician self-awareness. It can help clarify situations in which clinicians may experience a particular sense of wisdom or vulnerability with a family. At our Center, all trainees in the Families, Illness, and Collaborative Healthcare program complete and present their genograms with a specific focus on multigenerational illness and loss experiences and themes. Even seasoned marriage and family therapists often have not had an opportunity to examine their own family systems through this particular lens. Experiences or beliefs related to our bodies are typically neglected. Experiences with health care systems and practitioners that have shaped our own attitudes are overlooked. Much mental health training tends to attune providers to "dysfunction" in their personal history that leads to countertransference. The FSI model and genogram process gives equal weight to positive personal experiences that are can be sources of resilience and wisdom in clinical practice. The key question is how can we harness these experiences positively to enhance our connection to families and be more effective clinically.

Some important information to gather in a clinician genogram includes:

1. Types of illnesses
2. System(s) established to cope and adapt to these conditions over time
3. Timing of illness in your own individual and family development
4. Personal, practical, and emotional roles in the illness system(s)
5. Health-related beliefs and ethnocultural, gender-based, and spiritual values
6. Experience with health care providers and systems
7. What sources of resilience and vulnerability were derived from the experiences of illness and loss
8. The effect of these experiences on your work as a clinician

In training or continuing education, presentation of one's multigenerational history in the form of an illness- and loss-oriented genogram deepens individual or group case consultation. Using a systemic lens promotes discussion of the interface between the clinician's own family system(s) and that of a current case. It facilitates a greater awareness of how personal experiences and themes influence patient, family, and provider interactions. In this regard, *The Shared Experience of Illness: Stories of Patients, Families, and their Therapists*, is a wonderful and unique resource (McDaniel et al., 1997). Each colleague contributor describes a personal illness experience, followed by a presentation of an illness case and discussion of how his or her personal experience influences work with that case. At the end of this chapter, I include an excerpt from my own chapter in that book (Rolland, 1997) that describes how my own illness experience as a well spouse during early adulthood intersects with a case.

Any multigenerational history of unresolved loss, inadequate coping, or issues related to blame, shame, or guilt undoubtedly can compromise clinical effectiveness. These feelings will be intensified if the case involves the same illness or a condition similar to some aspect of the clinician's personal experience. It can elicit for the clinician something analogous to a sense of déjà vu, or, if extremely painful, a posttraumatic stress reaction. For instance, witnessing a family struggle with a decision to institutionalize a patient with an advanced dementia can rekindle painful memories of a beloved family member who needed nursing home placement. If this personal experience was tumultuous, the provider may feel off balance in her or his professional role in the current case. Just as family members' difficulties in coping with a particular illness phase are often explained by a multigenerational history of a similar traumatic or unresolved experience, so too may a clinician's sudden difficulty with a case be related to the surfacing of a multigenerational history related to a particular illness phase.

I have been impressed that clinicians working with particular kinds of disorders or specialty services have a disproportionately frequent personal history of experience with that condition. In working with the diabetes programs at both the University of Chicago and Yale University, I was struck by the number of staff who had diabetes themselves or in their families. Having parallel experiences can lead to greater understanding and sensitivity. However, certain patients' dilemmas can trigger emotions related to past or current illness. In these instances, we need mindfulness to the potential interplay of our personal histories with our professional roles.

Clinicians also need an awareness of the roles they have played in their family of origin or nuclear family with regard to illness and adversity. These roles can fuel identifications with particular cases or family members. For instance, a provider with a disabled spouse can show great empathy for the well spouse of a patient with a spinal cord injury. Yet, the clinician needs a thorough understanding of the strengths and vulnerabilities in his or her own illness system and marriage; otherwise dysfunctional triangular inclusion and interactions with the patient and spouse may occur. For instance, if providers have ambivalent feelings and harbor unexpressed escape fantasies in their personal situations, they might unconsciously project such "unacceptable" feelings onto the well spouse of a patient. This identification and projection process could become linked dysfunctionally with the ambivalent part of the well spouse. The need for respite time might become collusively encouraged in ways that get acted out in an affair or premature separation by the well spouse.

A provider, who was in an overresponsible position in his or her family of origin, might gravitate toward assuming too much responsibility for patients' well-being or overlook the needs of devoted caregivers for respite. Similarly, a clinician who was in a rescuer position or felt helpless as a child to assist a family member in a crisis could have difficulties in situations, such as terminal cancer, that cannot be controlled. A clinician would be particularly vulnerable if she or he felt like a failed rescuer (for instance, with an alcoholic parent) and needed to make up for it now through achieving successful outcomes with patients and their families. A provider's difficulty in letting go because of his or her personal background could be misinterpreted by the patient's family as a need to persevere with treatments in the face of inevitable loss.

LIFE-CYCLE TIMING

Clinicians are typically more affected by patients and families who are at the same phase of the individual and family life cycles. This is especially true for untimely conditions. A pediatric social worker who had worked closely with the oncology service noted that she had greater difficulty with distancing from her cases after the birth of her first child. This kind of reaction is natural but, if denied, can seriously affect one's clinical performance.

Providers who had illnesses or were involved in a family illness at a particular phase of their own development may identify strongly with a family or a family member whose situation occurs at the same developmental phase. For instance, clinicians who had a protracted illness in early adolescence that delayed his or her becoming more independent might identify with teenagers with disabling conditions. Similarly, a clinician exposed to early-onset dementia in a grandparent may feel more personally vulnerable at midlife when working with cognitively impaired geriatric patients. Such life-cycle synchronicities can help explain expressions of extraordinary empathy as well as distancing or overinvolvement in a case.

HEALTH PROFESSIONALS' BELIEF SYSTEMS

Clinicians need to become aware of how their own family background affects their health beliefs and their interactions with patients and families. It is useful for clinicians to take a personal inventory of the types of beliefs described in Chapter 8, or to try the following helpful exercise.

1. Think about an important experience with illness, adversity, or loss in your family. Recall this experience, how it unfolded, and your personal involvement on a practical and emotional level.
2. What beliefs did you and your family use in that situation? These entail health beliefs and core values related to family culture, ethnicity, race, religion, gender roles, and rituals.
3. How did that experience affect your beliefs about normative coping and adaptation, mastery, control, optimism, and fatalism, and the value of family efforts?

4. Did issues of blame, shame, or guilt surface in the family during this experience? How were they handled? Were they resolved? What helped?
5. How did that experience strengthen you, your family, and your core beliefs or values?
6. How does that experience influence your philosophy and work as a clinician?

An extension of this exercise is to consider a particular illness case and how one's belief system either enhanced or interfered with clinical effectiveness.

Practitioners need to understand how they define their own competence or success. The credo of medicine throughout history and during medical training has been, and continues to be, overcoming disease and saving lives. When patients do not get better, we tend to label them "treatment failures" and, as professionals, tell ourselves, "If we had been better clinicians, we would have saved the patient." As a result, we are vulnerable to labeling ourselves professional failures.

Only in recent years, with the advent of models of care for the chronically mentally and physically ill, have we begun to redefine our beliefs about successful outcomes. The caregiving philosophies of palliative care and hospice represent such a paradigm shift. As we professionals move beyond equating chronicity and dying with failure, we facilitate family acceptance and mastery of those realities. For instance, to the extent that pathological family transactions are believed to be the cause of disorders such as schizophrenia, both families and clinicians will see themselves as deficient if the condition becomes chronic. Fortunately, psychoeducational models are based on a belief that serious mental disorders are biologically based and that their cures, at present, are beyond the control of the family and the clinician. This frees patients, families, and clinicians from creating illness narratives that are marked by shame and failure.

ISSUES GENERATED IN THE CLINICIAN'S OWN FAMILY

Maintaining a functional boundary between one's professional and personal life is a common challenge when working with chronic disorders and loss. Clinicians often feel a disconnect developing between themselves and their families, particularly their partners or spouses. They can feel isolated and out of phase with their partners. Family members' reluctance to listen to the provider's intimate clinical experience is one example. They can feel overwhelmed by stories about disability, suffering, and loss that threaten well-sealed defenses against existential fears of infirmity and death. Reactive distancing by a partner can occur when a clinician, who has witnessed suffering and loss, has an intense need to share the experience and be nurtured. He or she is attempting to cope psychologically with issues often reserved for later life and may feel that no one can really understand. This sense of aloneness and isolation can be terribly disheartening to providers if they are not prepared for what is really a normative experience. All these processes are isomorphic with those experienced by families coping with chronic conditions, who can feel isolated and out of sync with peers and extended kin.

Another challenge may arise when spouses or other family members feel that clinicians give more time, attention, and nurturance to their patients than to their families. This is particularly true for families of physicians, but by no means exclusive to them. Often this pattern begins in training that entails working long hours at the hospital or being on call and prioritizing patients' needs. Spouses might tolerate sacrificing their own needs for the sake of the relationship goal of helping the clinician successfully finish professional training. Unfortunately, this skewed pattern often persists, fostering a long-term triangular pattern involving the provider, their patients, and the provider's family. Often providers' family members feel chronically neglected and, as a result, may resent listening to personal concerns generated by their cases.

If an illness occurs in the clinician's family, powerful family reactions, such as jealousy, may occur. In one situation, a terminally ill mother induced tremendous guilt in her daughter, a social worker, for caring and being concerned more for her patients than for her. The situation was further complicated by both the geographic distance separating the mother and daughter, which precluded regular visits, and the uncertain course of the mother's illness, which made it difficult to know when to take an extended leave. The daughter's conflict was further heightened by colleagues praising her for continuing to meet all her clinical responsibilities ("not missing a beat") at a time of her personal family crisis. Health care systems undoubtedly need to provide more opportunities for professionals to take time away from their duties to attend to caregiving needs in their own families. By adopting this self-caring approach providers can model for families the importance of balancing caregiving demands with the need for respite and the preservation of other relationships.

Providers and their family members benefit from talking frankly about expectations and limits. Each clinician needs to work out a level of sharing that is in tune with his or her values and family relationships. For the families we treat, a chronic condition may represent the first time family members have had to deal with caregiving expectations and limitations. The same holds true for clinicians working with chronic disorders, especially for younger clinicians/couples in which the subject of illness and loss may never have been broached.

Clinicians should anticipate that working with serious illness might test previously understood boundaries in their personal relationships, particularly with a partner or spouse. Typically, the limits of a couple's conversational comfort zone are tested. It is natural for the concerns confronting their patients to arouse similar concerns in clinicians about their own families. Often, clinicians' preoccupation with vulnerability, uncertainty, and/or loss in their own lives may be out at odds with their partner's. An early career clinician working with a young, terminally ill patient may become concerned about getting his or her own family affairs in order and drawing up an advance directive, just in case. Raising this subject in one's own family can be an opportunity for growth or precipitate intense conflict or a crisis.

Even for seasoned clinicians, exposure to a different type of disorder or one that is especially life threatening or disfiguring may evoke personal issues that remained dormant when working with more benign conditions. A seasoned female clinician working for the first time with a patient who had just had a mastectomy found personal fears about vulnerability and possibly being rejected by her spouse surface powerfully. A male clinician with the same patient might worry about his spouse's vulnerability to breast cancer.

Psychoeducation for Clinicians and Their Families

Just as families need to be prepared for what they will need to face over the course of an illness, clinicians and their families need guidance concerning common issues that may surface in their personal lives. From this vantage point, any psychosocial orientation for clinicians can be improved by including their families. This is analogous to the difference between interventions focused solely on the individual and those that include the broader family system. A preventive systemic approach geared to the quality of life for clinicians and their families can help reduce clinician turnover and loss of work time and optimize professionals' family functioning.

Clinicians and their families benefit from understanding how exposure to particular disorders can shape the kind of issues that become salient in their own lives. A preventive psychoeducational orientation format can include the typical psychosocial demands of the kind of disorders they will be working with. Alzheimer's disease, by example, involves moderate or severe cognitive impairment, dependency and loss of control, and possible institutionalization. Providers who care for patients and their families affected by this disease need to know the associated issues they will be sensitized to in their own family life. For clinicians and their spouses, learning about Alzheimer's disease can open up a discussion about their preferences, if ever one of them were affected by dementia. Like affected families, clinicians who work with them can gain a greater appreciation of living in the present for themselves and their family. Normalizing the powerful influences that chronic disorders can have on all clinicians' family members counteracts patterns of self-blame and clinician countertransference.

Consulting with one hospice program, I learned that significant staff turnover resulted, not from the clinicians' job satisfaction, but rather from the strain that working with terminal illness imposed on their personal lives. Together, we decided that staff members would invite their spouses, partners, or other close family members to attend a psychoeducational group meeting to discuss managing the common strains that hospice work placed on family relationships. It provided prevention-oriented and problem-solving information and stimulated networking among staff and their families. The resounding success of the meeting led to the formation of a psychoeducational orientation program for new staff and their families and periodic ongoing discussion opportunities geared to hospice worker and family well-being.

Clinician Psychotherapy and Mindfulness-Based Stress Reduction

Clinicians need to normalize the possibility that working with chronic disorders may stimulate the need for psychotherapy. Just as we strive to normalize such a need for average families coping with long-term conditions, we have to make room in our own experience for added support. Professional involvement with illness and loss is usually an added psychological strain, particularly with certain patients or at different junctures in our own or our family life cycles. Including psychotherapy or consultation as an acceptable option for support reduces anxieties about burdening family members or losing control in a professional situation. Ideally, self-exploration of personal issues related to illness and loss, in some form, should be included as part of one's training experience, regardless of discipline. Ultimately, one's level of comfort and effectiveness depends largely on the ability to accept one's own vulnerability and mortality and the inevitable loss of loved ones.

As discussed in Chapter 8, a variety of MBSR approaches can be enormously beneficial for health care provider stress and compassion fatigue. The techniques are user-friendly, as they can be woven into a daily schedule, even for 10 minutes, such as just before or after work or during a midday break. Relaxation, improved focus, and enhanced clinical efficiency and effectiveness are among the immediate benefits. An increasing number of health care systems now offer meditation and MBSR as part of their provider wellness programs.

GENERAL GUIDELINES FOR MEETING CLINICIAN NEEDS

The FSI model provides a framework for conceptualizing the needs of clinicians and the health care team.

- Clinicians will be more effective if they appreciate the culture and basic dynamics of the health care system they work in. This includes patterns of communication about practical and emotional issues, problem solving mechanisms, hierarchical structure, role differentiation, and so on.
- They need to understand the psychosocial demands over time of the different kinds of conditions they are treating.

- They need to understand the belief systems, multigenerational patterns, and life-cycle issues relevant to themselves and the program or institution in which they work.
- They need opportunities for sharing their personal experiences in working with chronic disorders. Generally, clinicians will function best when support can be achieved in a balanced way from both their professional and personal lives.

The effectiveness of psychoeducation or consultation depends largely on understanding the evolution of developmental strains for each clinician, the health care team, and any supporting institution. The FSI framework offers clinicians the same psychosocial map for their own experience as their patients and families have. It highlights common transitions and nodal points of strain for which cost-effective use of a consultant might be warranted.

For clinicians working in an institutional or collaborative team setting, I advocate incorporating opportunities in the program for processing personal experiences. An initial orientation phase for new staff can serve as a basis for ongoing discussion forums that further long-term adaptation and well-being. As in any group process, the willingness of clinician team members to disclose personal matters will need time to reach a comfortable level. However, the shared experience of working with particular disorders and their issues, such as loss, can facilitate this process.

Clinician Personal Involvement with the Patient's Family

Maintaining customary patient–clinician boundaries is often more complex in working with chronic disorders. Traditional mental health guidelines are frequently more difficult to establish and maintain. As discussed earlier, a "we–they" split between the clinician and the patient or family is illusory to the extent that we all inevitably have to face illness, death, and loss.

Self-Disclosure

We need to distinguish a therapeutic humility based on common human experience from professional boundaries designed to preserve a therapeutic function. Most forms of family consultation or therapy are not based on a traditional psychotherapeutic transference relationship, and therefore, relatively speaking, rules about boundaries and self-disclosure are less strict. The FSI model strongly advocates the use of normalization, which includes selective use of self-disclosure as an important therapeutic resource.

The most significant aspects of self-disclosure have to do with an awareness of its purpose and of who will benefit from it. It is ill advised for clinicians to use self-disclosure as a vehicle for working through unresolved personal issues. This should be distinguished from the use of disclosure, when appropriate, of issues not completely worked through. When revealing personal information, one should think about its effect on all family members, such as the impact on a couple of revealing that one has a chronic illness or is the healthy spouse of an ill partner. With a high-conflict couple, a triangle can be fostered, in which the couple can perceive the clinician to be allied with the spouse with whom they share a common history.

In New Haven, which is a small city, many families seeking my help knew I had lost my first wife to cancer. Initially I was concerned that this knowledge would interfere with my helping families. As I examined my own feelings of vulnerability, I realized my discomfort was connected to my professional training and my belief that to maintain a therapeutic position I had to keep significant, not completely worked through, personal experiences outside the therapy relationship. Because I was anxious about how this knowledge might affect the therapeutic relationship with families aware of my history, I asked directly about what it meant to them. I discovered that patients and families valued that I had "been there" and could probably empathize more directly with them. This connection was valuable in establishing rapport and making families feel comfortable. At the same time, I was aware that I maintained control over what I chose to disclose and that families were generally very respectful of my personal boundaries.

Provider Participation in Family Rituals

Families sometimes invite clinicians to participate in important family rituals. Clinicians may also need to participate in rituals, such as a memorial service, for their own as well as the family's sense of closure. Families are often appreciative when clinicians who have been involved in a family member's care take the time to join the family in saying good-bye. Providers often avoid this kind of participation because of fears of possibly "losing control" and crying. The fear often reflects a clinician's conflict about beliefs that professionalism dictates a certain level of objectivity and personal composure. This fear is usually not the family's concern. At the end of a protracted illness, family closure and healing are promoted by a transformation of the clinician's role from that of a health care provider to a more basic human one, by joining the family at the graveside or at the family's home.

In one family, in which the wife died after a bone marrow transplant for leukemia, the husband invited me to listen to a piano recital given by his two young daughters in the home, with friends and extended family present. This event affirmed the life of their wife and mother, who loved music. It also involved me in the family's expression of continuity and hope for the future, even in a time of great sadness. This poignant ritual facilitated their closure with me, and mine with them. It helped me witness their resilient belief in recovery, which would have been much more difficult if my last picture of them had been the scene of their mother's death in the intensive care unit.

CASE ILLUSTRATION*

The following case of Jim and Ann exemplifies how I needed to be mindful of my own personal history as I worked with them. I begin with my own story.

My and Essie's Story

At 27, illness struck in my personal life. Within a year, my mother had a stroke and my first wife, Essie, was diagnosed with an incurable form of cancer. Although I was a young physician in the second year of my residency in psychiatry and came from a highly educated, financially secure, and close-knit family, I was wholly unprepared for the strains of coping with my family members' life-threatening illnesses, particularly Essie's. Growing up, no one in my immediate family had ever been seriously ill. There were stories of tragedy and loss related to being part of a first-generation Jewish refugee family. But there were no family stories about how our family coped with life-threatening or terminal illness. My family's values stressed the ability to overcome adversity and the importance of an education.

Over the next 4 years, until Essie's death, I learned, mostly through trial and error, many of the excruciatingly painful issues that confront couples and families, when one partner or an aging parent becomes seriously ill. It was an eye-opening and humbling experience. Also, I became acutely aware of how little my own profession of psychiatry had to offer couples in our predicament. The tendency of psychiatric models to focus almost exclusively on pathological individual dynamics did not jibe with the many normative relationship issues we faced with each other or with our entire extended families.

Essie's diagnosis was delayed because her primary tumor was behind her kidney, and therefore difficult to feel on examination, and her primary complaint of back pain did not raise a suspicion of cancer in someone her age. Only when she developed fevers and intense pain did I somewhat frantically demand a second opinion by a renowned neurosurgeon, who quickly diagnosed the problem, which involved a near-collapsed vertebra affected by bone metastases. These events shattered any beliefs I held about youthful invulnerability and reinforced the conviction that assertiveness rather than passive acceptance with health professionals can spell the difference between life and death.

Essie was given 6 months to live and was offered palliative chemotherapy and radiation treatments. We sought out any and all possible treatments. This quest led us simultaneously to a very high-dose and risky experimental chemotherapy treatment given by a "maverick" physician researcher at Memorial Sloan Kettering Cancer Center in New York and to Carl and Stephanie Simonton. The Simontons' approach involved the use of visual imagery and encountering the patterns in one's life that facilitated the growth of cancer. These somewhat diametrically different approaches to healing became the central ways we as a

---

*Adapted and revised from Rolland (1997). Copyright © 1997. Reprinted by permission of Basic Books, an imprint of Perseus Books, LLC, a subsidiary of Hachette Book Group, Inc.

couple dealt with Essie's cancer. She improved markedly, although objective signs of cancer never completely disappeared. Essie ultimately lived for 4 years from the time of diagnosis, longer than anyone else had with her form of cancer, a disease usually only seen in children and rarely in adults.

As a couple, we encountered many of the relationship imbalances that can occur between the ill and well spouse. These skews surfaced more after the first year. Essie's main objectives were survival and living in the present; I found that my long-term dream for a family and career goals occupied more of my emotional life. I became more aware of ambivalence and the need to take better care of myself. Both of us became increasingly conscious of the toll that her struggle to continue living exacted. We felt out of phase with our age peers, many of whom were starting families and certainly not dealing with a situation like ours.

During Essie's illness and for several years after her death, I needed time for emotional healing before I began again to work with serious conditions. Where feasible, I avoided terminal illness cases that too closely resembled my personal situation for me to be clinically effective.

Jim and Ann

My work with Jim and Ann began 5 years after Essie's death, during a time when I started the Center for Illness in Families and began to draw on my personal experience with a family systems approach to serious health conditions.

Jim and Ann were both 31 when they found out Jim had lung cancer. Jim had been in good health until several weeks prior to diagnosis, when he first noticed a mild but persistent cough. An initial consultation with his internist soon led to the diagnosis. Giving the couple a guarded prognosis, the oncologist recommended surgery and aggressive chemotherapy.

My first consultation with Jim and Ann was about 6 weeks after the diagnosis. Jim had tolerated his surgery and initial chemotherapy extremely well. However, he had become viewed as an arrogant, demanding patient. Also, he and Ann had experienced growing marital discord; Jim had thrown and broken a vacuum cleaner during a recent argument. Their internist, with whom I had collaborated previously, was rightfully concerned and referred them to me. Before I met Jim and Ann, I spoke with his internist, who painted a tragic and relatively hopeless picture: Treatments, at best, could buy time but not a cure.

Jim and Ann, who had been married for 4 years, were both successful in the business world. Two years earlier, they had bought their first home, and they looked forward to having children. This was not Jim's first encounter with health problems. As a child and adolescent, he had had a number of allergies that required desensitization injections and the intermittent use of steroid medication to control symptoms of wheezing and shortness of breath. Fortunately, the treatments had been successful, and largely on his own, Jim had learned how to manage this condition effectively. By late adolescence, his allergies had gradually lessened and were well controlled with medication. From this experience, Jim had developed a faith in the ability of doctors to correct problems and in his own ability to control physical ailments effectively. His mastery over his allergies became a source of self-pride and a template for life in general: With a positive can-do attitude, life's challenges could be met and overcome.

Jim was suddenly confronted with a disease that had totally different psychosocial demands, was life threatening, and had a strong likelihood of becoming terminal. The odds of successful treatment were very uncertain. Jim, who was fiercely independent and needed to feel in control, found himself in a situation where it was very unclear what role he would have in his own healing. He found being in a more passive position and the disease uncertainties almost unbearable. Lashing out in anger toward his wife or dissecting the human shortcomings of health professionals became his only means of expressing his feelings of helplessness.

Family-of-Origin Legacies

Both Ann and Jim had family-of-origin legacies that complicated their ability to cope with the situation. Both their mothers had left and divorced their fathers, seeing them as weak and ineffectual men. Jim was the youngest of three siblings. His parents divorced when he was 6. His mother ended the relationship, seeing Jim's father as a failure, particularly in the business world. Several years after the divorce, the father's business completely failed. He became increasingly depressed and a heavy drinker and died in a car accident while intoxicated. Jim's mother viewed Jim as the "shining star" of the family who, unlike his father, would be a success.

Ann was the third of four daughters. When Ann was a teenager, her mother divorced her father. Ann's mother viewed her husband as a nice but ineffectual man. After the divorce, her father had a series of depressions that required hospitalization. Eventually, as Ann put it, he "groveled" his way back into the family home, living as a boarder, while her mother moved on with her life independently and developed her own successful business. Ann and her sisters had tried to rescue their father emotionally, but Ann felt that they had failed since their father continued to live a marginal existence. Ann saw in Jim a man completely unlike her father in that he had a take-charge, can-do, self-sufficient attitude about everything. Jim had been a star scholar-athlete, who excelled in athletics despite his chronic allergies. At the time of his diagnosis, at age 30, he was on the fast track to success.

Although the couple shared with me that the physician had given Jim a prognosis of 1-to-2 years, Jim maintained a strong belief that he would "beat cancer." As is typical during initial consultations, I spent some time with them individually to determine whether there were any topics, such as issues of shame, or any secrets, which were off-limits for discussion. Ann revealed that she privately believed Jim would die from his cancer, but said, "I think if anyone can beat this disease, it will be Jim."

Needless to say, I strongly identified with many aspects of this couple's situation: a young, well-educated, dual-career couple at the same stage of the family and individual life cycles as Essie and I had been, advancing in their careers, and also planning to have a family. Like us, they were coping with a terminal disease that was out of phase with their peer group, and they held a strong belief in a cure, despite the odds. An initial dilemma I faced was whether to reveal my own story. At that time, 5 years after Essie's death, I did not feel comfortable about even considering self-disclosure; I was concerned that disclosing would create an unhealthy triangle. An overt alliance between Ann and myself as well spouses might create problems in working effectively with Jim. Above all else, I felt like a kindred spirit to both of them as a fellow traveler on a very difficult road. I was painfully aware of the many challenges that would confront them as individuals and as a couple. I was particularly conscious of sensitive subjects in which open communication would be essential.

At this time, in this case, I decided to keep my own history private. I have found that I often use my own experience most effectively by thinking about what Essie or I would have found most useful in various situations that come up in my clinical work. Yet even with nondisclosure, I had to be careful not to align with Ann covertly because of our similar positions. As a former well spouse, I naturally found it easier to identify and empathize with Ann's role. This case challenged me most directly to remain mindful of possible imbalances of empathy expressed by clinicians who are in similar positions with regard to serious illness in their own families.

Initial Crisis Phase

Initially, I saw Ann and Jim weekly for several months. The internist's assessment of Jim's cancer contrasted sharply with my initial encounter with the couple. Jim in particular had developed a game plan based on seeking every possible avenue of treatment and expecting a cure. He had already researched physicians and places that were using experimental protocols. Jim accurately conveyed what doctors had told him about his chances for a cure and did acknowledge the possibility of death. As he put it, "It is important to consider any and all treatments. If you just sit here, you're going to die."

These interactions were like déjà-vu for me. Essie and I had been told the basic facts about her illness, although as a physician I had been given more blunt and sobering statistics about her chances of survival. Then we searched outside the Yale system to see what other treatments were available. The difference from my situation that concerned me, and that turned out to be a problem for the couple, was Jim's belief in a cure as the only acceptable outcome. Jim maintained a steadfast belief that he had to beat cancer to feel successful. The roots of this belief lay with the legacy of his father, who was portrayed as weak, and who ultimately died a shameful and "out of control" death. His mother's investment in Jim as the family star and the antithesis of his father fueled his belief that to die of cancer would be shameful, a repeat of the legacy of weak men. Ann understood this legacy but also wanted to believe in Jim. She needed to experience herself as an effective caregiver to make up for her legacy of failing to rescue her father. Jim's success and her support of him in his quest would free both from shameful legacies.

In the initial crisis phase, as Ann and Jim devoted themselves to fighting Jim's life-threatening cancer, I tried to help them understand its psychosocial demands and how to live with anticipatory loss. One important aspect of the intervention was to openly acknowledge the potentially fatal nature of Jim's illness and, while sustaining hope, build flexibility into their plans. This included a discussion of each partner's needs and wishes if the disease should become terminal. Since Jim expected a cure, I needed to frame discussion of "what-ifs" in terms of his being a strong and protective husband who would ensure the well-being of his spouse, just in case things didn't work out.

With this strategy and my personal experience of investigating all treatments, I was able to be supportive of Jim's desire to look further for treatment possibilities. He felt validated by my support. His doctors' skepticism and annoyance at his looking outside "the system" had been a major source of conflict with them. In joining with them as a couple, I wanted to position myself as a connection and facilitator between the biomedical and psychosocial worlds of living with serious illness.

Chronic Phase

Jim's good response to treatments enabled him to return to work. Ann and Jim entered a living-in-limbo chronic phase that lasted for almost 8 months. During this relative calm, many of the typical imbalances emerged. Ann and Jim had an extensive social network, but in the wake of the many visits and phone calls around the time of diagnosis, they experienced a lull in social contact. As is common for young couples, their age peers were uncomfortable and had fears about their own vulnerability. Jim and Ann became self-conscious, insecure, and somewhat tentative with their friends, thereby furthering their own isolation. As was true for me, they were dealing with issues normative for later in life and felt out of sync with their peers, whom they felt could not really understand their situation. To prevent escalating cycles of social distancing between them and their friends, I tried to help them begin to accept the inevitable differences. This acceptance allowed them to stay engaged with their friends and to discuss the impact of cancer on important outside relationships.

Ann became more aware that she and Jim were living in different psychosocial worlds. His life was focused on beating cancer; the marital relationship and Ann's needs became secondary to him. A crisis point was reached when he was hospitalized with pneumonia, when Ann felt that Jim treated her horribly, was demanding, and was totally preoccupied with his disease. As Ann once stated to me privately, "As long as Jim has cancer, we have no future." She maintained her life dreams that included having a career and raising children. During the first year, she had tried to live within his world, devoting herself to his mission of curing himself. Doing so required cutting corners at work whenever possible and basically denying her own needs. In the aftermath of his pneumonia, she realized that only she could take care of herself. As she put it, "I had to make room for me."

One conversation I had with them just before his discharge home crystallized this rebalancing of their relationship. On a particularly frustrating day, he suggested that they quit their jobs, stop all his treatments, and move to their favorite small island in the Caribbean. She was able to say, "If you go, you'll have to go without me." It was the first time that she set a limit that protected the one aspect of her life, her career, that would provide continuity if Jim died. He quickly dropped the subject and returned to immediate concerns. They were dealing with normative ambivalence. Jim was becoming ambivalent about his struggle to cure himself. Ann was experiencing the limits of being a selfless caregiver. Both were experiencing escape fantasies. I remembered these thoughts and feelings; Essie and I both had had them. I felt that I needed to be particularly careful with Jim and Ann at this juncture. I did not want to encourage Ann to take a path I had fantasized about but avoided. Also, as a man, I was aware that during Essie's illness that I had been supported by virtually all of our friends, family members, and colleagues in protecting my career by completing my medical training. I realized that I was very supportive of Ann's efforts to protect her career, but I wondered: Did I take this position to justify my own actions as a male caregiver, or was it a therapeutic position that any clinician would endorse? I had to revisit my own ambivalence and painful decisions. I became aware that in order to protect my own life I had to create more boundaries between Essie and me. We had had to acknowledge a fundamental difference in our lives.

In situations of anticipatory loss in the chronic phase, couples often need to confront a real, unavoidable gulf that has emerged between them. Particularly for young couples, the survival of the relationship requires a redefinition of togetherness and separateness in a balanced way that includes the life-cycle goals of the well spouse and respects the here-and-now focus demanded by the ill spouse's condition. Ann's response to Jim's fantasy of a Caribbean adventure was a poignant example of this process. It heightened Jim's awareness that he was the ill spouse and Ann the healthy one, and that he was clinging only tenuously to his goals. Memories of similar strains, in my and Essie's experience, helped me empathize with both Jim's and Ann's feelings. After this nodal conversation, Jim became more available and sensitive to Ann. Ann felt less trapped and more entitled to voice her own needs, regardless of the state of his cancer. They had, in a critical way, taken the cancer out of the center of their relationship.

Couples in young adulthood coping with illness are more likely to experience normative ambivalence and shame because so many dreams and phases of life lie ahead. Periodic individual sessions helped each of them speak about such topics.

Terminal Phase

Toward the middle of the second year, tests revealed that Jim's cancer had spread widely, including metastases to his brain. The transition to the terminal phase was particularly difficult because it meant relinquishing any lingering hopes for a cure. This transition was the most personally difficult in my work with Jim and Ann, because it brought back most vividly many painful memories. In the terminal phase, both Essie and I had felt some sense of defeat. Essie, in particular, felt that had her will power been stronger, she could have overcome her cancer. The part of me that felt we had not believed or tried hard enough saw in Jim the possibility to succeed for Essie and myself. On another level, Jim's "failure" validated that sometimes trying your hardest may not be enough to overcome a disease. It reminded me to redefine the criterion of success as participation in healing rather than as biological outcome.

During the latter phase of Jim's illness, my contact with them became more intermittent because of distance and was limited mostly to contact by phone. Increasingly, Ann would request consultations about Jim's worsening cognitive impairment or when she felt very alone in her role as primary caregiver. Unfortunately, Jim's dementia and almost single-minded mission to cure himself limited the usefulness of individual sessions for him. During more lucid periods, he was able to express his caring for Ann and convey his wishes about such practicalities as a memorial service. Jim was also able to express some of his suffering, particularly his sadness about the loss of his life and dreams and his anger about the injustice that others (including Ann) would survive.

With Jim's progressive dementia, the situation at home became increasingly unworkable. To die in a hospital or institution was anathema to Jim, who saw this as being weak like his father. I could understand his wish, remembering how important it had been to Essie to die at home and not in a hospital. Ann thought that Jim's going to an inpatient hospice was akin to abandoning him, replicating the shame of her own mother. Everyone, including all the health professionals involved, were reluctant to insist on Jim going to hospice. When he did finally agree to go, he became agitated and combative soon after admission and required heavy sedation. At that point, Jim became mute. Within days, he slipped into a coma, dying quietly a week later. During this time, I consulted with the hospice team and met every few days at hospice with Ann, sometimes sitting quietly with her at Jim's bedside. Although sad, her predominant feelings seemed to be exhaustion and relief. I identified with her feelings at the end of a protracted ordeal. I remembered how important and supportive it had felt to me when, during Essie's initial hospitalization, a senior residency supervisor had visited, joining me quietly at Essie's bedside while she slept.

Closure

After the funeral, I didn't see Ann again for 4 months. At that point, I called her to suggest one follow-up appointment, to which she readily agreed. The consultation offered a chance for her to recount her story and bring closure to our relationship. My main contribution was to suggest that we review sequentially the different phases of her illness experience. I was struck by her focus on the terminal phase of Jim's illness and on her own shortcomings; she sharply condensed the preceding 20 months. Ann revealed the issues concerning shame that emerged in the terminal phase and that she had since buried and not discussed with anyone.

When Jim required medication to control his combativeness, Ann had interpreted Jim's muteness as a response to her decision to put him into hospice. She felt that this decision propelled him downhill toward death. I was stunned to hear her framing of these events. In fact, Jim was close to death at the time of his admission to hospice. As his providers, we felt remiss that we had not insisted on hospice sooner. Part of her feeling was a repetition in her mind of her mother's shame in feeling that her departure caused her husband's depressions and psychiatric hospitalizations; moreover, Ann and her sisters were unable to rescue their disabled father.

As has been my experience with similar cases in young adults, survivor guilt feelings are often intense. There are so many dreams and life goals yet to be achieved. The awareness that the well spouse can continue on the journey, while the ill spouse forever relinquishes dreams, is an existential gap that widens as a disease progresses. Often fraught with anger, shame, and grief, it is one of the most agonizing issues for young couples to communicate about, yet it is at the heart of their reality. Ann and Jim had difficulty addressing this issue while Jim was alive, largely because he had his mission of finding a cure and she respected his need to pursue it.

Perhaps I had not pushed harder for them to deal with these issues when he was still able to because I also wanted to believe in his ability to "succeed" and make up for whatever feelings Essie and I had about "losing" her battle with cancer. Essie also had felt some shame in the terminal phase. In not beating cancer, she felt she wasn't living up to a model Simonton patient, who could will a cure.

In this last consultation with Ann, I intervened mostly by recalling vignettes of her tireless efforts and of their quality of life as a couple earlier in the illness. I recollected the sadness we all experienced at the end of a medically hopeless situation. It was in the context of this discussion that I revealed that I had lived through a similar situation and had encountered many of the same feelings. Self-disclosure during this last meeting seemed a natural part of my closure with Ann. It allowed her to reveal that she had at times in our work together felt an "uncommon understanding" for her plight. Without asking for details, she conveyed an appreciation for my sharing this information.

I used this personal disclosure as an opportunity to reinforce the typical life-cycle issues of being a young adult well spouse. I was also able to validate how difficult it is to affirm one's efforts as a caregiver when age peers are living out a very different version of life, moving ahead with life plans while many of one's own are on hold. Ann described how she felt permanently out of phase with her peers: She felt that she and Jim had lived a 30-year marriage during his 2-year illness, and that no one her age could really understand her experience and her feeling of being psychologically older because of it. I understood exactly what she meant, but I could speak to her from the perspective gained 6 years after a similar loss and could affirm that time would alter, but not entirely eliminate, her feelings. I find Ann's aftermath feelings very common in younger surviving spouses and usually try to introduce them psychoeducationally in my clinical work.

Several days later, Ann called to thank me, saying the session had been very therapeutic. She told me that this had been the first time since Jim's death that she had let herself recount the entire story. Now that sufficient time had elapsed since Jim's death, the session had rebalanced her final picture of the experience. The phone call turned out to be my last contact with Ann.

In retrospect over 25 years later, I view Jim and Ann's case, which closely mirrored my own, as one turning point in my professional growth. Not only did I become more conscious of the vulnerable areas I needed to be mindful of, but I also gained an awareness of some of the areas of personal resilience I could draw on therapeutically in helping other couples and families. Most significant, through my own experience I developed a deeper appreciation for and humility about the profound struggles of families and couples facing serious illness. Some key challenges that I personally encountered and have seen repeatedly are the need to keep relationship imbalances to a minimum, for well members to continue to feel like equals, and for all members to acknowledge personal limits. Addressing these challenges has further enabled me to find more collaborative ways to engage families therapeutically.

CHAPTER 18

Collaborative Health Care

Linking Families with Systems of Care

The quality of fit among families facing major health issues, providers, and systems of care is a major focus of this book. Using the FSI model as a guide, this chapter presents a brief overview of collaborative and integrated family-oriented care and describes some innovative examples of family-based programs in specialty care services and with consumer-based organizations. Then clinical interface issues related to the quality of fit between the patient, family, and provider system over a condition's course are addressed. Finally, key principles and policies for advancing family-oriented health care are discussed.

OVERVIEW

Integrated and collaborative health care are becoming the prevailing paradigms for health care delivery, particularly in primary care (Collins et al., 2015; McDaniel et al., 2005; McDaniel et al., 2014; Peek, 2015; Talen & Burke Valeras, 2013). *Integrated care* refers to models of unified care planning and on-site, colocated teams of biomedical and behavioral health care health (BHC) providers (Pomerantz et al., 2010). It includes financial, structural, and infrastructural components (Blount et al., 2007; Peek, 2015). The patient-centered medical home is one prime example that demonstrates cost containment and improved patient health access, outcomes, and satisfaction with care (Cohen, Davis, Hall, Gilchrist, & Miller, 2015; Nielsen, Gibson, Buelt, Grundy, & Grumbach, 2015). *Collaborative care* refers to ongoing communication and treatment planning among biomedical providers, behavioral specialists, patients, and families.

Mental health and behavioral specialists involved in delivering care bring unique perspectives and expertise from diverse disciplines and treatment philosophies, such as psychiatry, psychology, social work, medical family therapy, and pastoral care. Medical family therapists and other family systems-based mental health professionals emphasize the patient in the context of the family system and community. There is a vital need for this diverse and complementary system of biopsychosocial and spiritual approaches. Varying levels of collaboration are possible, based on such factors as the receptivity of a health care program and its leadership; the skills of the mental health providers; and the infrastructural, financial, and philosophical underpinnings of the health care institution or program. Doherty (1995) delineates five levels of involvement: (1) minimal collaboration; (2) basic collaboration from a distance (off-site); (3) basic collaboration on-site; (4) close collaboration in a partly integrated system; and (5) close collaboration in a fully integrated system (see Table 18.1).

Part of the current health care delivery transformation involves a rapid movement of clinical care to integrated health care teams comprising physicians, nurse practitioners, specialized therapists (e.g., nutrition, respiratory, physical, occupational), pharmacists, chaplains, and behavioral health specialists in community contexts (Etz et al., 2008). An ever-increasing body of research documents the efficacy of collaborative health care delivery (Butler et al., 2008; Miller, Kessler, Peek, & Kallenberg, 2011). This includes impressive data showing improvements for specific mental health issues, such as depression (Butler et al., 2011; Katon, Unutzer, Wells, & Jones, 2010); for chronic conditions, such as diabetes (Ell et al., 2010); and for delivering primary care to patients with severe and persistent mental illness in specialty care mental health settings (Druss et al., 2010).

The movement toward biopsychosocial integration varies significantly across the primary and specialty care spectrum. In family practice, providers may care for many family members and become personally acquainted with the family unit. In pediatrics, the dependency of a child naturally engages parents. The inevitable impact of a chronic illness on all key family members guides family-oriented specialty care. These differences need to be considered in designing and implementing integrated care in different contexts.

The Underutilized Potential of Families and Communities in Integrated Care

Most advances in collaborative practice have been taking place in models of *patient-centered care* emphasizing provider teamwork with the patient. The nature of the relationship with the patient is highly variable, ranging from a traditional hierarchical one to a more egalitarian, mutual relationship (Doherty, Mendenhall, & Berge, 2010). Despite the inclusion of "family" in the language of collaboration, in practice far less attention has been given to

TABLE 18.1. Levels of Systemic Collaboration between Therapists and Other Health Professionals

Level	Description	Location	Handles adequately	Handles inadequately
1. Minimal collaboration	• Separate facilities and systems • Rarely communicate	Private practice, most agencies	Routine medical or psychosocial problems	Refractory problems or those with biopsychosocial interplay
2. Basic collaboration, off-site	• Separate facilities and systems • Periodic communication about patients, linkages, and treatment planning	Setting with active referral linkages	Patients with moderate biopsychosocial interplay (e.g., diabetes, depression)	Problems with significant biopsychosocial interplay
3. Basic collaboration, on-site	• Separate mental health and other health care systems in the same facility • Regular communication and appreciation of each other's work • Ill-defined teams, no common language • Physicians have more power and influence than other providers, who may resent this	Some HMOs, rehabilitation settings, medical clinics, without systemic approaches to collaboration, mutual consultation, and team building	Patients with moderate biopsychosocial interplay who require occasional face-to-face interactions among providers and coordinated treatment plans	Problems with significant biopsychosocial interplay and ongoing, challenging management problems
4. Close collaboration in a partly integrated system	• Shared site and systems • Regular interaction, mutual consultations • Shared systemic and biopsychosocial paradigm • Routines difficult, some attention to team building • Unresolved tension over physicians' greater power and influence on the team	Some HMOs, CHCs, rehabilitation settings, hospice, family medicine, and other clinical settings that systematically build teams	Problems with significant biopsychosocial interplay and management problems (e.g., chronic illness, somatization)	Complex patients with multiple providers and multiple systems, especially with conflicting agendas among providers and triangulation by patients and families
5. Close collaboration in a fully integrated system	• Shared site, systems, and biopsychosocial vision • Shared expectations for team-based prevention and treatment • Regular team meetings • Conscious effort to balance power and influence among providers, according to patient need and provider expertise	Some large, closed health systems, primary care clinics, hospice, etc.	The most difficult and complex biopsychosocial problems with challenging management issues	Patients with insufficient team resources or breakdowns in collaboration with larger systems

Note. Data from Doherty (1995). CHC, community health center.

collaboration with the patient's family system (Peek, 2015; Rolland, 2015). The actual involvement of families and communities as valued resources and partners who collaborate with health care professionals remains far less common. One factor has been the concern in the traditional medical arena that including families and consumer-based organizations as equal partners could diminish professional identity and authority. In health care training and settings, a growing appreciation is needed of what it means to be a professional with special knowledge and skills, while also recognizing the limits of that expertise in forging optimal collaboration.

Individuals, families, and communities who deal with or are at high risk for major health conditions have extraordinary expertise and a willingness to share it. They are an enormous untapped resource for improving the quality of health for all. Their inclusion is a necessary component of the collaborative health care equation and of integrated care policy formulation and implementation (Mendenhall, Berge, & Doherty, 2014; Ooms, Rolland, Mintz, & Doppelt, 1996). The complementary value of professional knowledge and skills in tandem with those of consumers and their communities have the extraordinary potential of advancing better health care.

I believe that health and mental health professionals have the ethical responsibility, when possible, to challenge and change the systems we work in, particularly hierarchical power relationships that marginalize and subordinate the family. Challenging underlying assumptions and biases would help promote valuable strategic alliances that are so essential in achieving the next developmental phase of family-oriented, integrated health care.

Chronic Disorders: Linking Specialty Care with Primary Care

Chronic illness and disability generally call for specialty care medicine. There are many versions of how this happens, each with different implications for collaborative integrated care. Care may be provided in the primary care setting, with the primary care physician (PCP) or team still guiding treatment. A specialist might provide care in the medical home setting, often consulting with the PCP. Or, the patient may receive care in a specialty center or clinic. Specialty centers or services are prevalent for more common medical conditions in large urban areas. In these situations, the patient's specific disease care is generally taken over by the specialist, leaving the rest of routine medical care to the PCP. Once complex medical conditions and multiple chronic disorders come into play, however, the cast of specialists operating in their own "silos" can become bewildering to the patient and result in disconnected care applied to different body parts and systems. We can play an urgently needed role in facilitating coordination among different specialists and the PCP. I often act as a "bridge-builder" by contacting the patient's different providers, suggesting the need for improved networking, or by coaching patients to advocate for better communication and collaboration among their different providers.

Behavioral health care models within specialty-care medicine vary enormously from infrequent requests for individual psychiatric consultations to family-based consultation and integrated behavioral health care for any patient entering the specialty care setting. In each model, who is engaged (the patient, family, or extended network), at what phase in the illness, and in what manner can vary; each one conveys a different version of the collaborative relationship. As I have advocated throughout this book, a paradigm of early involvement of patients and their families in a prevention- and psychoeducation-oriented consultation model of care creates the best foundation for effective collaboration with consumers.

Ironically, with greater attention to the psychosocial component of chronic illness, parallel models of integrated care are developing, each in their own silo. I participated in a Mental Health Issues of Diabetes national initiative, which brought together prominent biomedical and behavioral diabetes care providers, consumer leaders, consumer-based organizations, such as the Juvenile Diabetes Research Foundation, and health care insurance representatives to discuss innovative models of integrated diabetes care. This gathering had many similarities to the annual meeting of the Collaborative Family Healthcare Association (CFHA) (of which I have been a longtime active member). The mission of CFHA is to "promote comprehensive and cost-effective models of healthcare delivery that integrates mind and body, individual and family, patients, providers and communities." Despite the fact that similar versions of integrated care were articulated at both national meetings, there was a lack of contact between the groups, one based in primary care and the other in specialty health care. This lack of connection mirrors the challenges experienced by patients and their families in their attempt to get their primary and specialty care providers to work effectively together. We desperately need cross-fertilization and linkage between primary and specialty care knowledge and services in providing optimal biopsychosocial–spiritual care for chronic conditions.

COLLABORATION IN DIFFERENT HEALTH CARE SETTINGS AND CONTEXTS

Working with Primary Care Programs

As noted earlier, the initiation and impressive growth of integrated and collaborative care has mainly occurred in primary health care. (See the excellent descriptions in Collins, Hewson, Munger, & Wade, 2010 and Talen & Burke Valeras, 2013.) Today integrated care programs far outnumber family systems-oriented programs. Almost all of these programs involve collaboration between university-affiliated family medicine departments (e.g., University of Rochester, University of Minnesota) and mental health departments (e.g., psychiatry), or graduate programs in medical family therapy (e.g., East Carolina University), or health psychology.

Over the past 25 years, the Chicago Center for Family Health (CCFH) has collaborated with two family medicine programs providing primary integrated care, one at MacNeal Hospital affiliated with the University of Chicago, and one at Advocate Illinois Masonic Family Practice Center. A lynchpin of these collaborations is the placement of full-time Families, Illness, and Collaborative Healthcare doctoral fellows on-site at these locations, who use the FSI model as a conceptual base for behavioral health care collaboration.

Working with Specialty Care Programs

My primary collaboration experiences in Chicago have been through the CCFH, which provides on-site short- and long-term consultation and training services to community-based health care and social service organizations. Collaborative program development is tailored to the specific health care setting. Consultation components might include any of the following:

- *Program development* to ensure the centrality of a family-oriented approach
- *Clinical case consultation* for difficult or complex individual and family cases
- *Staff education* regarding family systems and collaborative care
- *Family education* to develop multifamily groups for support and education regarding the specific illness or disability
- *Community education* and outreach to clergy, schools, and other community service organizations
- *Intensive training* to identify staff members who can become the on-site experts
- *Clinical services* that accept referrals for complex cases.

I describe two examples connected with large university-based medical centers, one a comprehensive diabetes center, the other a pediatric cystic fibrosis (CF) program. In both cases, the medical leadership and funders were believers in and committed to development of a systems- and family-oriented integrated collaborative care model. This starting point was essential in promoting a successful program that represented an advance over a complex-case referral model of collaborative care. Here, the collaboration began at the top of the administrative pyramid, where the medical director had substantial influence over clinical program philosophy and development. More typically, collaborative care begins with a mental health provider in a specialty service, who makes periodic referrals of complex cases. In these situations, the challenge is to move from a crisis-referral model toward one that implements integrated, preventive care for all patients and their families from the time of diagnosis.

University of Chicago Kovler Diabetes Center and CCFH

The Kovler Diabetes Center (KDC) is a comprehensive diabetes care center that services over 7,000 patients at all stages of the illness. Newly founded, the KDC and CCFH directors were brought together by a prominent diabetes patient, who became their first board chair, and who was deeply committed to an integrated biopsychosocial model of care. Essentially, he provided a mandate for a partnership between our two centers and the initial financial resources to launch the program.

The overall design of the family-based Behavioral Health and Wellness Program had four components: (1) family-centered clinical and psychoeducational services, (2) professional education and development, (3) community education and outreach, and (4) a family resource and network database (Rolland, Lister, Kelleher, & Williams, 2011). For the first 2 years, the behavioral program was staffed on-site 3 days a week by two CCFH Families, Illness, and Collaborative Healthcare doctoral fellows (medical family therapists) and a part-time health psychologist. I provided overall program oversight, supervision, and needed psychiatric consultation. I will briefly describe these components.

FAMILY-CENTERED CLINICAL AND PSYCHOEDUCATIONAL SERVICES

A protocol was developed that included a behavioral health component for all patients at the time of initial diagnosis at the KDC. In the waiting area, the patient and family members were given a brochure describing the Behavioral Health and Wellness Program. Their initial appointment included a meeting with the endocrinologist, nurse practitioner, diabetes educator, and BHC specialist, followed by a team discussion with the patient and family members. At this first meeting, the BHC specialist gave a brief 10- to 15-minute description of the overall behavioral health service component, explaining how diabetes affects all family members and the importance of the family as a resource and partner in care. The specialist then negotiated a more in-depth family screening consultation to coincide with the first follow-up medical appointment. Short individual and family psychological screening instruments were given to the patient and key family members to complete and bring to the first follow-up appointment.

The screening consultation utilized the key dimensions of the FSI model, emphasizing family organization, communication, belief systems, and multigenerational themes within an illness, individual, and family developmental framework. Additional consultations or referrals for brief or more intensive treatment were offered on an as-needed basis. The KDC's lifespan model dovetailed very well with the developmental orientation of the FSI model.

This initial screening consultation benefited families in four ways.

1. It engaged the patient and their families.
2. It provided orientation and psychoeducation about treatment plans and the family's caregiving role.
3. It identified family strengths as a resource for optimal diabetes care.
4. It facilitated early identification of high-risk cases.

Periodic psychosocial checkups and consultations were available at regular medical appointments or at key diabetes-related transitions or disruptive individual or family transitions.

The BHC specialist also handled cases involving poor medical adherence or patient and family stress or dysfunction. The health care team decided in advance of a medical appointment which cases could benefit from a behavioral consultation; patients and families in crisis could be seen for follow-up sessions or more intensive therapy.

Psychoeducational services included an initial multifamily workshop for newly diagnosed patients and their families (see Chapter 4). Topical psychosocial workshops targeted major developmental transitions, such as the transition to early adulthood; common family challenges, such as communication, problem solving or caregiving in advanced diabetes situations; and disruptive life changes (e.g., divorce, job loss, relocation). Large group presentations and discussions were followed by breakout sessions, facilitated by a behavioral specialist.

Additionally, we organized conferences that addressed the biomedical and psychosocial aspects of diabetes as an integrated whole. They covered the most recent clinical application research about diabetes; individual and family psychosocial issues and interventions; and diet, lifestyle, and wellness information for diabetes prevention or optimal disease management. One very successful half-day conference for patients and families was held on Chicago's south side. Featuring a program entitled "Living Well with Diabetes," it attracted over 300 patients and largely minority family members on a snowy March day! It included the following presentations: "Diabetes Research Update: Lessons from Recent Clinical Trials" (KDC medical director); "Diabetes and the Family: Mastering the Challenges" (myself); and "To Be or Not to Be: Practical Changes to Your Eating and Activity That Will Last" (diabetes educator).

PROFESSIONAL EDUCATION AND DEVELOPMENT

Continuing education programs were offered for physicians, social workers, dieticians, diabetes educators, and other allied providers. One program, called "Resilience: Supporting Individuals and Families Facing the Challenges of Diabetes," provided information and skills training needed for facilitating family resilience, as well as screening/evaluation, identification, intervention, and appropriate referral of persons with diabetes and families at a high risk for maladaptation, depression, anxiety, and other mental health difficulties.

We developed monthly *Psychosocial Rounds* involving collaborative presentation of several complex cases that were jointly selected by an endocrinologist and BHC specialist. The presentations were followed by a group discussion. The collaborative preparation and presentation process by a biomedical and BHC provider, in which the primary purpose was biopsychosocial, furthered close-range cooperation and helped consolidate a family systems-based approach to diabetes care. The Rounds quickly became very popular and were attended by both senior providers and trainers from a broad range of health and mental health care disciplines.

COMMUNITY EDUCATION AND OUTREACH

This component offered free educational events to members of the community. Programs were marketed through community organizers, church leaders, and advocacy organizations that reach out to individuals with diabetes and their families. Distinct educational programs were aimed at individuals with diabetes and their families, those at a higher risk for developing diabetes, and community leaders. One family forum called "Getting Ready for Summer!" was held at the end of the school year for children and adolescents, and combined family psychoeducation, nutritional guidelines, and the latest advances in type 1 diabetes-care management.

FAMILY RESOURCE AND NETWORK DATABASE

A database was developed to link families in the program who had successfully mastered diabetes challenges and who were willing to serve as resource volunteers with newly diagnosed families or families going through a difficult transition, such as deciding to have children or launching an adolescent into adulthood. "Veteran" families are typically very willing to participate and share their collective experiences and wisdom with other families. It effectively promotes a closer collaborative relationship between the health care providers and consumers.

Cystic Fibrosis Program

Our Center was approached by the new medical director of the CF program at Chicago's Children's Memorial Hospital (affiliated with the Northwestern Feinberg School of Medicine). During her pediatric residency training, she acquired basic family systems knowledge and interviewing skills, an experience that led her to advocate for a family-centered model. She described the CF program's needs as twofold: staff and program development geared toward more family-centered services and help with two specific populations: (1) parents who recently learned that they have an infant with CF and were themselves carriers of the CF mutation and (2) adolescents with CF who had difficulties with disease management. Funding was secured from a pharmaceutical firm that provides medications for CF patients.

To develop a knowledge base about a family systems approach, we first conducted a series of in-service case presentations for the entire CF staff, including physicians, nurses, social workers, consulting health psychologists, respiratory therapists, and nutritionists. They provided a common baseline for the staff that was essential for delivering future care services. At the same time, we recommended that the CF social worker take the 1-year intensive Families, Illness, and Collaborative Healthcare advanced certificate program at our Center, which ensured an on-site family-oriented psychosocial expert was within the CF program.

This initial in-service training transitioned into a monthly family-centered "difficult case" conference, for which I served as a consulting family psychiatrist. Everyone involved in the care of a particular child participated in the presentation of the case and follow-up discussion. Our collaborative relationship and the inclusion of all relevant staff were crucial in solidifying family knowledge and skills and implementing other programmatic changes. The case conference also led to referrals of complex cases to our Center and educated CF staff about which cases warranted more intensive family or couple therapy.

General service delivery changes for all CF families were implemented next. The changes included a family intake assessment and consultation with a staff nurse for all parents with a child newly diagnosed with CF or for families who were transferring care from another health care institution. This initial contact laid the foundation for working together with families and introducing at the outset of a family's relationship with the CF program a family-oriented biopsychosocial care model and identifying high-risk families. Second, we designed a four-session prevention-oriented psychoeducational multifamily discussion group for families with a newly diagnosed infant. A new group of four to seven families was begun approximately every 2 months. Participation was encouraged by the primary physician at the initial intake appointment and presented as a standard part of entry into the program. A descriptive pamphlet about the groups was given to parents at this time as well. This approach yielded approximately a 75% rate of participation.

During the first year, the groups were jointly led by either myself or another senior CCFH faculty member, along with either the CF head nurse or social worker (who was in advanced training at our Center). This "apprenticeship period" was a time of learning how to facilitate multifamily groups. The medical director or head nurse was the featured person at the first meeting, which bolstered the rate of family participation. The first group meeting focused on the integration of the biomedical with the psychosocial aspects of CF. The four meetings dealt with other topics, such as a family systems orientation, initial family challenges of coping with CF, illness-related communication and problem solving, living with future uncertainty, and ways for families to create meaning with CF.

These initial families took the initiative of developing an ongoing monthly family support group in which the CF social worker served as facilitator. Topics were decided together by participating families and various staff members. CCFH faculty members were invited as guest experts to lead discussions on specific topics (e.g., enriching marriage when raising a child with chronic illness). A family from the ongoing support group came to the fourth (and last) meeting of each initial multifamily group to provide information about the monthly group.

It proved far more challenging to implement a psychoeducational group that included adolescents with CF and their families. Ultimately, an afternoon program was piggybacked onto periodic Saturday gatherings sponsored by the CF foundation. Traditionally, these meetings are designed to give the latest information about advances in CF research and treatment, and they serve a social-networking function for CF families in the Chicago region. Scheduling a social event for adolescents in the late afternoon offered an incentive to attend the educational program.

Rehabilitation Medicine, Palliative Care, and Hospice and Residential Care Settings

The rapid expansion of rehabilitation medicine, palliative and hospice care, and geriatric health care offers huge opportunities for family-oriented integrated care. Overall, collaboration with these settings suits a family systems-oriented model. Because they do not involve acute, cure-oriented health care, these settings emphasize quality of life, meaning-making, and achieving optimal functioning in the chronic or terminal phase. Collaborative teams are the norm and often involve patients and their families, and mental health staffing tends to be more generous. Many of these services routinely include a family meeting at the time of admission to the service, yet family systems knowledge and skills training are often limited. So there is a tremendous unmet need and opportunity for mental health professionals with family systems expertise (e.g., medical family therapists) to provide consultation and seek hiring opportunities.

Collaboration with Consumer-Based Organizations and Communities

Most chronic illnesses have consumer-based organizations that provide essential resources to the affected person and family caregivers. They range from education about disease symptoms, treatment options, and promising research information to networking and support for patients and families through blogs, patient and caregiver support groups and advocacy, and disease-related fundraising. These organizations are key players in empowering families and counteracting isolation. Information is disseminated mainly through an organization's website and public educational events. Health care provider involvement includes participation on medical advisory boards, as invited speakers, and on the organization's specialist provider referral lists, but generally, these organizations do not provide direct clinical services. Many organizations have large memberships; they disseminate information on a regular basis to all members and maintain relationships with medical centers and specialist physicians.

Collaboration between health care institutions and community and consumer-based organizations is vastly underutilized, but has enormous potential, especially in the psychosocial domain. For instance, a number of cities have developed professional–consumer coalitions to address end-of-life clinical care, public education, advocacy, and policy issues. The Chicago End-of-Life Care Coalition is one excellent example.

As yet, most groups do not employ a systems-based approach for couples and families. Most concentrate on patient and caregiver role functions, but systemic and relational challenges for couples and families are often neglected. The FSI model can provide a useful resource for purposes of collaboration. Here is one example of what is possible.

Resilient Partners Program: MS Society—Chicago Center for Family Health Collaboration

In collaboration with the National Multiple Sclerosis Society, Illinois chapter, the Chicago Center for Family Health (CCFH) developed the Resilient Partners Program for couples facing MS (Rolland, McPheters, & Carbonell, 2008; see also Chapter 4). (Funding for 3 years was provided through the MS Society's education budget.) Our focus on couple and family resilience rather than on deficit and dysfunction was essential to forming this joint project.

Forming a collaborative partnership was essential in developing the Resilient Partners Program. To establish the project and formulate a contract, meetings were held over several months that involved CCFH leadership, MS Society staff and Board of Directors (BOD) members, and three couples coping with MS, who were either on the Society BOD or active leaders in the Illinois chapter. The program's content was codeveloped by CCFH staff (myself, senior faculty, medical family therapist, and psychologist fellows); the MS Society Director of Educational Programs (a social worker with advanced training in family therapy from CCFH); and six couples of diverse ages, life-cycle phases, ethnic and cultural groups, and stages of MS disease. The entire project development and implementation process drew upon my own background and models in public health-based community psychiatry. The model was similar in many respects to the excellent Families & Democracy and Citizens Health Care Project model (Doherty et al., 2010).

Given the larger urban and suburban population, offerings could be tailored to either the illness or life-cycle phase. CCFH provided in-service and advanced continuing-education training to the mental health professional staff in charge of MS Society educational programs. The collaboration extended into research projects by two CCFH doctoral fellows: one on the association of depression with couples functioning and MS disease status, and the other on an MBSR program for couples using a multicouple group format. Access to a large database greatly facilitated recruitment of participants.

While we collaborated, it was essential to be mindful of the relationship between consumers and providers of health care. The traditional hierarchical model that marginalizes consumers leads to a mistrust of health care providers and systems. Deference to the MS Society's needs and balanced coleadership were vital to success. At its core, this required an outlook that equally validated the unique wisdom and expertise of consumers and professionals.

Inclusion of Clinicians and Health Care Systems in the Patient's Family Life

Information and Community Resources

Families usually depend on health care providers to give them useful information about potentially helpful community resources and services. Clinicians should gain some familiarity with resources available for the management of long-term conditions. They includes a range of primary and tertiary medical, rehabilitation, respite, transportation, housing, institutional, and financial entitlement services. Friends, neighbors, self-help groups, and religious, cultural, or community organizations are also potential resources.

Since belief systems, ethnocultural values, and family dynamics influence a family's willingness to utilize available resources, it is useful to inquire about a family's prior experiences with providers and community resources. Have they been affirming or alienating? Is the family adequately informed about potential outside sources of help? Lack of awareness may reflect family isolation due to factors such as geographic distance, education or language barriers, poverty, and racial, ethnic, and religious marginalization.

A chronic disorder presents a dilemma for families with rigid boundaries and tendencies to view the outside world as threatening. Despite a family's preference for handling life crises themselves and relying minimally on outsiders, the condition may necessitate including professionals in disease management. Establishing a viable family and health care team relationship requires exquisite sensitivity to these family patterns and values. When ongoing professional involvement or sustained care is warranted, such families will need active assistance and links to potential supports, along with help in overcoming mistrust.

Mutual Accommodation

Ongoing functional relationships with health care team and treatment procedures are essential. The continual need for medical interventions can vary from a daily but momentary reminder to take medications with breakfast to round-the-clock care in a nursing home. Highly uncertain and life-threatening conditions tend to foster a greater dependence on professionals as permanently involved not only in medical care, but also as part of the psychosocial life of a family, regardless of day-to-day medical needs. Disorders differ tremendously in terms of their inherent intrusion on family life, and families vary in their capacity for or comfort with these inclusion processes.

At the time of a hospital admission, the patient and family must adapt to a time-limited shift to a foreign turf. Control issues often center on the degree to which the health care setting allows or encourages families to maintain aspects of their identity. They involve both the permissible options of the hospital or unit and patient and family assertiveness in personalizing the hospital room and the overall experience. How family rituals, such as bedside vigils, mesh with rules of the hospital system for patient and family behavior is one example. Conflicting norms often occur at key illness junctures and frequently surface as issues of control that can severely impair the relationship between the health care and family systems, as the following case vignette illustrates.

A family and close friends had gathered at the hospital the day after the patient had been diagnosed with inoperable cancer. It was a very emotional time for all concerned. Late in the day, several family members and friends had to leave. In the hospital lobby, as the father and son were saying good-bye to a male friend, the emotions that had been contained erupted, and the three men began to cry and hug each other. Within moments, the lobby receptionist had two male hospital security guards tell these three grieving men that they would have to move on. They were hastily ushered into an examining room adjacent to the lobby.

The family never forgot that incident and never forgave the hospital. The hospital was making a statement about acceptable behavior: crying was not permitted in public areas. And the fact that it involved three men was considered particularly disruptive. The meta-message was that men should not display their feelings because it expressed a lack of control, a weakness that undermined the image of normality the hospital wished to convey. This experience impaired the family's collaboration with the physician and health care system, expressed in heightened conflict and control issues about treatment decisions.

Prior Family Experiences with Health Care Systems and Providers

Just as it is vital to understand a family's multigenerational illness and loss experiences in an initial assessment (see Chapter 6), so too is understanding their history of encounters with health and mental health systems and professionals. Useful questions include: "What did you like best about your relationship with Dr. Jones or about your past hospital experiences?" and "What would you have changed about it?" Acknowledgment of past negative experiences is a first step in forming a more productive alliance. Sometimes it is useful for families to write to or re-contact professionals with whom they have had particularly disappointing or traumatic encounters.

Dilemmas of Home-Based Care

When extensive home-based care is vital to basic survival, nurses or other professional caregivers may need to be incorporated into daily family life on the home turf. It is important to explore with families what this change will mean for them. For an elderly couple, a live-in professional caregiver can be both a source of desperately needed respite and a first-time intrusion on their longstanding privacy. Reluctance by other family members may reflect difficulties with accepting a transition to a new illness phase. Often the need for home-based or 24-hour care signals the transition to a terminal phase, and helping families accept this fact can reduce tensions among family members and with clinicians.

Working with Shifting Treatment Settings

Caring for families dealing with chronic conditions often requires clinicians to adapt flexibly to a number of settings, such as office, hospital, specialty services, intensive care unit, family home, extended-care facility, or hospice. With some conditions having medical crises that require frequent hospitalizations, such as kidney failure, the family needs to adapt to unavoidable transitions and health care involvements. It is crucial not to rigidly hold to the traditional boundary around the therapeutic process to help families navigate multiple junctures.

Typically, different treatment settings have designated mental health providers, such as a medical social worker, health psychologist, and consulting psychiatrist. As patients and families alternate between specialty care settings, their available mental health care providers change. As integrated care continues to grow, this scenario will become increasingly common. Like biomedical care, behavioral health care can become fragmented, and patients and families may need a coordinating mental health care provider, who can ensure continuity and collaboration in all health care settings over the illness course. This is especially needed when a number of specialists are involved in continuing care. A family systems-oriented BHC clinician is ideally suited for this role. For example, a medical family therapist may provide behavioral health care to a patient and family dealing with heart disease in a primary care setting. When the disease progresses and requires cardiac bypass surgery, followed by inpatient and outpatient cardiac rehabilitation, this therapist can be proactive with the associated mental health care providers in these settings. Since specialty care providers, such as medical social workers and nurses, are typically overextended, this proactive collaboration is typically appreciated.

BELIEFS AND EXPECTATIONS: FIT AMONG CLINICIANS, HEALTH CARE SYSTEMS, AND FAMILIES

As health care providers, we need to be aware of three kinds of beliefs that are important to both effective collaboration and our own well-being: personal beliefs about illness and its meaning, beliefs adopted from our diverse professional disciplines, and the beliefs and regulations of the institutional setting. Personal beliefs include all the same values described in Chapter 8.

The mission, values, and norms of varied health care settings overlap, yet differ. Generally, as health care services change from intensive, acute care to recovery, rehabilitation, or palliative care, relationships become more balanced between providers and patient families. The relative emphasis shifts from biomedical intervention toward biopsychosocial–spiritual care. The relative meshing of our personal belief systems with our professional disciplines' guiding principles can vary, depending on the setting.

The same questions about beliefs asked of families are relevant questions for each of us on the health care team. Here are a few examples.

1. What key values and health beliefs guide you in life (see Chapter 8)?
2. What professional discipline values guide you as a clinician?
3. What values guide your work in your particular health care setting(s)?
4. What are your attitudes about your contribution and the family's ability to influence the illness course and outcome?
5. How do you see the balance between your and the family's participation in the treatment process?
6. How can important differences in beliefs be bridged?

Belief Fit and Differences

In systemic practice, we must stay mindful of multiple levels of meaning from the individual, interpersonal, and larger systems levels in which we and the patients and families are embedded. This means attending to the fit between patient and family members' beliefs and those of providers and systems (see Figure 18.1).

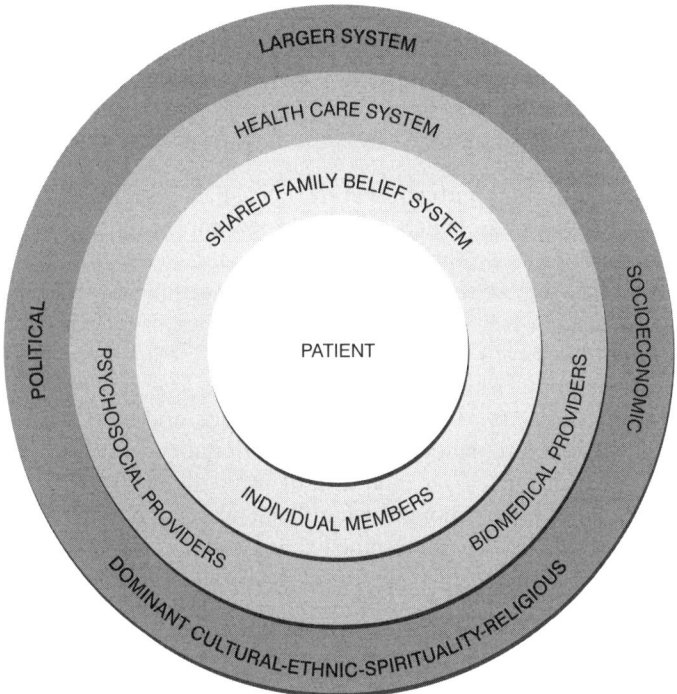

FIGURE 18.1. Fit of beliefs: Mutual influences within and across levels.

Belief differences should generally be acknowledged and addressed. Pseudo-mutuality with a family can be as harmful as disregarding their beliefs. Normative differences among family members, families and providers, or families and institutions may erupt into destructive conflicts during a health crisis, as shown in the following case.

The head nurse for an intensive care unit (ICU) contacted me to intervene with a patient and his mother who were disrupting the unit because the mother insisted on remaining at her son's bedside. The unit's customary rules limited family visits to 10 minutes. Also, the highly emotional arguing among the patient, his wife, and his mother about this issue was a further annoyance that was impossible to manage.

The patient, Stavros H., a teacher in his early forties, had been admitted to the ICU with symptoms of intractable angina. A first-generation Greek American, he had been married for 12 years to Dana, who was from a Scandinavian background. A long-standing, smoldering triangular conflict regarding divided loyalties between himself, his mother, and his spouse now flared up. When Stavros was admitted to the hospital with heart disease, his mother began a 24-hour vigil by her son's hospital bed, so she could tend to him at any hour. Dana greatly resented her mother-in-law's seemingly intrusive behavior. Mrs. H. criticized what she perceived as Dana's emotional coldness and relative lack of concern. Stavros felt caught between his warring mother and wife and complained of increased symptoms.

Called in to consult with this family, I became acutely aware of the multiple layers of conflicting beliefs and positions, including my own, at issue in this situation. Because the consultation request was in my capacity as a consultation–liaison psychiatrist, I realized that my primary loyalty was to the hospital. This meant restoring an optimal environment for the unit to conduct its normal medical task of providing state-of-the-art technological care to acutely ill patients. From that perspective, the mother was interfering with the unit's basic mission. Her continuous presence and emotional behavior constituted the problem, whereas the "unemotional" wife, who felt comfortable keeping her distance, was seen as a healthy ally of the unit. Therefore, in the triangular conflict among the family members, the unit's staff inadvertently had chosen sides. It was assumed that I should intervene in the situation accordingly—from the perspective of the unit's primary purpose and the family beliefs and behaviors that would support that mission.

This crisis brought the family's longstanding tensions to professional attention for the first time. They saw me as a powerful tie-breaking vote in resolving their long-standing feud. Both his mother and wife lobbied for my vote, while Stavros looked on in torn dismay.

Differing cultural norms needed to be acknowledged. It is normative in Greek culture for parents and their children to maintain close ties after marriage, and it is expected that a good mother would tend to her son in a health crisis. A son would be disloyal not to allow his mother to fulfill that role. This norm sharply differed from the wife's Scandinavian traditions and normative expectation that a wife's position should take primacy over her mother-in-law's. Each side pathologized the other, escalating this conflictual triangle with the patient caught in the middle.

In this situation it was vital first to affirm normative multicultural differences that had reached an emotional crescendo during a health crisis. Essentially, I announced there was no need for a vote since I saw everyone behaving normatively. My affirmation promoted a shift from blaming and pathologizing to one of accommodating different, equally legitimate cultural preferences. This intervention allowed the beliefs and values of all family members to be affirmed, which then facilitated mutual acceptance.

The mother accurately perceived that the medical team was siding with her daughter-in-law, which heightened her reactivity to the unit, which, in turn, increased the unit's reactive attempts to control her in a mutually escalating cycle. Further, she assumed that I would have undivided loyalty to the hospital and would side with the unit and Dana. Abandoning the idea of identifying the source of family pathology allowed a team solution-focused approach. I was able to address Stavros and his mother in the following manner: "The unit and I really understand how important your being together at this time is for both of you. Do you think you could help the unit out by compromising a little so that it can give you the best medical care possible?"

My intervention in this case involved psychosocial shuttle diplomacy. Discussion with the staff about my view of the family was coupled with requests for some flexibility on its part to allow biomedical care to be delivered without significant compromise. I suggested that affirming the mother's values would enable her to work with the unit staff rather than in opposition to it. The staff made some accommodations by extending the mother's visitation time and arranged a sleeping cot in a nearby utility room, allowing her to be close should any crisis emerge.

Interestingly, my position of impartiality and normalization sparked discussion among the staff about their own personal and family values. Some unacknowledged cultural differences among the staff were openly communicated for the first time, which increased the cultural sensitivity and flexibility of the unit in subsequent cases.

In this case my own personal and professional belief system was an important consideration. My cultural background was more in sync with the Greek side of this family, in the sense that bedside rituals are a common Jewish tradition. Awareness of my own values was important in maintaining a balanced position with family members, and averting problems in my relationship to the ICU. My tendency to ally with the Greek side of the family was also influenced by my professional beliefs about optimal mental health and the value of open communication and expression of feelings, here displayed in the mother–son relationship. Reinforcement of that value in this situation could have been easily interpreted as an alliance with the mother-in-law against the wife, so it was also important to validate Dana's position and her importance to Stavros as his loving wife.

If Stavros had been a patient in a hospice service, his traditional Greek values would have fit relatively seamlessly with those of palliative care. Family members staying at the bedside or conducting rituals are welcome and common. The participation of family and health care providers together in nonmedical care or rituals is part of the hospice culture, fostering more holistic collaborative care than that in an intensive care unit. It's important to remember that with chronic illness, patients and their families move between these different health care environments and cultures, sometimes frequently and during the same illness phase or episode, where multiple components of care are provided in tandem, for example, in surgery, rehabilitation, and physical therapy.

Illness Phase-Related Issues

There is an ongoing evolution in the fit between clinicians and families in different contexts, at different illness phases, and in relation to individual and family development. During the initial crisis phase, when the typical aim of a medical workup is a diagnosis, the meaning of symptoms is often objectified as narrowly biological. For providers, family belief systems can appear to be an extraneous distraction from the central medical task. Unfortunately, having a strictly technological imperative can become synonymous with professionalism. Failing to acknowledge the patient's and family members' beliefs or explanations about illness can signify disrespect for the patient and family.

During a health crisis, the patient may undergo care in the most technologically sophisticated part of a health system, such as the intensive care unit. For all concerned, there is a heightened focus on the competition between technology and disease, and providers can easily adopt a battlefield mentality in their efforts to achieve success. In such situations it requires the utmost skill for clinicians and families to remain sensitive to issues of quality of life, personal dignity, and compassionate care as core beliefs that need to be sustained throughout a chronic illness, not left at the doors to the intensive care unit. Typically, the patient's room is so full of high-tech equipment that there is little space to personalize. One hurried, normally sensitive physician exclaimed bluntly, "Get that picture [which happened to be a family photo] out of the way so I can see the monitor." In this pressured instant, an imperative for competency superseded all others at the expense of family well-being and of the physician's relationship with the patient and family members.

Transition Points

It is common for differences in beliefs or attitudes to erupt at major treatment or illness transition points. For instance, the murky boundary between the chronic and terminal phase highlights the potential for professionals' beliefs to collide with those of the patient and family. We can either facilitate or hinder this process. A health care team that persists in its heroic efforts to prevent the death of the patient can convey confusing messages. Families may not know how to interpret continued lifesaving efforts, assuming real hope when virtually none exists. Providers can feel bound to a technological imperative that requires them to exhaust all possibilities at their disposal, regardless of the odds of success.

Often physicians feel committed to this course for ethical reasons or concerns about legal liability. Is the medical team having its own difficulties letting go? Strong relationships with certain patients can be fueled by losses, often unresolved, in health care professionals' own lives (see Chapter 17). Endless treatment can represent the medical team's inability to separate their general value of controlling diseases from their beliefs about participation (separate from cure) in a patient's total care, which includes biopsychosocial and spiritual well-being.

Multiple Providers and Health Care Systems Interface Issues

An initial family consultation should include an assessment of the various interlocking layers of clinicians and systems that are currently involved or may become involved over the anticipated course of the condition. Regarding this complex interface, a systems-oriented BHC provider can act as a bridge between the patient, family, and health care system, functioning flexibly as psychosocial interpreter, shuttle diplomat, mediator, and advocate.

Clinicians need to be particularly attuned to emotionally charged situations in which family members may have differences about important decisions. For instance, if family members disagree about the need for nursing home placement of a deteriorating aging parent, clinicians or services may argue by proxy about the same subject and become isomorphically aligned, sometimes dysfunctionally, with different family member's viewpoints. Conversely, a family given inconsistent advice about the need for a placement may wind up having a family debate that mirrors issues that providers have not resolved.

PRINCIPLES FOR FAMILY-ORIENTED PROGRAMS AND POLICIES

Any family that has lived with illness and disability understands at some basic level that clinical care, effective coping, and adaptation can best occur within a healing environment that is family-oriented, contextual, and, above all, collaborative. I strongly believe that the future of our profession lies in our ability to envision and translate systemic thinking and issues related to social justice into the larger society. Systemic thinking that transcends the boundaries of the patient and family can best guide our involvement with families and promote healing and health. To this end, we need family-oriented health policies and programmatic initiatives. The following principles are essential in supporting families coping with illness and disability.

- *Health care reform should provide universal care that includes reimbursable, prevention-oriented family and relational-centered mental health services.* Psychosocial care needs to be reimbursed on the same basis as physical health care.

- *The definition of family should be broad enough to encompass the diversity of family forms and kin networks in contemporary society.*

- *Cost-effective family-oriented integrated care models need to be further developed and researched.* They should include the entire range of biomedical and mental health care providers. Collaborative care models that include health care institutions, families, and communities can significantly reduce direct and indirect costs and enhance overall family well-being.

- *Professional education and service delivery models need to better address the psychosocial needs of families facing major health conditions.* Basic knowledge about family systems and the normative psychosocial demands of various health disorders throughout illness phases should be included in the education of all health and mental health care professionals.

- *More resources must be directed toward preventing the psychosocial difficulties associated with chronic disorders.* The efficacy of routinely offering a family behavioral health consultation at the time of diagnosis or early in the initial crisis phase of a serious health condition needs further research documentation.

- *Policies that advocate comprehensive home and community-based care should be advanced*, thereby reducing the need for institution-based health care. They include expanded provisions for rehabilitation and long-term care that supports family caregiving roles, while protecting families' job and economic security.

- *Policies concerning continuing life support and end-of-life decisions, including physician-assisted dying to support patients' rights, dignity, and control in the dying process, need further advancement.* These complex decisions need to be addressed, not just from technological and ethical perspectives, but also in terms of the profound impact on patient and family well-being and resources.

- *Innovative programs should be implemented to address workplace and family caregiving needs.* These should include more flexible work arrangements that accommodate the immediate and long-term demands of illness and disability, while maintaining the continuity of home and work life equitably for both men and women. This includes adequate insurance coverage for home health care.

- *Programs should be sensitive and flexible so that families of many different cultural orientations and at various life-cycle phases* can be accommodated.

In conclusion, in the next phase of evolution of integrated health care, I believe we need to (1) recommit ourselves to a partnership with patients and their families as essential resources and equal partners in collaborative, integrated health care, (2) forge relationships between integrated primary and specialty health care, and (3) promote the involvement of the consumer, patient, family, and community in both health care services and in strategic planning at the advocacy and policy levels. Above all, we must advocate for a humane, responsive system of health care that provides this vision of care not as a privilege, but as a basic right for all patients and their families.

References

Ablitt, A., Jones, G. V., & Muers, J. (2009). Living with dementia: A systematic review of the influence of relationship factors. *Aging & Mental Health, 13*(4), 497–511.
Agronin, M. E. (2015). Sexuality and aging. In D. Steffens, D. Blazer, & K. Thakur (Eds.), *The American Psychiatric Publishing textbook of geriatric psychiatry* (5th ed., pp. 389–415). Washington, DC: American Psychiatric Publishing.
Alderfer, M., Nausaria, N., & Kazak, A. (2009). Family functioning and post-traumatic stress disorder in adolescent survivors of childhood cancer. *Journal of Family Psychology, 23*(5), 717–725.
Alderfer, M., Stanley, C., Conroy, R., Long, K., Fairclough, D., Kazak, A., et al. (2014). The social functioning of siblings of children with cancers: A multi-informant investigation. *Journal of Pediatric Psychology, 40*(3), 309–319.
Aldwin, C. M., & Igarashi, H. (2012). An ecological model of resilience in later life. In B. Hayslip & G. Smith (Eds.), *Emerging perspectives on resilience in adulthood and later life. Annual Review of Gerontology and Geriatrics, 22*, 115–130. New York: Springer Publishing.
Alzheimer's Association. (2015). 2015 Alzheimer's disease facts and figures. *Alzheimer's and Dementia, 11*(3), 332–384.
Anderson, C. M., Reiss, D., & Hogarty, G. (1986). *Schizophrenia and the family*. New York: Guilford Press.
Antonovsky, A. (1998). The sense of coherence: An historical and future perspective. In H. McCubbin, E. Thompson, A. Thompson, & J. Fromer (Eds.), *Stress, coping and health in families: Sense of coherence and resiliency* (pp. 3–20). Thousand Oaks, CA: SAGE.
Asen, E., & Scholz, M. (2010). *Multi-family therapy: Concepts and techniques*. New York: Routledge.
Badr, H., & Acitelli, L. K. (2005). Dyadic adjustment in chronic illness: Does relationship talk matter? *Journal of Family Psychology, 19*(3), 465–469.
Barakat, L., Alderfer, M., & Kazak, A. (2005). Posttraumatic growth in adolescent survivors of cancer and their mothers and fathers. *Journal of Pediatric Psychology, 31*(4), 413–419.

Barlow, J. H., & Ellard, D. R. (2006). The psychosocial well-being of children with chronic disease, their parents and siblings: An overview of the research evidence base. *Child, Care, Health, and Development, 32*, 19–31.

Bateson, G. (1979). *Mind and nature: A necessary unity.* New York: Dutton.

Batsch, N., & Mittelman, M. (2012). *World Alzheimer Report, 2012: Overcoming the stigma of dementia.* London: Alzheimer's Disease International.

Beck, T., & Haigh, E. (2014). Advances in cognitive theory and therapy: The generic cognitive model. *Annual Review of Clinical Psychology, 10*, 1–24.

Becker, E. (1973). *The denial of death.* New York: Free Press.

Belle, S. H., Burgio, L., Burns, R., Coon, D., Czaja, S. C., Gallagher-Thompson, D., et al. (2006). Enhancing the quality of life of dementia caregivers from different ethnic or racial groups: A randomized, controlled trial. *Annals of Internal Medicine, 145*, 727–738.

Benbow, S., & Sharman, V. (2014). Review of family therapy and dementia: Twenty-five years on. *International Psychogeriatrics, 26*(12), 2037–2050.

Berg, C. A., & Upchurch, R. (2007). A developmental-contextual model of couples coping with chronic illness across the adult life span. *Psychological Bulletin, 133*, 920–954.

Blount, A., Kathol, R., Thomas, M., Schoenbaum, M., Rollman, B. L., O'Donohue, W., et al. (2007). The economics of behavioral health services in medical settings: A summary of the evidence. *Professional Psychology: Research and Practice, 38*(3), 290–297.

Bolier, L., Haverman, M., Westerhof, G., Riper, H., Smit, F., & Bohlmeijer, E. (2013). Positive psychology interventions: A meta-analysis of randomized controlled studies. *BMC Public Health, 13*, 119.

Borden, W. (1991). Stress, coping, and adaptation in spouses of older adults with chronic dementia. *Social Work Research and Abstracts, 27*, 14–22.

Boss, P. (2005). *Loss, trauma, and resilience: Therapeutic work with ambiguous loss.* New York: Norton.

Boss, P. (2010). The trauma and complicated grief of ambiguous loss. *Pastoral Psychology, 59*, 137–145.

Boss, P. (2011). *Loving someone who has dementia.* San Francisco: Jossey-Bass.

Boszormenyi-Nagy, I., & Sparks, G. (2013). *Invisible loyalties: Reciprocity in intergenerational family therapy.* New York: Routledge. (Original work published 1984)

Bowen, M. (1993). *Family therapy in clinical practice.* New York: Jason Aronson.

Bowen, M. (2004). Family reaction to death. In F. Walsh & M. McGoldrick (Eds.), *Living beyond loss: Death in the family* (pp. 47–60). New York: Norton.

Brody, E. (2004). *Women in the middle: Their parent-care years.* New York: Springer.

Brouwer-Dudokdewit, A. C., Savenije, A., Zoeteweij, M., Maat-Kievit, A., & Tibben, A. (2002). A hereditary disorder in the family and the family life cycle: Huntington disease as a paradigm. *Family Process, 41*(4), 677–692.

Butler, M., Kane, R. L., McAlpine, D., Kathol, R., Fu, S. S., Hagedorn, H., et al. (2011). Does integrated care improve treatment for depression?: A systematic review. *Journal of Ambulatory Care Management, 34*(2), 113–125.

Byng-Hall, J. (2004). Loss and family scripts. In F. Walsh & M. McGoldrick (Eds.), *Living beyond loss: Death in the family.* New York: Norton.

Cameron, L., & Muller, C. (2009). Psychological aspects of genetic testing. *Current Opinion in Psychiatry, 22*, 218–223.

Campbell, T. (2003). The effectiveness of family interventions for physical disorders. *Journal of Marital and Family Therapy, 29*(2), 263–281.

Carr, A. (2013). *Positive psychology: The science of happiness and human strengths* (2nd ed.). New York: Routledge.

Carr, D., & Springer, K. W. (2010). Advances in families and health research in the 21st century. *Journal of Marriage and the Family, 72*(3), 743–761.

Centers for Disease Control and Prevention. (2014). *Report to Congress on traumatic brain injury in the United States: Epidemiology and rehabilitation.* Atlanta, GA: National Center for Injury Prevention and Control, Division of Unintentional Injury Prevention.

Centers for Disease Control and Prevention (CDC) and National Institutes of Health (NIH) in collaboration with the Department of Defense and Department of Veterans Affairs Leadership Panel. (2013). *Report to Congress on traumatic brain injury in the United States: Understanding the public health problem among current and former military personnel.* Washington, DC: Authors.

Cheavans, J. S., Michael, S. T., & Snyder, C. R. (2005). The correlates of hope: Psychological and physiological benefits. In J. A. Eliott (Ed.), *Interdisciplinary perspectives on hope* (pp. 119–132). Hauppauge, NY: Nova Science.

Choosing death: Health quarterly special. (1993). [Television series episode] In *Frontline*. Boston: WGBH Educational Foundation.

Clarke, T., Black, L., Stussman, B., Barnes, P., & Nahin, R. (2015, February). Trends in the use of complementary health approaches among adults: United States, 2002–2012. *National Health Statistics Reports, 79*, 1–16.

Cohen, D. J., Davis, M. D., Hall, J., Gilchrist, E., & Miller, B. F. (2015). *A guidebook of professional practices for behavioral health and primary care integration: Observations from exemplary sites.* Rockville, MD: Agency for Healthcare Research and Quality.

Collins, C., Hewson, D. L., Munger, R., & Wade, T. (2010). *Evolving models of behavioral health integration in primary care.* New York: Milbank Memorial Fund.

Collins, F. S., Green, E., Guttmacher, A. E., & Guyer, M. S. (2003). A vision for the future of genomic research. *Nature, 422*, 835–847.

Collins, S., Rasmussen, P., Beutel, S., & Doty, M. (2015). *The problem of underinsurance and how rising deductibles will make it worse—Findings from the Commonwealth Fund Biennial Health Insurance Survey.* New York: Commonwealth Fund.

Combrinck-Graham, L. (1985). A developmental model for family systems. *Family Process, 24*, 139–150.

Compas, B., Jaser, S., Dunn, M., & Rodriguez, E. (2012). Coping with chronic illness in childhood and adolescence. *Annual Review of Clinical Psychology, 8*, 455–480.

Coon, D. W. (2012). Resilience and family caregiving. *Annual Review of Gerontology and Geriatrics, 32*(1), 231–249.

Cousino, M. K., & Hazen, R. A. (2013). Parenting stress among caregivers of children with chronic illness: A systematic review. *Journal of Pediatric Psychology, 38*(8), 809–828.

Cousins, N. (2001). *Anatomy of an illness as perceived by the patient: Reflections on healing and regeneration.* New York: Norton. (Original work published in 1979)

Coyne, J. C., Rohrbaugh, M. J., Shoham, V., Sonnega, J. S., & Nicklas, J. M. (2001). Prognostic importance of marital quality for survival of congestive heart failure. *American Journal of Cardiology, 88*, 526–529.

Csikszentmihalyi, M. (2014). *Flow and the foundations of positive psychology.* New York: Springer.

Daneshpour, M. (1998). Muslim families and family therapy. *Journal of Marital and Family Therapy, 24*, 355–390.

Daniels, K. J., Lamson, A. L., & Hodgson, J. (2007). An exploration of the marital relationship and Alzheimer's disease: One couple's story. *Families, Systems, and Health, 25*(2), 162–177.

Davey, M., Kissl, K., & Lynch, L. (2016). *Helping children and families cope with parental illness.* New York: Routledge.

Didonna, F. (Ed.). (2009). *Clinical handbook of mindfulness.* New York: Springer.

Dixon, L., McFarlane, W. R., Lefley, H., Luckstead, A., Cohen, M., Falloon, I., et al. (2001). Evidence-based practices for services to families of people with psychiatric disabilities. *Psychiatric Services, 52,* 903–910.

Doherty, W. J. (1995). The whys and levels of collaborative family healthcare. *Family Systems Medicine, 13,* 275–281.

Doherty, W. J., & Baird, M. A. (1983). *Family therapy and family medicine: Towards the primary care of families.* New York: Guilford Press.

Doherty, W. J., & Baird, M. A. (1986). Developmental levels in family-centered medical care. *Family Medicine, 18,* 153–156.

Doherty, W. J., McDaniel, S., & Baird, M. A. (1996). Five levels of primary care/behavioral healthcare collaboration. *Behavioral Healthcare Tomorrow, 5,* 25–27.

Doherty, W. J., Mendenhall, T. J., & Berge, J. M. (2010). The Families & Democracy and Citizens Health Care Project. *Journal of Marital and Family Therapy, 36,* 389–402.

Doka, K. (2002). *Disenfranchised grief.* Champaign, IL: Research Press.

D'Onofrio, B. M., & Lahey, B. B. (2010). Biosocial influences on the family: A decade review. *Journal of Marriage and Family, 72*(3), 762–782.

Driver, J., Tabares, A., Shapiro, A., & Gottman, J. (2012). Interaction in happy and unhappy marriages: Gottman Laboratory studies. In F. Walsh (Ed.), *Normal family processes* (4th ed., pp. 57–77). New York: Guilford Press.

Druss, B. G., von Esenwein, S. A., Compton, M. T., Rask, K. J., Zhao, L., & Parker, R. M. (2010). A randomized trial of medical care management for community mental health settings: The Primary Care Access, Referral, and Evaluation (PCARE) study. *American Journal of Psychiatry, 167*(2), 151–159.

Elder, G. H., & Shanahan, M. J. (2006). The life course and human development. In R. M. Lerner & W. Damon (Eds.), *Handbook of child psychology* (6th ed., Vol. 1, pp. 665–715). Hoboken, NJ: Wiley.

Ell, K., Katon, W., Xie, B., Lee, P., Kapetanovic, S., Guterman, J., et al. (2010). Collaborative care management of major depression among low-income, predominantly Hispanic subjects with diabetes: A randomized control trial. *Diabetes Care, 33*(4), 706–713.

Ellis, D., Naar-King, S., Templin, T., Frey, M., Cunningham, P., & Sheidow, A. (2008). Mulitsystemic therapy for adolescents with poorly controlled type 1 diabetes: Reduced diabetic ketoacidosis admissions and related costs over 24 months. *Diabetes Care, 31,* 1746–1747.

Engel, G. L. (1977). The need for a new medical model: A challenge for biomedicine. *Science, 196,* 129–136.

Etz, R. S., Cohen, D. J., Woolf, S. H., Holtrop, J. S., Donahue, K. E., Isaacson, N. F., et al. (2008). Bridging primary care practices and communities to promote healthy behaviors. *American Journal of Preventive Medicine, 35*(Suppl. 5), S390–S397.

Falicov, C. J. (2009). Religion and spiritual tradition in immigrant families: Significance for Latino health and mental health. In F. Walsh (Ed.), *Spiritual resources in family therapy* (2nd ed., pp. 156–173). New York: Guilford Press.

Falicov, C. J. (2013). *Latino families in therapy: A guide to multicultural practice* (2nd ed.). New York: Guilford Press.

Feinberg, L., Reinhard, S., Houser, A., & Choula, R. (2011). *Valuing the invaluable: 2011 update the growing contributions and costs of family caregiving.* Washington, DC: AARP Public Policy Institute.

Fekete, E. M., Stephens, M., Mickelson, K. D., & Druley, J. (2007). Couples' support provision during illness: The role of perceived emotional responsiveness. *Families, Systems, and Health, 25*(2), 204–217.

Fisher, L., & Lieberman, M. A. (1994). Alzheimer's disease: The impact of the family on spouses, offspring, and in-laws. *Family Process, 33*(3), 305–325.

Forgeard, H., & Seligman, M. (2012). Seeing the glass half full: A review of the causes and consequences of optimism. *Practiques Psychologiques, 18*(2), 107–120.

Frank, A. W. (1998). Just listening: Narrative and deep illness. *Families, Systems, and Health, 16*(3), 197–212.

Franks, H. M., & Roesch, S. C. (2006). Appraisals and coping in people living with cancer: A meta-analysis. *Psycho-oncology, 15*(12), 1027–1037.

Fredriksen-Goldsen, K. I., Kim, H. J., Barkan, S. E., Muraco, A., & Hoy-Ellis, C. P. (2013). Health disparities among lesbian, gay, and bisexual older adults: Results from a population-based study. *American Journal of Public Health, 103*(10), 1802–1809.

Freedman, J., & Combs, G. (1996). *Narrative therapy: The social construction of preferred realities.* New York: Norton.

Gaugler, J., Anderson, K., Zarit, S., & Pearlin, L. (2004). Family involvement in the nursing home: Effects on stress and well-being. *Aging and Mental Health, 8*, 65–75.

Gaugler, J., Gallagher-Winkler, K., Kehrberg, K., Lund, A., Marsolek, C., Ringham, K., et al. (2011). The Memory Club: Providing support to persons with early stage dementia and their care partners. *American Journal of Alzheimer's Disease and Other Dementias, 26*, 218–226.

Gawande, A. (2014). *Being mortal: Medicine and what matters in the end.* New York: Henry Holt.

Gelhert, S., & Browne, T. (Eds.). (2018). *Handbook of health social work* (3rd ed.). Hoboken, NJ: Wiley.

Gerrard-Morris, A., Taylor, H. G., Yeates, K. O., Walz, N. C., Stancin, T., Minich, N., et al. (2010). Cognitive development after traumatic brain injury in young children. *Journal of the International Neuropsychological Society, 16*(1), 157–168.

Godwin, E., Kreutzer, J., Arango-Lasprilla, J., & Lehan, T. (2012). Marriage after brain injury. Review, analysis, and research recommendations. *Journal of Head Trauma Rehabilitation, 26*(1), 43–55.

Goins, R. T., Spencer, M., & Byrd, J. (2009). Research on rural caregiving: A literature review. *Journal of Applied Gerontology, 28*(2), 139–170.

Gold, K., Sen, A., & Schwenck, T. (2013). Details on suicide among US physicians: Data from the National Violent Death Reporting System. *General Hospital Psychiatry, 35*(1), 45–49.

Gonzalez, S., Steinglass, P., & Reiss, D. (2002). Application of multifamily groups in chronic medical disorders. In W. F. McFarlane (Ed.), *Multifamily groups in the treatment of severe psychiatric disorders* (pp. 315–340). New York: Guilford Press.

Gottman, J. M. (2011). *The science of trust: Emotional attunement for couples.* New York: Norton.

Grabiak, B., Bender, C., & Puskar, K. (2007). The impact of parental cancer on the adolescent: An analysis of the literature. *Psycho-Oncology, 16*, 127–137.

Greef, A., & Nolting, C. (2013). Resilience in families of children with developmental disabilities. *Families, Systems, and Health, 31*, 396–405.

Green, R. J. (2012). Gay and lesbian couples and families. In F. Walsh (Ed.), *Normal family processes: Growing complexity and diversity* (4th ed., pp. 172–195). New York: Guilford Press.

Green, R. J., & Werner, P. (1996). Intrusiveness and closeness-caregiving: Rethinking the concept of family enmeshment. *Family Process, 35*, 115–136.

Griffith, J., & Griffith, M. (1994). *The body speaks*. New York: Basic Books.

Groleau, D., Young, A., & Kirmayer, L. (2006). The McGill Illness Narrative Interview (MINI): An interview schedule to elicit meanings and modes of reasoning related to illness experience. *Transcultural Psychiatry, 43*(4), 671–691.

Hagedoorn, M., Sanderman, R., Bolks, H. N., Tuinstra, J., & Coyne, J. C. (2008). Distress in couples coping with cancer: A meta-analysis and critical review of role and gender effects. *Psychological Bulletin, 134*(1), 1–30.

Halfon, N., & Newacheck, P. W. (2010). Evolving notions of childhood chronic illness. *Journal of the American Medical Association, 303*, 665–666.

Hall, M. J., & Olopade, O. I. (2006). Disparities on genetic testing: Thinking outside the BRCA box. *Journal of Clinical Oncology, 24*(14), 2197–2203.

Hansson, K., & Cederblad, M. (2004). Sense of coherence as a meta-theory for salutogenic family therapy. *Journal of Family Psychotherapy, 15*, 39–54.

Hartling, L., Milne, A., Tjosvold, L., Wrightson, D., Gallivan, J., & Newton, A. S. (2014). A systematic review of interventions to support siblings of children with chronic illness or disability. *Journal of Paediatrics and Child Health, 50*(10), E26–E38.

Hartmann, M., Bazner, E., Wild, B., Eisler, I., & Herzog, W. (2010). Effects of interventions involving the family in the treatment of adult patients with chronic physical diseases: A meta-analysis. *Psychotherapeutics and Psychosomatics, 79*, 136–148.

Heron, M. (2012). Deaths: Leading causes for 2008. *National Vital Statistics Reports, 60*(6).

Heru, A. (2013). *Working with families in medical settings: A multidisciplinary guide for psychiatrists and other health professionals*. New York: Routledge.

Himmelstein, D., Thorne, D., Warren, E., & Woolhandler, S. (2009). Medical bankruptcy in the United States, 2007: Results of a national study. *American Journal of Medicine, 122*, 741–746.

Hodgson, J., Lamson, A., Mendenhall, T., & Crane, R. (Eds.). (2014). *Medical family therapy: Advance applications*. New York: Springer.

Hoffman, L. (1990). Constructing realities: An art of lenses. *Family Process, 29*, 1–13.

Holtkamp, S. C. (2000). Anticipatory mourning and organ donation. In T. A. Rando (Ed.), *Clinical dimensions of anticipatory mourning: Theory and practice in working with the dying, their loved ones, and their caregivers* (pp. 511–535). Champaign, IL: Research Press.

Hood, R. W., Hill, P. C., & Spilka, B. (2009). *The psychology of religion: An empirical approach* (4th ed.). New York: Guilford Press.

Hughes, A., Hertlein, K., & Hagey, D. (2011). A MedFT-informed sex therapy for treating sexual problems associated with chronic illness. *Journal of Family Psychotherapy, 22*, 114–127.

Hurd, M., Martorell, P., Delavande, A., Mullen, K., & Langa, K. (2013). Monetary costs of dementias in the United States. *New England Journal of Medicine, 368*, 1326–1334.

Hurley, K., Miller, S., Rubin, L., & Weinberg, D. (2006). The individual facing genetic issues. In S. Miller, S. McDaniel, J. Rolland, & S. Feetham (Eds.), *Individuals, families, and the new era of genetics: Biopsychosocial perspectives* (pp. 79–117). New York: Norton.

Hurt, C., Burn, D., Hindle, J., Samuel, M., Wilson, K., & Brown, R. (2014). Thinking positively about chronic illness: An exploration of optimism, illness perceptions, and well-being in patients with Parkinson's disease. *British Journal of Health Psychology, 19*(2), 363–379.

Imber-Black, E. (2012). The value of rituals in family life. In F. Walsh (Ed.), *Normal family processes* (4th ed., pp. 483–497). New York: Guilford Press.

Imber-Black, E. (2014). Will talking about it make it worse?: Facilitating family conversations in the context of chronic and life-shortening illness. *Journal of Family Nursing, 20*(2), 151–163.

Imber-Black, E., Roberts, J., & Whiting, R. (Eds.). (2003). *Rituals in families and family therapy* (2nd ed.). New York: Norton.

Jacobs, B. (2006). *The emotional survival guide for caregivers: Looking after yourself and your family while helping an aging parent.* New York: Guilford Press.

Jacobs, B., & Mayer, J. (2016). *Meditations for caregivers: Practical, emotional, and spiritual support for you and your family.* Boston: Da Capo Press.

Jaremka, L. M., Derry, H. M., & Kiecolt-Glaser, J. K. (2014). Psychoneuroimmunology of interpersonal relationships. In D. Mostofsky, *The handbook of behavioral medicine: Assessment and methodology.* New York: Wiley-Blackwell.

Jessop, D., & Stein, R. (1985). Uncertainty and its relations to psychological and social correlates of chronic illness in children. *Social Science in Medicine, 20*, 993–999.

Joling, K., van Marwijk, H., Smit, F., van der Horst, H., & Scheltens, P. (2012). Does a family meetings intervention prevent depression and anxiety in family caregivers of dementia patients?: A randomized trial. *PLOS ONE, 7*, e30936.

Kabat-Zinn, J. (2003). Mindfulness-based interventions in context: Past, present, and future. *Clinical Psychology: Science and Practice, 10*(2), 144–156.

Kasper, J., Freedman, V., & Spillman, B. (2014). Disability and care needs of older Americans by dementia status: An analysis of the 2011 National Health and Aging Trends Study. Available from *https://aspe.hhs.gov/daltcp/reports/2014/NHATS-DS.cfm.*

Katon, W., Unutzer, J., Wells, K., & Jones, L. (2010). Collaborative depression care: History, evolution and ways to enhance dissemination and sustainability. *General Hospital Psychiatry, 32*(5), 456–464.

Kayser, K., Watson, L. E., & Andrade, J. T. (2007). Cancer as a "we-disease": Examining the process of coping from a relational perspective. *Families, Systems, and Health, 25*(4), 404–418.

Kazak, A. (2005). Evidence-based interventions for survivors of childhood cancer and their families. *Journal of Pediatric Psychology, 30*(1), 47–49.

Kazak, A. (2006). Pediatric Psychosocial Preventative Health Model (PPPHM): Research, practice and collaboration in pediatric family systems medicine. *Families, Systems, and Health, 24*, 381–395.

Khoury, B., Lecomte, T., Fortin, G., Masse, M., Therien, P., & Bouchard, V. (2013). Mindfulness-based therapy: A comprehensive meta-analysis. *Clinical Psychology Review, 33*, 763–771.

Kiecolt-Glaser, J. K., & Newton, T. L. (2001). Marriage and health: His and hers. *Psychological Bulletin, 27*, 472–503.

King, D. A., & Quill, T. (2006). Working with families in palliative care: One size does not fit all. *Journal of Palliative Care, 9*(3), 704–715.

King, D. A., & Wynne, L. C. (2004). The emergence of "family integrity" in later life. *Family Process, 43*(1), 7–21.

Kirmayer, L. J. (2004). The cultural diversity of healing: Meaning, metaphor and mechanism. *British Medical Bulletin, 69*(1), 33–48.

Kirmayer, L. J., Guzder, J., & Rousseau, C. (2014). *Cultural consultation: Encountering the other in mental health care*. New York: Springer.

Kissane, D., & Parnes, F. (Eds.). (2014). *Bereavement care for families*. New York: Routledge.

Klass, D. (2009). Bereavement narratives: Continuing bonds in the twenty-first century. *Mortality, 14*, 305–306.

Kleinman, A. (1988). *The illness narratives: Suffering, healing, and the human condition*. New York: Basic Books.

Kleinman, A. (2009). Caregiving: The odyssey of becoming more human. *The Lancet, 373*, 292–293.

Knudsen-Martin, C. (2012). Changing gender norms in families and society. In F. Walsh (Ed.), *Normal family processes* (4th ed., pp. 324–346). New York: Guilford Press.

Kochanek, K., Arias, E., & Anderson, R. (2013). *How did cause of death contribute to racial differences in life expectancy in the United States in 2010?* (NCHS Data Brief, no 125). Washington, DC: National Center for Health Statistics, U.S. Department of Health and Human Services.

Koenig, H. (2012). Religion, spirituality, and health: The research and clinical implications. *ISRN Psychiatry*, Article ID 278730.

Kreutzer, J., Stejskal, T., Godwin, E., Powell, V., & Arango-Lasprilla, J. (2010). A mixed methods evaluation of the Brain Injury Family Intervention. *NeuroRehabilitation, 27*, 19–29.

Kübler-Ross, E. (Ed.). (1975). *Death: The final stage of growth*. Englewood Cliffs, NJ: Prentice-Hall.

Kuijer, R. G., Buunk, B. P., de Jong, G. M., Ybema, J. F., & Sanderman, R. (2004). Effects of a brief intervention program for patients with cancer and their partners on feelings of inequity, relationship quality and psychological distress. *Psycho-Oncology, 13*, 321–334.

Kunzler, A., Nussbeck, F., Moser, M., Bodenmann, G., & Kayser, K. (2014). Individual and dyadic development of personal growth in couples coping with cancer. *Supportive Care in Cancer, 22*(1), 53–62.

Kushner, H. S. (1981). *When bad things happen to good people*. New York: Random House.

Landau, J., & Hissett, J. (2008). Mild traumatic brain injury: Impact on identity and ambiguous loss in the family. *Families, Systems, and Health, 26*(1), 69–85.

Lattanzi-Licht, M., Maloney, J. J., & Miller, G. W. (1998). *The hospice choice: In pursuit of a peaceful death*. New York: Simon & Schuster.

Law, D., & Crane, R. (2007). The influence of individual, marital, and family treatment on high utilizers of health care. *Journal of Marital and Family Therapy, 29*(3), 353–363.

Lebow, J., & Stroud, C. (2012). Assessment of effective couple and family functioning: Prevailing models and instruments. In F. Walsh (Ed.), *Normal family processes: Growing diversity and complexity* (3rd ed., pp. 501–529). New York: Guilford Press.

Ledesma, D., & Kumano, H. (2009). Mindfulness-based stress reduction and cancer: A meta-analysis. *Psycho-Oncology, 18*(6), 571–579.

Lee, M. Y., & Mjelde-Mossey, L. (2004). Cultural dissonance among generations: A solution-focused approach among elders and their families. *Journal of Marital and Family Therapy, 30*(4), 497–513.

Leeman, J., Crandell, J. L., Lee, A., Bai, J., Sandelowski, M., & Knafl, K. (2016). Family functioning and the well-being of children with chronic conditions: A meta-analysis. *Research in Nursing and Health, 39*(4), 229–243.

Lefcourt, H. M. (1982). *Locus of control* (2nd ed.). Hillsdale, NJ: Erlbaum.

Lefley, H. (2009). *Family psychoeducation for serious mental illness.* New York: Oxford University Press.

Lerman, C., Croyle, R., Tercyak, K., & Hamann, H. (2002). Genetic testing: Psychological aspects and implications. *Journal of Consulting and Clinical Psychology, 70,* 784–797.

Levine, S. (1987). *Healing into life and death.* New York: Doubleday.

Levinson, D. J. (1986). A conception of adult development. *American Psychologist, 41,* 3–13.

Lifton, R. J. (1975). Preface. In A. Mitscherlich & M. Mitscherlich (Eds.), *The inability to mourn.* New York: Grove Press.

Lifton, R. J. (1982). Beyond psychic numbing: A call to awareness. *American Journal of Orthopsychiatry, 52*(4), 619–629.

Limbers, C., & Skipper, S. (2014). Health-related quality of life measurement in siblings of children with physical chronic illness: A systematic review. *Families, Systems, and Health, 32*(4), 408–415.

Lindquist, L. K., Love, H. C., & Elbogen, E. (2017). Traumatic brain injury in Iraq and Afghanistan veterans: New results from a National Random Sample Study. *Journal of Neuropsychiatry and Neurosciences, 29*(3), 254–259.

Lobato, D., & Kao, B. (2005). Family-based group intervention for young siblings of children with chronic illness and developmental disability. *Journal of Pediatric Psychology, 30*(8), 678–682.

Long, K., & Marsland, L. (2011). Family adjustment to childhood cancer: A systematic review. *Clinical Child and Family Psychology Review, 14*(1), 57–88.

Lucksted, A., McFarlane, W., Downing, D., Dixon, L., & Adams, C. (2012). Recent developments in family psychoeducation as an evidence-based practice. *Journal of Marital and Family Therapy, 1,* 101–121.

Ludwig, D. S., & Kabat-Zinn, J. (2008). Mindfulness in medicine. *Journal of the American Medical Association, 300,* 1350–1352.

Lum, T. Y., Kane, R. A., Cutler, L. J., & Yu, T. C. (2008). Effects of Green House nursing homes on resident's families. *Health Care Financing Review, 30,* 35–51.

Lynn, J., Schuster, J. L., Wilkinson, A., & Simon, L. N. (2007). *Improving care for the end of life: A sourcebook for health care managers and clinicians* (2nd ed.). New York: Oxford University Press.

Madsen, W. (2011). Collaborative helping maps: A tool to guide thinking and action in family-centered services. *Family Process, 50*(4), 529–543.

Manne, S., & Badr, H. (2008). Intimacy and relationship processes in couples' psychosocial adaptation to cancer. *Cancer, 112,* 2541–2555.

Marks, L. (2006). Religion and family relational health: Overview and conceptual model. *Journal of Religion and Health, 45*(4), 603–618.

Martire, L., Lustig, A., Schulz, R., Miller, G., & Helgeson, V. (2004). Is it beneficial to involve a family member?: A meta-analysis of psychosocial interventions in chronic illness. *Health Psychology, 23,* 599–611.

Martire, L. M., Schulz, R., Helgeson, V. S., Small, B. J., & Saghafi, E. M. (2010). Review and meta-analysis of couple-oriented interventions for chronic illness. *Annals of Behavioral Medicine*, 40(3), 325–342.

McDaniel, S., Campbell, T., Hepworth, J., & Lorenz, A. (2005). *Family-oriented primary care: A manual for medical providers* (2nd ed.). New York: Springer-Verlag.

McDaniel, S., Doherty, W., & Hepworth, J. (2014). *Medical family therapy and integrated care* (2nd ed.). Washington, DC: American Psychological Association Press.

McDaniel, S., Hepworth, J., & Doherty, W. (Eds.). (1997). *The shared experience of illness: Stories of patients, families, and their therapists*. New York: Basic Books.

McEwan, J. (2006). Genetic testing: Legal and policy issues for individuals and their families. In S. Miller, S. McDaniel, J. Rolland, & S. Feetham (Eds.), *Individuals, families, and the new era of genetics: Biopsychosocial perspectives* (pp. 506–530). New York: Norton.

McFarlane, W. F. (Ed.). (2002). *Multifamily groups in the treatment of severe psychiatric disorders*. New York: Guilford Press.

McGoldrick, M., Garcia Preto, N., & Carter, B. (Eds.). (2016). *The expanded family life cycle: Individual, family, and social perspectives* (5th ed.). New York: Pearson.

McGoldrick, M., Gerson, R., & Petry, S. (2008). *Genograms: Assessment and intervention* (3rd ed.). New York: Norton.

McGoldrick, M., Giordano, J., & Garcia-Preto, N. (2005). *Ethnicity and family therapy* (3rd ed.). New York: Guilford Press.

Mendenhall, T., Berge, J., & Doherty, W. (2014). Engaging communities as partners in research: Advancing integrated care through purposeful partnerships. In J. Hodgson, A. Lamson, T. Mendenhall, & R. Crane (Eds.), *Medical family therapy: Advance applications* (pp. 259–283). New York: Springer.

Miller, B. F., Kessler, R., Peek, C. J., & Kallenberg, G. A. (2011). *A national agenda for research in collaborative care* (AHRQ Publication No. 11-0067) (Presented at the Collaborative Care Research Network Research Development Conference). Rockville, MD: Agency for Healthcare Research and Quality.

Miller, S., McDaniel, S., Rolland, J., & Feetham, S. (Eds.). (2006). *Individuals, families, and the new era of genetics: Biopsychosocial perspectives*. New York: Norton.

Minuchin, S., Rosman, B. L., & Baker, L. (1978). *Psychosomatic families: Anorexia nervosa in context*. Cambridge, MA: Harvard University Press.

Mishel, M. (2014). Theories of uncertainty in illness. In M. J. Smith, & P. Liehr (Eds.), *Middle range theory for nursing* (3rd ed., pp. 53–87). New York: Springer.

Mittelman, M. (2013). Psychosocial interventions to address the emotional needs of caregivers of individuals with Alzheimer's disease. In S. Zarit & R. Talley (Eds.), *Caregiving for Alzheimer's disease and related disorders*. New York: Springer.

Mittelman, M., Brodaty, H., Wallen, A., & Burns, A. (2008). A three-country randomized controlled trial of a psychosocial intervention for caregivers combined with pharmacological treatment for patients with Alzheimer's disease: Effects on caregiver depression. *American Journal of Geriatric Psychiatry*, 16, 893–904.

Nadeau, J. W. (2008). Meaning-making in bereaved families: Assessment, intervention, and future research. In M. Stroebe, R. Hansson, H. Schut, & W. Stroebe (Eds.), *Handbook of bereavement research: 21st century perspectives* (pp. 511–530). Washington, DC: American Psychological Association.

National Alliance for Caregiving (NAC) & AARP Public Policy Institute (2015, June). *Caregiving in the U.S. 2015*. Bethesda, MD: NAC & Washington, DC: AARP.

Navon, S. (1999). The non-illness intervention model: Psychotherapy for physically ill patients and their families. *American Journal of Family Therapy, 27*(3), 251–270.

Neimeyer, R. A. (Ed.). (2001). *Meaning reconstruction and the experience of loss.* Washington, DC: American Psychological Press.

Neimeyer, R. A., Burke, L. A., Mackay, M. M., & van Dyke Stringer, J. G. (2010). Grief therapy and the reconstruction of meaning: From principles to practice. *Journal of Contemporary Psychotherapy, 40*(2), 73–83.

Nielsen, M., Gibson, A., Buelt, L., Grundy, P., & Grumbach, K. (2015). The patient-centered medical home's impact on cost and quality: Annual review of evidence 2013–2014. Available from *www.pcpcc.org/resource/patient-centered-medical-homes-impact-cost-and-quality.*

Northouse, L., Kershaw, T., Mood, D., & Schafenacker, A. (2005). Effects of a family intervention on the quality of life of women with recurrent breast cancer and their family caregivers. *Psycho-Oncology, 14,* 478–491.

Northouse, L., Mood, D., Schafenacker, A., Montie, J., Sandler, H. M., Forman, J. D., et al. (2007). Randomized clinical trial of a family intervention for prostate cancer patients and their spouses. *Cancer, 110,* 2809–2818.

Nussbaum, R. L., McInnes, R. R., & Willard, H. F. (2016). *Thompson & Thompson genetics in medicine* (8th ed.). Philadelphia: Elsevier Health Sciences.

O'Brien, I., Duffy, A., & Nicholas, H. (2009). Impact of childhood chronic illnesses on siblings: A literature review. *British Journal of Nursing, 18*(22), 1358–1365.

O'Donnell, E. H., Eddy, K., & Rauch, P. (2013). Parenting with chronic and life-threatening illness: A parent guidance model. In A. Heru (Ed.), *Working with families in medical settings: A multidisciplinary guide for psychiatrists and other health professionals.* New York: Routledge.

Ogden, C. L., Carroll, M. D., Kit, B. K., & Flegal, K. M. (2014). Prevalence of childhood and adult obesity in the United States, 2011–2012. *Journal of the American Medical Association, 311*(8), 806–814.

Okie, S. (2005). Physician-assisted suicide—Oregon and beyond. *New England Journal of Medicine, 352*(16), 1627–1630.

Olkin, R. (1999). *What psychotherapists should know about disability.* New York: Guilford Press.

Ooms, T., Rolland, J., Mintz, S., & Doppelt, L. (1996) Families and the collaborative process. *Families, Systems, and Health, 13*(3–4), 299–313.

Ormond, K., & Ross, L. F. (2006). Ethical issues in reproductive genetics. In S. Miller, S. McDaniel, J. Rolland, & S. Feetham (Eds.), *Individuals, families, and the new era of genetics: Biopsychosocial perspectives* (pp. 465–486). New York: Norton.

Osborn, T. (2007). The psychosocial impact of parental cancer on children and adolescents: Asystematic review. *Psycho-Oncology, 16,* 101–126.

Pai, A. L., & Ostendorf, H. M. (2011). Treatment adherence in adolescents and young adults affected by chronic illness during the health care transition from pediatric to adult health care. *Children's Health Care, 40*(1), 16–33.

Paniagua, C. T., & Taylor, R. E. (2008). The cultural lens of genomics. *OJIN: Online Journal of Issues in Nursing, 13*(1).

Paris, M., & Hogue, M. (2010). Burnout in the mental health workforce: A review. *Journal of Behavioral Health Services and Research, 37,* 519–528.

Parkes, C. M., Laungani, P., & Young, B. (Eds.). (2015) *Death and bereavement across cultures* (2nd ed.). New York: Routledge.

Patterson, J. M., Holm, K., & Gurney, J. (2004). The impact of childhood cancer on the family: A qualitative analysis of strains, resources, and coping behaviors. *Psycho-Oncology, 13*, 390–407.

Peek, C. J. (2015). Don Bloch's vision for collaborative family health care: Progress and next steps. *Families, Systems, and Health, 33*(2), 86–99.

Penchaszadeh, V. (2001). Genetic counseling issues in Latinos. *Genetic Testing, 5*(3), 193–199.

Penn, P. (1983). Coalitions and binding interactions in families with chronic illness. *Family Systems Medicine, 1*(2), 16–25.

Penn, P. (2001). Chronic illness: Trauma, language, and writing: Breaking the silence. *Family Process, 40*(1), 33–52.

Perry, A., & Rolland, J. (2008). The therapeutic benefits of a justice-seeking spirituality: Empowerment, healing, and hope. In F. Walsh (Ed.), *Spirituality resources in families and family therapy* (2nd ed.). New York: Guilford Press.

Peters, N., Rose, A., & Armstrong, K. (2004). The association between race and attitudes about predictive genetic testing. *Cancer Epidemiology, Biomarkers and Prevention, 13*(3), 361–365.

Pew Research Center. (2013). *Views on end-of-life medical treatments.* Washington, DC: Author.

Picoraro, J., Womer, J., Kazak, A., & Feudtner, C. (2014). Posttraumatic growth in parents and pediatric patients. *Journal of Palliative Care, 17*(2), 209–218.

Pinsof, W. M. (2002). The death of "Till death us do part": The transformation of pair-bonding in the 20th century. *Family Process, 41*, 135–157.

Pomerantz, A. S., Shiner, B., Watts, B. V., Detzer, M. J., Kutter, C., Street, B., et al. (2010). The White River model of colocated collaborative care: A platform for mental and behavioral health care in the medical home. *Families, Systems, and Health, 28*(2), 114–129.

Proulx, C. M., & Snyder, L. A. (2009). Families and health: An empirical resource guide for researchers and practitioners. *Family Relations, 58*(4), 489–504.

Qualls, S. H., & Williams, A. A. (2013). *Caregiver family therapy: Empowering families to meet the challenges of aging.* Washington, DC: American Psychological Association.

Qualls, S. H., & Zarit, S. H. (Eds.). (2009). *Aging families and caregiving.* New York: Wiley.

Rakel, D. (2012). *Integrative medicine* (3rd ed.). Philadelphia: Elsevier.

Rando, T. A. (1984). *Grief, dying, and death.* Champaign, IL: Research Press.

Rando, T. A. (Ed.). (2000). *Clinical dimensions of anticipatory mourning: Theory and practice in working with the dying, their loved ones, and their caregivers.* Champaign, IL: Research Press.

Rasmussen, H., Scheier, M., & Greenhouse, J. (2009). Optimism and physical health: A meta-analytic review. *Annals of Behavioral Medicine, 37*(3), 239–256.

Redfoot, D. L., Feinberg, L., & Houser, A. (2013). *Insight on the Issues: The aging of the baby boom and the growing care gap: A look at future declines in the availability of family caregivers.* Washington, DC: AARP Public Policy Institute.

Reibstein, J. (2004). Staying alive: My family inheritance of breast cancer. In F. Walsh & M. McGoldrick (Eds.), *Living beyond loss: Death in the family* (2nd ed., pp 406–413). New York: Norton.

Reiss, D. (1981). *The family's construction of reality.* Cambridge, MA: Harvard University Press.

Reiss, D., Neiderhiser, J. M., & Hetherington, E. M. (2009). *The relationship code:*

Deciphering genetic and social influences on adolescent development (Vol. 1). Cambridge, MA: Harvard University Press.

Robison, L., Armstrong, G., Boice, J., Chow, J., Davies, S., Donaldson, S., et al. (2009). The childhood cancer survivor study: A National Cancer Institute-supported resource for outcome and intervention research. *Journal of Clinical Oncology, 14,* 2308–2318.

Rodrigues, N., & Patterson, J. M. (2007). Impact of severity of a child's chronic condition on the functioning of two-parent families. *Journal of Pediatric Psychology, 32,* 417–426.

Roesch, S., & Weiner, B. (2001). A meta-analytic review of coping with illness: Do causal attributions matter? *Journal of Psychosomatic Research, 50,* 205–219.

Rohrbaugh, M. J., Shoham, V., Skoyen, J. A., Jensen, M., & Mehl, M. R. (2012). "We"-talk, communal coping, and cessation success in a couple-focused intervention for health-compromised smokers. *Family Process, 51*(1), 107–121.

Rolland, J. S. (1984). Toward a psychosocial typology of chronic and life-threatening illness. *Family Systems Medicine, 3*(2), 245–262.

Rolland, J. S. (1987a). Chronic illness and the life cycle: A conceptual framework. *Family Process, 26,* 203–221.

Rolland, J. S. (1987b). Family systems and chronic illness: A typological model. *Journal of Psychotherapy and the Family, 3*(3), 143–168.

Rolland, J. S. (1990). Anticipatory loss: A family systems developmental framework. *Family Process, 29,* 229–244.

Rolland, J. S. (1994a). *Families, illness, and disability: An integrative treatment model.* New York: Basic Books.

Rolland, J. S. (1994b). In sickness and in health: The impact of illness on couples' relationships. *Journal of Marital and Family Therapy, 20*(4), 327–347.

Rolland, J. S. (1997). A journey with hope, fear, and loss: Young couples and cancer. In S. McDaniel, J. Hepworth, & W. Doherty (Eds.), *The shared experience of illness: Stories of patients, families, and their therapists* (pp. 139–151). New York: Basic Books.

Rolland, J. S. (1999). Families and genetic fate: A millennial challenge. *Families, Systems, and Health, 17*(1), 123–133.

Rolland, J. S. (2004). Helping families with anticipatory loss and terminal illness. In F. Walsh & M. McGoldrick (Eds.), *Living beyond loss: Death in the family* (2nd ed., pp. 213–237). New York: Norton.

Rolland, J. S. (2006a). Living with anticipatory loss in the new era of genetics: A life cycle perspective. In S. Miller, S. McDaniel, J. Rolland, & S. Feetham (Eds.), *Individuals, families, and the new era of genetics: Biopsychosocial perspectives* (pp. 139–173). New York: Norton.

Rolland, J. S. (2006b). Genetics, family systems, and multicultural influences. *Families, Systems, and Health, 24*(4), 425–442.

Rolland, J. S. (2012). Mastering family challenges in illness, disability, and genetic conditions. In F. Walsh (Ed.), *Normal family processes,* (4th ed., pp. 452–482). New York: Guilford Press.

Rolland, J. S. (2013). Family adaptation to chronic medical illness. In A. Heru (Ed.), *Working with families in medical settings: A multidisciplinary guide for psychiatrists and other mental health professionals.* New York: Routledge.

Rolland, J. S. (2015). Advancing family involvement in collaborative health care: Next steps. *Families, Systems, and Health, 33*(2), 104–108.

Rolland, J. S. (2016). Chronic illness and the life cycle. In M. McGoldrick, N. Garcia-Preto,

& B. Carter (Eds.), *The expanding family life cycle: Individual, family, and social perspectives* (5th ed., pp. 430–454). Boston: Pearson.

Rolland, J. S. (2017). Neurocognitive impairment: Addressing couple and family challenges. *Family Process, 56*(4), 799–818.

Rolland, J. S., Emanuel, L., & Torke, A. (2017). Applying a family systems lens to proxy decision making in clinical practice and research. *Families, Systems, and Health, 35*(1), 7–18.

Rolland, J., Lister, Z., Kelleher, M., & Williams, I. (2011). *A model program for integrated family-centered collaborative healthcare: Chicago Center for Family Health and University of Chicago Kovler Diabetes Center.* Presentation at the 13th annual meeting of the Collaborative Family Healthcare Association.

Rolland, J., McPheters, J., & Carbonell, E. (2008). *Resilient partners: A collaborative project with the MS Society.* Paper presented at the 10th annual conference of the Collaborative Family Healthcare Association.

Rolland, J. S., & Walsh, F. W. (2005). Systemic training for healthcare professionals: The Chicago Center for Family Health Approach. *Family Process, 44*(3), 283–301.

Rolland, J. S., & Walsh, F. W. (2006). Facilitating family resilience with childhood illness and disability. *Pediatric Opinion, 18*, 1–11.

Rolland, J. S., & Williams, J. K. (2005). Toward a biopsychosocial model for 21st century genetics. *Family Process, 44*(1), 3–24.

Rosenberg, T., & Pace, M. (2006). Burnout among mental health professionals: Special considerations for the marriage and family therapist. *Journal of Marital and Family Therapy, 32*, 87–99.

Rosenblatt, P. (2013). Family grief in cross-cultural perspective. *Family Science, 4*(1), 12–19.

Ross, L. F., & Fost, N. (2006). Ethical issues in pediatric genetics. In S. Miller, S. McDaniel, J. Rolland, & S. Feetham (Eds.), *Individuals, families, and the new era of genetics: Biopsychosocial perspectives* (pp. 486–506). New York: Norton.

Roth, D., Haley, W., Hovater, M., Perkins, M., Wasley, V., & Judd, S. (2013). Family caregiving and all-cause mortality: Findings from a population-based propensity-matched analysis. *American Journal of Epidemiology, 178*(10), 1571–1578.

Rowland, E., & Metcalfe, A. (2012). Communicating inherited genetic risk between parent and child: A meta-thematic analysis. *International Journal of Nursing Studies, 50*(6), 870–880.

Ryan, C., Epstein, N., Keitner, G., Miller, I., & Bishop, D. (2005). *Evaluating and treating families: The McMaster Approach.* New York: Routledge.

Saucier, J. B., Johnston, D., Wicklund, C. A., Robbins-Furman, P., Hecht, J. T., & Monga, M. (2005). Racial-ethnic differences in genetic amniocentesis uptake. *Journal of Genetic Counseling, 14*(3), 189–195.

Schaie, K. W., & Willis, S. (Eds.). (2012). *Handbook of the psychology of aging* (7th ed.). San Diego, CA: Academic Press.

Scheinkman, M. (2008). A multi-level approach: A roadmap for couples therapy. *Family Process, 47*(2), 197–213.

Schermerhorn, A. C., D'Onofrio, B. M., Turkheimer, E., Ganiban, J. M., Spotts, E. L., Lichtenstein, P., et al. (2011). A genetically informed study of associations between family functioning and child psychosocial adjustment. *Developmental Psychology, 47*(3), 707–725.

Schover, L. R., & Jensen, S. B. (1988). *Sexuality and chronic illness.* New York: Guilford Press.

Schulz, R., & Beach, S. (1999). Caregiving as a risk factor for mortality: The Caregiver and Health Effects Study. *Journal of the American Medical Association, 282*(23), 2215–2219.

Schulz, R., & Martire, L. M. (2004). Family caregiving of persons with dementia: Prevalence, health effects, and support strategies. *American Journal of Geriatric Psychiatry, 12,* 240–249.

Scott, J. L., Halford, W. K., & Ward, B. G. (2004). United we stand?: The effects of couple-coping interventions on adjustment to early stage breast or gynecological cancer. *Journal of Consulting and Clinical Psychology, 72,* 1122–1135.

Seabum, D., Lorenz, A., & Kaplan, D. (1992). The transgenerational development of chronic illness meanings. *Family Systems Medicine, 10,* 385–395.

Seaburn, D., Gunn, W., Mauksh, L., Gawinski, A., & Lorenz, A. (Eds.). (1996). *Models of collaboration: A guide for mental health professionals working with physicians and health care providers.* New York: Basic Books.

Seagraves, R. T., & Balon, R. (2003). *Sexual pharmacology: Fast facts.* New York: Norton.

Seligman, M., & Darling, R. B. (2009). *Ordinary families, special children: A systems approach to childhood disability* (3rd ed.). New York: Guilford Press.

Sherman, K., Miller, S., Shaw, L.-K., Cavanagh, K., & Gorin, S. (2014). Psychosocial approaches to participation in BRCA1/2 genetic risk assessment among African American women: A systematic review. *Journal of Community Genetics, 5*(2), 89–98.

Shields, C., Finley, M., Chawla, N., & Meadors, P. (2012). Couple and family interventions in health problems. *Journal of Marital and Family Therapy, 38*(1), 265–281.

Siegel, B., & Sander, J. (2009). *Faith, hope, and healing: Lessons learned from people living with cancer.* Hoboken, NJ: Wiley.

Sipski, M. L., & Alexander, C. J. (Eds.). (1997). *Sexual function in people with disability and chronic illness: A health professional's guide.* Silver Springs, MD: Aspen.

Skerrett, K. (2003). Couple dialogues with illness: Expanding the "we." *Families, Systems, and Health, 21*(1), 69–80.

Smith, G. E., & Lunde, A. (2013). Early diagnosis of Alzheimer's disease, caregiving, and family dynamics. In *Caregiving for Alzheimer's disease and related disorders* (pp. 3–16). New York: Springer.

Smith, G. R., Williamson, G. M., Miller, L. S., & Schulz, R. (2011). Depression and quality of informal care: A longitudinal investigation of caregiving stressors. *Psychology and Aging, 26*(3), 584–591.

Sobel, S., & Cowan, C. B. (2003). Ambiguous loss and disenfranchised grief: The impact of DNA predictive testing on the family as a system. *Family Process, 42*(1), 47–59.

Sontag, S. (1978). *Illness as metaphor.* New York: McGraw-Hill.

Spotts, E. (2012). Unraveling the complexity of gene-environmental interplay and family processes. In F. Walsh (Ed.), *Normal family processes* (4th. ed., pp. 529–552). New York: Guilford Press.

Steinglass, P., Ostroff, J., & Steinglass, A. (2011). Multiple family groups for adult cancer survivors and their families: A 1-day workshop model. *Family Process, 50,* 393–409.

Stewart, J., & Mishel, M. (2000). Uncertainty in childhood illness: A synthesis of the parent and child literature. *Research and Theory for Nursing Practice, 14*(4), 299–319.

Stroebe, M., & Schut, H. (2010). The Dual Process Model of coping and bereavement: A decade on. *Omega: Journal of Death and Dying, 61*(4), 273–289.

Stroebe, M., Schut, H., & Boerner, K. (2010). Continuing bonds in adaptation to bereavement: Toward theoretical integration. *Clinical Psychology Review, 30,* 259–268.

Stroebe, M., Schut, H., & Finkenauer. C. (2013). Parents coping with the death of their child: From individual to interpersonal, to interactive perspectives. *Family Science, 4*(1), 28–36.

Sue, D. W., & Sue, D. (2012). *Counseling the culturally diverse: Theory and practice* (6th ed.). New York: Wiley.

Talen, M. R., & Burke Valeras, A. (Eds.). (2013). *Integrated behavioral health in primary care: Evaluating the evidence, identifying the essentials.* New York: Springer.

Taylor, S., Kemeny, M., Reed, G., Bower, J., & Gruenwald, T. (2000). Psychological resources, positive illusions, and health. *American Psychologist, 55*(1), 99–109.

Thompson, S., & Kyle, D. (2000). The role of perceived control in coping with the losses associated with chronic illness. In J. Harvey & E. Miller (Eds.), *Loss and trauma: General and close relationship perspectives.* Philadelphia: Brunner-Routledge.

Tienari, P., Wynne, L. C., Sorri, A., Lahti, I., Laksy, K., Moring, J., et al. (2004). Genotype-environment interaction in schizophrenia-spectrum disorder: Long-term follow-up study of Finnish adoptees. *British Journal of Psychiatry, 184*(3), 216–222.

Traa, M. J., De Vries, J., Bodenmann, G., & Den Oudsten, B. L. (2015). Dyadic coping and relationship functioning in couples coping with cancer: A systematic review. *British Journal of Health Psychology, 20*(1), 85–114.

Tse, C., Chong, A., & Fok, S. (2003). Breaking bad news: A Chinese perspective. *Palliative Medicine, 17,* 339–343.

U.S. Census Bureau. (2015). *Health insurance coverage in the United States: 2014.* Washington, DC: U.S. Government Printing Office.

Van Cleave, J., Gortmaker, S., & Perrin, J. (2010). Dynamics of obesity and chronic health conditions among children and youth. *Journal of the American Medical Association, 303,* 623–630.

Vermaes, I. P., van Susante, A. M., & van Bakel, H. J. (2012). Psychological functioning of siblings in children with chronic health conditions. *Journal of Pediatric Psychology, 37,* 166–184.

Verschuren, J. E., Enzlin, P., Dijkstra, P. U., Geertzen, J. H., & Dekker, R. (2010). Chronic disease and sexuality: A generic conceptual framework. *Journal of Sex Research, 47*(2–3), 153–170.

Wade, S. L., Taylor, H. G., Yeates, K. O., Drotar, D., Stancin, T., Minich, N. M., et al. (2006). Long-term parental and family adaptation following pediatric brain injury. *Journal of Pediatric Psychology, 31*(10), 1072–1083.

Wailoo, K. (2001). *Dying in the city of the blues: Sickle cell anemia and the politics of race and health.* Chapel Hill: University of North Carolina.

Wallston, K. A. (2004). Control and health. In N. Anderson (Ed.), *Encyclopedia of health and behavior* (Vol. 1, pp. 217–220). Thousand Oaks, CA: SAGE.

Walsh, F. (2009). *Spiritual resources in family therapy* (2nd ed.). New York: Guilford Press.

Walsh, F. (2012). The "new normal": Diversity and complexity in 21st century families. In F. Walsh (Ed.), *Normal family processes* (4th ed., pp. 4–27). New York: Guilford Press.

Walsh, F. (2016a). Families in later life: Challenges, opportunities, and resilience. In M. McGoldrick, N. Garcia-Preto, & E. Carter (Eds.), *The expanded family life cycle: Individual, family, and social perspectives* (5th ed., pp. 339–359). Boston: Allyn & Bacon.

Walsh, F. (2016b). *Strengthening family resilience* (3rd ed.). New York: Guilford Press.
Walsh, F., & McGoldrick, M. (Eds.). (2004). *Living beyond loss: Death in the family* (2nd ed.). New York: Norton.
Walsh, F., & McGoldrick, M. (2013). Bereavement: A family life cycle perspective (Special issue). *Family Science, 4,* 20–27.
Wang V. O. (2001). Multicultural genetic counseling: Then, now and in the 21st century. *American Journal of Medical Genetics, 106,* 208–215.
Watts-Jones, D. (1997). Toward an African-American genogram. *Family Process, 36,* 375–383.
Weihs, K., Fisher, L., & Baird, M. (2002). Families, health, and behavior: A section of the commissioned report by the Committee on Health and Behavior: Research, Practice and Policy, Division of Neuroscience and Behavioral Health and Division of Health Promotion and Disease Prevention, Institute of Medicine, National Academy of Sciences. *Families, Systems, and Health, 20*(1), 7–47.
Weil, A. (2004). *Health and healing: The philosophy of integrative medicine.* New York: Barnes & Noble.
Weingarten, K. (1991). The discourses of intimacy: Adding a social constructionist and feminist view. *Family Process, 30*(3), 285–305.
Weingarten, K. (2010). Reasonable hope: Construct, clinical applications, and supports. *Family Process, 49,* 5–25.
Weingarten, K. (2012). Sorrow: A therapist's reflections on the inevitable and the unknowable. *Family Process, 51*(4), 440–455.
Weingarten, K. (2013). The "cruel radiance of what is": Helping couples live with chronic illness. *Family Process, 52,* 83–101.
Werner, P., Karnieli-Miller, O., & Eidelman, S. (2013). Current knowledge and future directions about the disclosure of dementia: A systemic review of the first decade of the 21st century. *Alzheimers Dementia, 9*(2), e74–e88.
Werner-Lin, A. (2008). Beating the biological clock: The compressed family life cycle of young women with BRCA gene alterations. *Social Work in Health Care, 47,* 416–437.
Werner-Lin, A., & Moro, T. (2004). Unacknowledged and stigmatized losses. In F. Walsh & M. McGoldrick (Eds.), *Living beyond loss: Death in the family* (2nd ed.). New York: Norton.
Werth, Jr., J. L., Blevins, D., Toussaint, K. L., & Durham, M. R. (2002). The influence of cultural diversity on end-of-life care and decisions. *The American Behavioral Scientist, 46*(2), 204–219.
White, M., & Epston, D. (1990). *Narrative means to therapeutic ends.* New York: Norton.
Williams, J. K., Schutte, D. L., Evers, C., & Holkup, P. A. (2000). Redefinition: Coping with normal results from predictive gene testing for neurodegenerative disorders. *Research in Nursing and Health, 23,* 260–269.
Wilper, A., Woolhandler, S., Lasser, K., McCormick, D., Bor, D., & Himmelstein, D. (2009). Health insurance and mortality in US adults. *American Journal of Public Health, 99*(12), 2289–2295.
Wood, B. L., Lim, J., Miller, B., Cheah, P., Zwatch, T., Ramesh, S., et al. (2008). Testing the biobehavioral family model in pediatric asthma: Pathways of effect. *Family Process, 47,* 21–40.
Wright, L. (2009). Spirituality, suffering, and beliefs: The soul of healing with families. In F. Walsh (Ed.), *Spiritual resources in family therapy* (2nd ed., pp. 65–80). New York: Guilford Press.

Wright, L. M. (2017). *Spirituality, suffering, and illness.* Calgary, Alberta, Canada: 4th Floor Press.

Wright, L. M., & Bell, J. M. (2009). *Beliefs and illness: A model for healing.* Calgary, Alberta, Canada: 4th Floor Press.

Wynne, L. C., & Wynne, A. R. (1986). The quest for intimacy. *Journal of Marital and Family Therapy, 12,* 383–394.

Wysocki, T., Lochrie, A., Harris, M., Mauras, N., Buckloh, L., White, N., et al. (2007). Randomized trial of behavioral family systems therapy for diabetes: Maintenance of effects on diabetes outcomes in adolescents. *Diabetes Care, 30,* 555–560.

Zarit, S., & Talley, R. (2013). *Caring for Alzheimer's disease and related disorders: Research, practice, policy.* New York: Springer.

Zentner, M., & Shiner, R. L. (Eds.). (2015). *Handbook of temperament.* New York: Guilford Press.

Index

Note. *f* or *t* following a page number indicates a figure or a table.

Acceptance
  clinicians and, 326
  couple functioning and, 244
  determining chronicity and, 43
  phases of illness and, 39, 179
  psychosocial map and, 14–15
  siblings and, 215
Acute onset, 21–22, 29, 30t–31t, 49f, 303–304. *See also* Onset
Adaptation
  family and couple functioning and, 79–81, 82, 266–267
  Family Systems Illness (FSI) model and, 5
  genetic factors and, 292–293
  health beliefs and, 145
  illness phase transitions and, 46
  life-cycle issues and, 127
  modalities of treatment and, 69
  neurocognitive conditions and, 311–312
  normative illness experience, 132–134
  uncertainty and, 29, 32
Adolescents
  aging parents and caregiving and, 231–232
  chronic conditions and, 17, 79–80, 200–201, 206–217, 292–293
  family functioning and, 79–80, 81
  life-cycle issues and, 114–115
  neurocognitive conditions and, 304
  parental illness and disability and, 227
Adulthood, 173–174, 217–220, 228–239, 230, 304. *See also* Onset
Advance directives, 194–197, 230
Adversity, 89, 98
Affective issues, 14f, 21, 97

Agency, 14–15, 143–145
Aging parents, 228–239
Alzheimer's disease
  anticipatory loss and, 165–166
  caregiving and, 62
  couple functioning and, 258
  course of disorders and, 22
  diagnosis and, 307
  disability and, 28
  onset and, 21
  overview, 301, 302, 305
  uncertainty and, 31
Ambiguous loss, 311–312. *See also* Loss
Ambivalence, 160, 164–165, 212, 249
Anger
  anticipatory loss and, 160
  case examples of, 215–216
  couple functioning and, 248, 257
  siblings and, 214–216
  terminal phase of illness and, 188
Anticipatory loss. *See also* Loss
  aging parents and caregiving and, 236–237
  belief systems and, 175–176
  case examples of, 163, 168, 169, 171, 173, 175
  childhood and adolescent conditions and, 201–202, 209
  family life cycle and, 168–175
  outcome and, 26
  overview, 159–161, 161t
Anticipatory suffering, 26, 159–161, 161t
Anxiety
  aging parents and caregiving and, 233–234
  genetic factors and, 290, 292–293

387

Anxiety *(cont.)*
  parental illness and disability and, 222
  terminal phase of illness and, 177, 188
Arrival period of the terminal phase, 186–189. *See also* Terminal phase of illness
Arthritis, 21, 22, 23, 25, 31, 32, 46, 216, 235, 238, 261, 316
Assessment
  course of disorders and, 23
  family functioning and, 77, 85–86, 87–88
  Family Systems Illness (FSI) model and, 5, 15
  genetic factors and, 272–273, 291, 295, 297
  genograms and, 91
  of health beliefs, 131–132
  illness characteristics and, 32
  levels of systems-based involvement and, 59–60
  life-cycle issues and, 112
  multigenerational factors and, 90, 106–107
  normative illness experience, 132
  overview, 17
  phases of illness and, 40, 50–51
  principles of intervention and, 61
Assisted dying, 197–199. *See also* Terminal phase of illness
Assisted living, 239, 357. *See also* Facility placement
Asthma
  anticipatory loss and, 167
  case examples of, 99–100
  childhood and adolescent conditions and, 200
  course of disorders and, 24
  expectations and, 36
  family functioning and, 79
Attachment, 224–225
Autism, 217–220
Autonomy
  aging parents and caregiving and, 234–235
  assisted dying and, 197
  childhood and adolescent conditions and, 201, 209–210
  family and couple functioning and, 82, 242–243
  life-cycle issues and, 111, 112–113, 114–115
Avoidance, 107, 329
Awareness phase, 277, 278*f*, 279*t*, 280–281, 294*f*

Behavioral health care (BHC), 65, 351, 361–362, 367
Belief systems. *See also* Health beliefs; Spirituality; Values
  agency and course of illness and, 143–145
  anticipatory loss and, 162–163, 175–176
  assessment and, 61, 131–132
  case examples of, 140–143, 144, 148, 149–150, 152–153, 154, 175, 267, 298
  causes of illness and disability and, 139–140
  childhood and adolescent conditions and, 202–203
  clinicians and, 18, 332–333, 337

collaborative care and, 362–367, 363*f*
couple functioning and, 267–268
ethnocultural and spiritual influences on, 134–136
experience of illness and, 129–131, 130*f*
Family Systems Illness (FSI) model and, 13–14
fit among family members and, 153–154
gender-based, 136–137
genetic factors and, 289–291
genograms and, 92–93
hope and optimism and, 145–146
illness narratives and metaphors, 146–151
integrative practices and, 154–156
mastery and control and, 137–139
multigenerational factors and, 89
normative illness experience and, 132–134
overview, 128–129
parental illness and disability and, 222–224
psychosocial map and, 15
rituals and, 151–153
terminal phase of illness and, 196
therapeutic triangle and, 53
Bereavement, 11, 44, 70, 94, 141, 176, 178–180, 312
Biological factors, 19, 21, 23–24
Biomedical factors, 15, 129–130, 130*f*, 362
Biopsychosocial understanding, 129, 134–135, 366
Blame
  beliefs regarding, 139–140, 141–143
  case examples of, 140–142, 175, 203–204
  childhood and adolescent conditions and, 203–204, 211–212
  clinicians and, 331
  family system and, 63
  neurocognitive conditions and, 315
  terminal phase of illness and, 180
Boundaries
  case examples of, 264–265
  clinicians and, 333–335, 337–338
  collaborative care and, 359
  couple functioning and, 240, 242–243, 258–261, 264–265
  family functioning and, 82–83
  life-cycle issues and, 115
  multigenerational factors and, 96
Boundary ambiguity, 311
Brain Injury Family Intervention model, 304
Breast disorders, 252–253, 303
Burnout, 328–329

Cancer
  case examples of, 223–224, 250, 298, 339–346
  childhood and adolescent conditions and, 200
  couple functioning and, 248–249, 260
  course of disorders and, 22, 23, 24
  disability and, 28
  genetic factors and, 290
  group-oriented services and, 73

Index   389

health beliefs and, 139
neurocognitive conditions and, 303
normative illness experience, 132
outcome and, 25
quality of life and, 3
sexuality and, 252–253
uncertainty and, 31
Cardiovascular disease. *See also* Heart attack
  anticipatory loss and, 167
  case examples of, 107, 118–119, 250–251
  disability and, 28
  genetic factors and, 290
  multigenerational factors and, 94
  outcome and, 25
  overview, 302–303
  quality of life and, 3
  treatment regimes and, 35
Caregiving system. *See also* Family factors; Support
  adulthood challenges and, 217–220
  aging parents and, 228–239
  anticipatory loss and, 164–165
  case examples of, 185–186, 262–263, 264–265
  childhood and adolescent conditions and, 205–206
  clinicians and, 256–257
  couple functioning and, 243, 248–249, 261–265
  dementia and, 301
  diagnosis and, 307–308
  extramarital affairs and, 255
  identifying, 62–63
  impact of caregiving, 229–230
  limits on, 264–265
  neurocognitive conditions and, 302, 312, 322
  role functioning and, 136–137
  siblings and, 214–216
  terminal phase of illness and, 184–186
Causation, 139–142
Celebrations, 152, 190–191, 191, 213
Cerebral palsy, 28, 217–220
Chicago Center for Family Health (CCFH), 358
Childhood conditions
  anticipatory loss and, 175–176
  case examples of, 203–204, 215–217
  communication and, 204–206
  developmental issues, 206–213
  modalities of treatment and, 68
  onset and, 172–173. *See also* Onset
  outcome and, 26
  overview, 6, 17, 200–201
  phases of illness and, 188–189, 201–204
  siblings and, 213–217
  terminal phase of illness and, 140–142
Child-rearing phases in the family life cycle. *See also* Life-cycle issues
  aging parents and caregiving and, 235–236
  anticipatory loss and, 170, 174–175
  case examples of, 115, 120–124, 223–224, 236

genetic factors and, 292
illness development and, 114–116
overview, 111
parental illness and disability and, 221–228
Children, 231–232, 292–293. *See also* Childhood conditions
Chronic conditions, 3–4, 108–109, 149, 350–351. *See also* Chronic phase of illness; *individual conditions*
Chronic phase of illness. *See also* Illness time phases
  anticipatory loss and, 164–165
  case examples of, 343–344
  couple functioning and, 243–244, 263–264
  developmental tasks associated with, 46*t*
  family functioning and, 84
  genetic factors and, 294*f*
  illness phase transitions and, 45–48, 46*t*
  integrated care and, 65–66
  life-cycle issues and, 125
  neurocognitive conditions and, 310–316
  overview, 37*f*, 42–44
  psychosocial developmental model and, 48–50, 49*f*
  sexuality and, 251–256
  triangulation and, 83
Clarity, 78*t*, 85–86
Clinical applications, 15, 50–51, 112–120, 124–127
Clinician factors. *See also* Health care professionals or providers; Health care team
  belief systems and, 332–333
  case examples of, 338, 339–346
  collaborative care and, 359–362, 362–367, 365
  couple functioning and, 249, 256–257
  engaging the family system and, 63–64
  expectations and, 36
  family functioning and, 81–82
  levels of systems-based involvement and, 57–60, 58*t*–59*t*
  life-cycle issues and, 332
  loss and limits and, 325–329
  meeting the needs of clinicians, 336–338
  multigenerational factors and, 330–332
  overview, 17–18, 325
  personal issues and, 333–336
  self-care and, 199
  treatment regimes and, 35
Clinician personal themes
  belief systems, 332–333
  case example, 339–346
  facing loss and personal limits, 325–329
  guidelines for meeting clinician needs, 336–338
  issues in clinician's own family, 333–336
  life-cycle timing, 332
  multigenerational legacies with illness and loss, 330–332
Cognitive-behavioral interventions, 6, 74, 75

Cognitive impairment. *See also* Neurocognitive
    impairment
  anticipatory loss and, 165–166
  case examples of, 262–263, 305–306
  couple functioning and, 258, 266–267
  threat of future cognitive impairment, 305–306
  uncertainty and, 32
Cognitive interventions, 6
Cognitive psychology, 13
Cohesion, 47–48, 81, 82, 89, 117–118
Collaborative Family Healthcare Association
    (CFHA), 351
Collaborative health care or practice, 347–367
  belief systems fit with patients and families
    362–367
  case examples of, 360, 363–364
  consumer-based organizations, 357–359
  combining mental health approaches, 74–75
  family functioning and, 78*t*, 85
  family-oriented programs and policies, 367–368
  genetic factors and, 295–296
  health care settings and contexts and, 351–362
  initial crisis phase of illness and, 39
  integrated care and, 64–66
  levels of collaboration, 348, 349*t*
  levels of systems-based involvement and, 58*t*
  modalities of treatment and, 70
  overview, 17–18, 347–351, 349*t*
  principles of intervention and, 60
  religious and spiritual beliefs and, 136
Communication
  assessment and intervention and, 50
  case examples of, 223–224
  childhood and adolescent conditions and,
    204–206
  clinicians and, 336
  combining mental health approaches and,
    74–75
  couple functioning and, 245–248, 253–254,
    264–265, 271
  determining chronicity and, 42–43
  examples of, 40–41
  family functioning and, 77–78, 78*t*, 85–88
  genetic factors and, 289–290
  initial crisis phase of illness and, 38–39, 40–41
  integrated care and, 64–66
  memory loss and, 313
  multigenerational factors and, 97
  parental illness and disability and, 221–224
  principles of intervention and, 61
  sexuality and, 251–252
  terminal phase of illness and, 177, 189
  treatment regimes and, 35
Community resources
  assessment and intervention and, 50
  collaborative care and, 348, 350, 355, 368
  life-cycle stages and, 110

  multigenerational factors and, 96
  neurocognitive conditions and, 309–310
Compassion, 185, 190
Compassion fatigue, 328–329
Complementary and alternative medicine (CAM),
    154–156
Conflict, 89, 167, 185–186, 259
Conjoint sessions, 241–242
Connectedness, 78*t*, 81–82
Constancy
  childhood and adolescent conditions and, 202
  chronic phase of illness and, 44
  overview, 23–24
  psychosocial developmental model and, 49*f*
  psychosocial typology matrix and, 29, 30*t*–31*t*
Consultation
  clinicians and, 329, 337
  collaborative care and, 352
  course of disorders and, 23
  disability and, 29
  family functioning and, 63–64, 77
  Family Systems Illness (FSI) model and, 5, 15
  health beliefs and, 131–132
  modalities of treatment and, 68
  neurocognitive conditions and, 315
  overview, 16
  principles of intervention and, 60–63
  timing of, 66–67
Continuity, 39, 79
Control, 127, 137–139, 204, 234–235, 261
Coping
  anticipatory loss and, 159–160
  assessment and intervention and, 50
  childhood and adolescent conditions and, 202
  clinicians and, 331, 334
  family and couple functioning and, 76, 82, 243,
    244, 249–250
  health beliefs and, 131
  life-cycle issues and, 114–115
  multigenerational factors and, 89, 94, 94–95
  neurocognitive conditions and, 311–312
  normative illness experience, 132–134
  onset and, 21
  outcome and, 27
  phases of illness and, 39, 45, 46, 177, 187
Core beliefs, 129, 130, 131, 151–153. *See also* Belief
    systems; Health beliefs
Couple functioning. *See also* Family functioning;
    Intimacy issues; Marital functioning,
    parental; Relationships; Rebalancing couple
    relationship
  adapting to diagnosis or crisis and, 266–267
  anticipatory loss and, 174–175
  belief systems and, 267–268
  boundaries and, 258–261
  case examples of, 250–251, 262–263, 264–265,
    266, 267, 269–270

Index

clinicians and, 256–257, 334
conjoint and individual sessions and, 241–242
genetic factors and, 273, 291–292
intimacy and, 242–256
LGBTQ couples, 256
life-cycle issues and, 268–271
neurocognitive conditions and, 312, 317–318, 321–322
overview, 240
relationship repair, 62, 179, 181–185
roles of patient and caregiver and, 261–265
separateness and togetherness needs and, 265
treatment regimes and, 35
younger couples, 243, 268–270, 304, 317–318
Course. *See also* Psychosocial typology of illness
anticipatory loss and, 165–168
beliefs regarding, 143–145
neurocognitive conditions and, 304–305
overview, 20, 21*f*, 22–25
psychosocial developmental model and, 49*f*
psychosocial typology matrix and, 29, 30*t*–31*t*
Crisis management. *See also* Initial crisis phase of illness
assessment and intervention and, 50
couple functioning and, 241–242
family psychoeducation and, 70
illness characteristics and, 33–34
life-cycle issues and, 119–120
multigenerational factors and, 89, 98
onset and, 21
parental illness and disability and, 226–227
Cultural factors. *See also* Ethnocultural factors
aging parents and caregiving and, 232–233, 239
assessment and, 61
case examples of, 154, 295–296
clinicians and, 336
collaborative care and, 359, 363–365
couple functioning and, 248–249
family functioning and, 81–82, 85–86
Family Systems Illness (FSI) model and, 12*f*
genetic factors and, 289–291
genograms and, 91, 92–93
health beliefs and, 134–136, 150–151, 153–154
intimacy and, 242
levels of meaning and, 130, 130*f*
life structures and, 110
life-cycle stages and, 110
modalities of treatment and, 69
outcome and, 27
principles of intervention and, 62
psychosocial map and, 15
psychosomatic label and, 8
role functioning and, 225
sharing of information and, 41
systems theory and, 9–10
terminal phase of illness and, 196

Cystic fibrosis
childhood and adolescent conditions and, 200, 207, 211, 213
collaborative care and, 355–357
genetic factors and, 290
outcome and, 25

Death, 17, 44–45, 192–194, 197–199, 227. *See also* Loss; Outcome; Terminal phase of illness
Decision making, 125, 208–209, 283, 289–290, 315
Deformities, 147–148
Denial, 145–146, 148, 160, 202, 210, 243, 260, 266
Dementia
anticipatory loss and, 165–166
case examples of, 237–238, 262–263, 319, 320, 344–345
diagnosis and, 307–308
family challenges related to, 318–321
Family Systems Illness (FSI) model and, 17
long-term facility placement and, 315–316
overview, 301, 302–303
threat of future cognitive impairment, 305–306
Departure period of the terminal phase, 192–194, 193. *See also* Terminal phase of illness
Depression
aging parents and caregiving and, 233–234
case examples of, 100–103, 101*f*, 107, 116–117, 149–150
overview, 302
Developmental factors. *See also* Life-cycle issues
age at onset and, 35
anticipatory loss and, 168–175
case examples of, 210–211
childhood and adolescent conditions and, 206–213
couple functioning and, 268–271
disability and, 217–220
Family Systems Illness (FSI) model and, 12, 12*f*, 14*f*
genetic factors and, 300
illness-related developmental tasks, 38, 45–48, 46*t*
overview, 50
parental illness and disability and, 222
role functioning and, 225–226
skews, 12. *See also* Relationship imbalances or skews
systems theory and, 9–10
Diabetes
anticipatory loss and, 172–173, 174–175
caregiving and, 62
case examples of, 103–105, 104*f*, 116–117
childhood and adolescent conditions and, 200, 205, 211
collaborative care and, 353–357
course of disorders and, 23
crisis management skills and, 34

Diabetes *(cont.)*
  family functioning and, 79–80
  genetic factors and, 290
  outcome and, 25
  quality of life and, 3
  treatment and, 6, 35
  uncertainty and, 32
Diagnosis
  couple functioning and, 266–267
  determining chronicity and, 42–43
  family functioning and, 85
  genetic factors and, 290, 291
  health beliefs and, 147–148
  labeling, 147
  levels of meaning and, 130
  life-cycle issues and, 124
  neurocognitive conditions and, 307–309
  sharing of information and, 40–41
  uncertainty following, 159
Disability. *See also* Psychosocial typology of illness
  adulthood challenges and, 217–220
  aging parents and caregiving, 228–229
  anticipatory loss and, 159, 170, 176
  caregiving and, 62–63
  childhood and adolescent conditions and, 200
  course of disorders and, 22, 23–25
  family beliefs regarding, 139–140
  health beliefs and, 149–150
  life-cycle issues and, 127
  neurocognitive conditions and, 306–307
  overview, 20, 21*f*, 28–29
  psychosocial developmental model and, 49*f*
  psychosocial typology matrix and, 29, 30*t*–31*t*
  therapeutic triangle and, 52
  triangulation and, 83–84
Disfigurement, 28, 72
Divorced families, 83, 89, 92
Do-not-resuscitate (DNR) orders, 194–195, 196
Dysfunctional patients and families, 61, 92, 106–107, 205–206, 236–238. *See also* Family functioning

Early adulthood, 120, 149–150, 209–213, 218–219, 284, 293, 296, 317–318, 339–346, 354
Educational resources, 309–310
Emotional expression
  anticipatory loss and, 160
  childhood and adolescent conditions and, 205
  couple functioning and, 248
  family functioning and, 78*t*, 86–87
  terminal phase of illness and, 188
Emphysema, 22, 23, 118–119
Enmeshed patterns, 114–115, 236–238
Epigenetics, 272, 275*t*. *See also* Genetic factors
Episodic course, 24–25, 29, 30*t*–31*t*, 44. *See also* Course

Ethical issues, 194–199, 239, 296–299, 366
Ethnicity
  aging parents and caregiving and, 232–233
  family functioning and, 85
  Family Systems Illness (FSI) model and, 12*f*
  genetic factors and, 290
  life-cycle stages and, 110
  principles of intervention and, 62
  psychosocial map and, 15
  social context of illness and disabilities and, 4–5
Ethnocultural factors, 110, 134–136, 289, 359. *See also* Cultural factors
Euthanasia, 197–199. *See also* Terminal phase of illness
Exhaustion, 160, 313–314
Expectations
  aging parents and caregiving and, 233–234, 239
  case examples of, 267
  childhood and adolescent conditions and, 207–209
  clinicians and, 334
  collaborative care and, 362–367, 363*f*
  couple functioning and, 261
  family functioning and, 80–82
  health beliefs and, 134
  life-cycle issues and, 125
  outcome and, 25–26
  overview, 36
Extended family, 62, 68–69, 77, 91–92, 105–106, 226, 228, 273, 282, 289
Externalization, 213–214, 260
Extramarital relationship or affair, 167, 254–256

Facility placement, 239, 309, 315–316, 331. *See also* Hospice care; Long-term care
Family factors. *See also* Caregiving system; Family functioning; Multigenerational factors; Roles within the family
  assessment and, 61
  collaborative care and, 348, 350, 355, 362–367, 363*f*, 367–368
  expectations and, 36
  family organization and communication, 21, 77–78, 78*t*
  family patterns, 26–27, 103–105, 104*f*, 106–107
  Family Systems Illness (FSI) model and, 12, 12*f*
  genograms and. *See* Genogram
  health beliefs and, 151
  levels of meaning and, 130, 130*f*
  life-cycle issues and, 111
  overview, 96
  resilience and, 6–7. *See also* Resiliency
  rituals and, 152
  systems theory and, 9–10
  therapeutic triangle and, 52–53, 52*f*
  timing of consultation and, 67

Index

Family functioning. *See also* Dysfunctional patients and families; Family factors; Multigenerational factors
   aging parents and caregiving and, 231–232, 236–238
   case examples of, 319, 320, 341–342
   childhood and adolescent conditions and, 200–201, 202–203
   clinicians and, 334
   collaborative care and, 359–362
   family organization and communication, 77–88, 78t
   genograms and, 90–93, 92f
   modalities of treatment and, 68
   multigenerational family processes and, 96–98
   neurocognitive conditions and, 312, 312–313, 318–321
   normative perspective of, 76–77
   overview, 11–14, 12f, 14f, 76, 88
   service delivery and, 54
   terminal phase of illness and, 189–190
   treatment regimes and, 35
Family life cycle. *See* Life-cycle issues
Family life review, 151, 237. *See also* Life review
Family meetings, 69–70, 107, 357
Family of choice, 62, 84
Family of origin. *See* Multigenerational factors
Family psychoeducation, 70, 71–72. *See also* Psychoeducation
Family rituals. *See* Rituals
Family Systems Genetics Illness (FSGI) model
   genetic factors and, 293–295, 294f
   overview, 273, 274–288, 275t, 278f, 279t
Family Systems Illness (FSI) model
   anticipatory loss and, 161
   clinicians and, 330–332, 336–338
   concepts and components of, 9–15, 11f, 12f, 14f
   couple functioning and, 240
   expanding on, 17
   genetic factors and, 273, 293–295, 294f, 300
   initial crisis phase of illness and, 38–39
   levels of systems-based involvement, 57–60, 58t–59t
   modalities of treatment and, 67–75
   need for, 5–9
   overview, 5, 8–9
   principles of intervention and, 60–66
   service delivery applications, 53–54
Family systems theory, 7–8, 9–10, 355–357
Family therapy, 59t, 62, 68–70, 179
Family–community networks, 84. *See also* Resources
Family-focused model, 5–9, 16
Family system reorganization process, 179, 183–184
Fatal outcome, 25, 29, 30t–31t, 49f. *See also* Outcome

Fear
   childhood and adolescent conditions and, 209–210
   clinicians and, 329
   couple functioning and, 265
   genetic factors and, 287
   outcome and, 26, 27
   parental illness and disability and, 222, 224
Flare-ups, 24–25, 44, 66–67
Flexibility
   family functioning and, 76, 78t, 79–81
   health beliefs and, 143–144
   initial crisis phase of illness and, 39
   role functioning and, 225
   treatment regimes and, 35
Framing events, 39–41, 77, 162
Frontotemporal dementia (FTD), 302
Funeral planning, 191, 230

Gender
   aging parents and caregiving and, 233–234, 239
   case examples of, 140–142, 250–251
   childhood and adolescent conditions and, 203–204
   family and couple functioning and, 86, 248–251, 261, 264–265
   Family Systems Illness (FSI) model and, 12f
   genetic factors and, 283
   genograms and, 92
   health beliefs and, 136–137
   intimacy and, 242
   life structures and, 110
   life-cycle issues and, 110, 125
   psychosocial map and, 15
Genetic factors
   anticipatory loss and, 172–173
   case examples of, 285, 288, 293, 295–296, 298, 299
   cultural meanings and beliefs and, 289–291
   ethical and legal issues and, 296–299
   Family Systems Genetics Illness (FSGI) model and, 273, 274–288, 275t, 278f, 279t, 293–295, 294f
   genetic mutations, 274–277, 275t
   illness time phases and, 277–288, 278f, 279t
   integrated collaborative practice and, 295–296
   life-cycle issues and, 291–293
   overview, 16–17, 272–274, 275t, 300, 302
Genetic Information Nondiscrimination Act (GINA), 297
Genogram
   case examples of, 101, 101f
   clinicians and, 330–331
   family health genogram, 93
   overview, 89, 91–93, 92f
   uses of, 90–91

Genomics, 272, 275t. *See also* Genetic factors
Goals, 39, 132–133, 201, 207–209
Gradual onset. *See also* Onset
   neurocognitive conditions and, 303
   overview, 21–22
   psychosocial developmental model and, 48, 49f
   psychosocial typology matrix and, 29, 30t–31t
Grief, 26, 165–166, 201–202, 312, 315. *See also* Loss
Group-oriented services, 16, 54, 71–74, 211, 335–336. *See also* Support groups
Guilt
   aging parents and caregiving and, 237
   anticipatory loss and, 160, 176
   case examples of, 203–204, 215–216, 262–263
   childhood and adolescent conditions and, 203–204, 212
   clinicians and, 331
   genetic factors and, 286
   health beliefs and, 142–143
   modalities of treatment and, 68
   neurocognitive conditions and, 315
   principles of intervention and, 61
   siblings and, 214
   terminal phase of illness and, 182, 188

Head injury. *See* Traumatic brain injury
Health beliefs. *See* Belief systems
Health care. *See also* Health care professionals or providers; Health care team
   aging parents and caregiving, 229
   childhood and adolescent conditions and, 212–213
   collaborative care and, 351–367, 363f
   family functioning and, 84–85
   genetic factors and, 281
   lack of access to, 4–5
   life-cycle stages and, 110
   overview, 3–4, 15
   phases of illness and, 39, 180, 195
   settings for, 361–362
   triangulation and, 84
Health care professionals or providers. *See also* Clinician factors; Health care; Health care team
   aging parents and caregiving and, 239
   assessment and intervention and, 198–199
   case examples of, 185–186
   childhood and adolescent conditions and, 211–212
   chronic conditions and, 350–351
   collaborative care and, 347–348, 359–362
   couple functioning and, 262–263
   genetic factors and, 286
   multigenerational factors and, 97
   multiple providers, 367
   neurocognitive conditions and, 307–308
   physicians, 40–41, 42–43, 51, 64–66
   terminal phase of illness and, 185–186
Health care team. *See also* Clinician factors; Health care; Health care professionals or providers; Physicians
   collaborative care and, 359–362
   integrated care and, 64–66
   multigenerational factors and, 96
   psychosocial checkups and, 54
   therapeutic triangle and, 51–53, 52f
   triangulation and, 84
Heart attack. *See also* Cardiovascular disease
   case examples of, 118–119
   couple functioning and, 253
   course of disorders and, 23
   life-cycle issues and, 125
   multigenerational factors and, 94
   onset and, 21
   outcome and, 25
   therapeutic triangle and, 53
   uncertainty and, 31
Helplessness, 61, 188
Hemophilia, 25, 172–173, 200, 280–281
Here-for-now period of the terminal phase, 189–191. *See also* Terminal phase of illness
HIV/AIDS
   anticipatory loss and, 176
   case examples of, 148
   disability and, 28
   family functioning and, 84
   group-oriented services and, 72
   overview, 302
   quality of life and, 3
   support and, 8
Holistic approaches, 8–9, 184
Home-based medical care, 50, 361
Hope, 145–146
Hospice care. *See also* Facility placement; Palliative care
   case examples of, 187, 345
   clinicians and, 327, 333, 335–336
   collaborative care and, 357
   terminal phase of illness and, 184–188, 195
Human experience level of meaning, 129, 130, 130f
Huntington's disease, 25, 302, 305–306
Hypertension, 31, 34, 42, 290

Illness narratives, 146–147, 148, 206, 318, 333
Illness time phases
   anticipatory loss and, 162–165
   assessment and intervention and, 50–53, 52f
   beliefs regarding, 138–139
   case examples of, 118–119, 154, 295–296
   childhood and adolescent conditions and, 207
   collaborative care and, 365–366

Index

couple functioning and, 261–262
Family Systems Illness (FSI) model and, 14f
genetic factors and, 277–288, 277f, 278f, 279t
group-oriented services and, 72–73
health beliefs and, 143–144, 146, 154
life-cycle issues and, 112–120
multigenerational factors and, 93–95
neurocognitive conditions and, 307–316
overview, 10–11, 12f, 16, 37, 37f
psychosocial developmental model and, 48–50, 49f
service delivery applications, 53–54
therapeutic triangle and, 51–53, 52f
transition periods and, 45–48, 46t
Illness typology. *See* Psychosocial typology of illness
Illness-related developmental tasks, 38, 45–48, 46t
Imbalances. *See* Relationship imbalances or skews
Individual sessions, 68–70, 179, 241–242
Infertility, 152–153, 209
Information sharing, 40–41, 42, 58t. *See also* Communication; Psychoeducation
Initial crisis phase of illness. *See also* Crisis management; Illness time phases
 case examples of, 203–204, 342–343
 childhood and adolescent conditions and, 201–204
 collaborative care and, 366
 determining chronicity and, 42–44
 developmental tasks associated with, 46t
 family and couple functioning and, 79, 241–242, 245, 249–251, 259, 263–264, 266–267
 genetic factors and, 294f
 health beliefs and, 131
 illness phase transitions and, 45–48, 46t
 life-cycle issues and, 117–118, 125
 neurocognitive conditions and, 307–310
 overview, 37f, 38–41
 psychosocial developmental model and, 48–50, 49f
 timing of consultation and, 66–67
Integrated family systems illness model, 5–9, 67–75, 154–156. *See also* Family Systems Illness (FSI) model
Integrated treatment approaches, 8–9, 74, 154–156, 295–296, 310, 367–368. *See also* Collaborative practice
Intervention. *See also* Treatment
 case examples of, 288
 Family Systems Illness (FSI) model for, 5
 genetic factors and, 290
 modalities of treatment and, 67–75
 phases of illness and, 50–53, 52f
 principles of, 60–66
 service delivery applications, 53–54
 therapeutic triangle and, 51–53

Intimacy issues, 240, 242–256, 265, 321–322. *See also* Couple functioning
Invisible symptoms, 33, 83–84. *See also* Symptoms

Kidney disease, 34, 200, 302
Kovler Diabetes Center (CDC), 353–357

Labeling, diagnosis and, 147
Later life, 221, 228–239, 270–271
Legal issues, 194–199, 296–299, 366
Leukemia, 23, 200
LGBTQ community, 62, 78, 84, 110, 256
Life course, 9. *See also* Developmental factors; Life-cycle issues
Life expectancy, 25, 230, 243, 313. *See also* Outcome
Life review, 151, 237
Life structures, 110–111, 119–120
Life-cycle issues. *See also* Developmental factors; Family life cycle; Transitions
 adult disabilities and, 217–220
 age at onset and, 35
 anticipatory loss and, 168–175
 caregiving and, 62
 case examples of, 107, 112–114, 115, 116–117, 118–119, 120–124, 169, 171, 269–270, 293, 316–318
 child-rearing and non-child-rearing stages, 111
 clinicians and, 18, 332, 337
 core life-cycle concepts, 109–111
 couple functioning and, 268–271
 genetic factors and, 276, 283–284, 291–293
 genograms and, 92
 health beliefs and, 150, 151
 illness development and, 112–120
 intimacy and, 242
 multigenerational factors and, 95–96
 neurocognitive conditions and, 304, 316–318
 overview, 108–110, 124–127
 psychosocial map and, 15
 psychosocial typology and, 116–117
 rituals and, 152
Living wills, 194–197
Long-term adaptation phase, 278f, 279t, 286–288, 294f
Long-term care, 229, 315–316. *See also* Facility placement
Loss. *See also* Anticipatory loss
 assessment and intervention and, 50
 case examples of, 100–103, 101f, 152–153
 childhood and adolescent conditions and, 201–202
 clinicians and, 325–329, 330–332
 couple functioning and, 244
 genograms and, 92
 initial crisis phase of illness and, 38–39

Loss (cont.)
  integrated care and, 65–66
  intimacy and, 243–244
  multigenerational factors and, 89
  neurocognitive conditions and, 311–312, 315, 320–321
  outcome and, 26
  rituals and, 152
  terminal phase of illness and, 44–45, 178
Low-income populations, 4–5, 23, 227–228
Lung disease and cancer, 21, 23, 31, 303, 340–346

Manipulation, 83–84, 205
Marital functioning, parental, 79, 167, 291–292. *See also* Couple functioning; Relationships
Mastery, 14–15, 137–139, 143–144, 287
Meaning-making
  childhood and adolescent conditions and, 202–203
  Family Systems Illness (FSI) model and, 13, 14f
  genetic factors and, 289
  health beliefs and, 131
  initial crisis phase of illness and, 39
  labeling language and, 147–148
  levels of meaning and, 129–131
  terminal phase of illness and, 179–181
Medical treatments, 3–4, 208–209, 252, 302
Medications, 34–35, 70, 302, 310, 357
Mental health care, 64, 65–66, 67–75, 361–362
Mental illness, 28, 302
Metaphors, 148–151, 260
Migraine headaches, 24, 32
Mild cognitive impairment, 302, 307, 310–311. *See also* Neurocognitive impairment
Mindfulness-based cognitive behavioral therapy (MCBT), 156
Mindfulness-based stress reduction (MBSR), 75, 155–156, 336
Mourning, 44–45, 180–181
Multicultural factors, 9–10, 110, 363–365
Multifamily group (MFG) approaches, 71–74, 211, 354, 356. *See also* Group-oriented services
Multigenerational factors. *See also* Family factors; Family functioning
  aging parents and caregiving and, 230–233
  anticipatory loss and, 168–170
  assessment and intervention and, 50
  case examples of, 99–107, 101f, 104f, 288, 341–342
  clinicians and, 18, 330–332, 337
  dysfunctional family patterns and, 106–107
  experiences with crisis and adversity and, 98
  family functioning and, 82–83, 96–98
  Family Systems Illness (FSI) model and, 13
  genetic factors and, 280–281
  genograms and, 90–93, 92f
  health beliefs and, 153–154
  levels of meaning and, 130, 130f
  life-cycle coincidences and, 95–96
  multiple chronic disorders and, 105–106
  overview, 89–90
  psychosocial typology and time phases and, 93–95
  systems theory and, 9–10
  time lines and, 93
Multiple sclerosis (MS)
  case examples of, 120–124, 267, 316–317
  collaborative care and, 358–359
  course of disorders and, 24
  disability and, 28
  group-oriented services and, 74
  labeling language and, 147–148
  life-cycle issues and, 127
  overview, 302
  threat of future cognitive impairment, 305–306
  uncertainty and, 29, 31
Multiple Sclerosis Society, 358
Muscular dystrophy, 202, 282, 299

Narratives, 13, 180, 181, 202–203
Neurocognitive impairment. *See also* Cognitive impairment
  anticipatory loss and, 165–166
  case examples of, 305–306, 314, 315–318, 319, 320–321
  couple functioning and, 321–322
  family challenges related to, 318–321
  Family Systems Illness (FSI) model and, 17
  life-cycle issues and, 316–318
  overview, 301–303
  psychosocial typology of, 303–307
  time phase-related issues and, 307–316
Non-child-rearing phases in the family life cycle. *See also* Life-cycle issues
  anticipatory loss and, 170, 174–175
  case examples of, 120–124
  couple functioning and, 268–270
  illness development and, 112–114
  overview, 111
Nonfatal outcome, 29, 30t–31t, 49f. *See also* Outcome
Normative experience of illness
  clinicians and, 335
  collaborative care and, 365
  couple functioning and, 264–265, 266–267
  extramarital affairs and, 255–256
  neurocognitive conditions and, 312, 315
  overview, 132–134

Obesity, 200, 290
Onset. *See also* Psychosocial typology of illness
  age at onset, 35
  anticipatory loss and, 172–174

Index   397

case examples of, 173
genetic factors and, 276
life-cycle issues and, 119–120
neurocognitive conditions and, 303–304
overview, 20, 21–22, 21f
psychosocial developmental model and, 49f
psychosocial typology matrix and, 29, 30t–31t
Optimism. *See* Hope
Outcome. *See also* Psychosocial typology of illness
health beliefs and, 143–144
overview, 17, 20, 21f, 25–27
psychosocial developmental model and, 49f
psychosocial typology matrix and, 29, 30t–31t

Pain, 33, 83–84, 149–150, 192
Palliative care, 184–188, 333, 357. *See also* Facility placement; Hospice care
Paradigm, 14f
Parental illness and disability, 221–228. *See also* Parents
child attachment, 224–225
communication, 221–224
grandparents and extended kin, 226
role functioning, 225–226
Parents
blame and, 203
childhood and adolescent conditions and, 201, 206–207, 208–209, 210–212
guilt and, 212
illness and disability of, 114–116, 221–228
terminal phase of illness and, 189
Parkinson's disease
case examples of, 262–263, 319
labeling language and, 147–148
multigenerational factors and, 94
onset and, 21–22
overview, 302–303
Permanency, chronicity and, 42–43, 99–100, 264
Pharmacological treatment. *See* Medications
Phases of illness. *See* Illness time phases
Physicians, 40–41, 42–43, 51, 64–66. *See also* Health care professionals or providers; Health care team
Policy principles, 367–368
Positive illusions. *See* Hope
Predictability, 29, 31–32, 79. *See also* Uncertainty
Preparedness, 26–27, 178, 194–197. *See also* Terminal phase of illness
Pretesting phase, 278f, 279t, 281–284, 294f
Prevention
anticipatory loss and, 174–175
collaborative care and, 356
Family Systems Illness (FSI) model and, 5
genetic factors and, 276–277, 291
health beliefs and, 142
psychosocial map and, 14–15

Primary care system, 350–352. *See also* Health care
Privacy, 282–283
Problem solving
assessment and intervention and, 50
childhood and adolescent conditions and, 211
family functioning and, 78t, 87–88
family psychoeducation and, 70
onset and, 21
terminal phase of illness and, 193–194
treatment regimes and, 35
uncertainty and, 29
Professional education and development, 354–355, 356, 368
Prognosis. *See also* Outcome
anticipatory loss and, 175
determining chronicity and, 42–44
hospice care and, 184–185
initial crisis phase of illness and, 38, 40–41
life-cycle issues and, 125
overview, 26
Progressive conditions. *See also* Course
anticipatory loss and, 165–166
case examples of, 120–124
communication and, 309
family functioning and, 85
family psychoeducation and, 70
health beliefs and, 139
life-cycle issues and, 125
neurocognitive conditions and, 305, 311
overview, 22–23
phases of illness and, 44, 195
psychosocial developmental model and, 49f
psychosocial typology matrix and, 29, 30t–31t
timing of consultation and, 66–67
Protection patterns, 68, 242
Psoriasis, 28, 147–148
Psychic numbing, 327
Psychodynamic psychotherapy, 75
Psychoeducation
clinicians and, 333, 335–336, 337
collaborative care and, 353–354, 356
course of disorders and, 25
disability and, 29
expectations and, 36
family psychoeducation, 70
Family Systems Illness (FSI) model and, 15
Family Systems Illness (FSI) model for, 5
group-oriented services and, 71–72
neurocognitive conditions and, 304
overview, 16
principles of intervention and, 61
service delivery and, 54
sexuality and, 252–253
Psychosocial adaptation. *See* Adaptation
Psychosocial checkups, 53–54, 61, 66
Psychosocial developmental model, 48–50

Psychosocial factors
  childhood and adolescent conditions and, 201–202, 211–212
  clinicians and, 336
  collaborative care and, 351, 354
  couple functioning and, 252–253
  developmental model and, 48–50, 49f
  Family Systems Illness (FSI) model and, 3–4, 19
  overview, 36
  parental illness and disability and, 225
  support and, 8
Psychosocial map, 3–4, 14–15, 38
Psychosocial typology of illness
  aging parents and caregiving and, 235
  anticipatory loss and, 162–165
  assessment and intervention and, 50–51
  case examples of, 116–117
  childhood and adolescent conditions and, 207
  collaborative care and, 368
  couple functioning and, 245, 261–262
  Family Systems Illness (FSI) model and, 12f, 14f
  genetic factors and, 274–277, 275t, 277, 285
  group-oriented services and, 72–73
  life-cycle issues and, 116–117
  matrix for, 29–35, 30t–31t
  modalities of treatment and, 69
  multigenerational factors and, 93–95
  neurocognitive conditions and, 303–307
  overview, 10, 12f, 16, 19–29, 21f
  psychosocial developmental model and, 48–50, 49f
  timing of consultation and, 66–67
  uncertainty and, 31
Psychosomatic patterns, 8–9, 106–107, 169–170, 205–206

Quality of life
  assisted dying and, 197
  childhood and adolescent conditions and, 201, 208–209
  clinicians and, 327
  genetic factors and, 298
  support and, 8

Race
  Family Systems Illness (FSI) model and, 12f
  genetic factors and, 290
  intimacy and, 242
  life structures and, 110
  life-cycle stages and, 110
  principles of intervention and, 62
  social context of illness and disabilities and, 4–5
Rebalancing couple relationship, 258–271. *See also* Relationship imbalances or skews

Relapsing course. *See also* Course
  anticipatory loss and, 167
  life-cycle issues and, 125
  overview, 24–25
  psychosocial developmental model and, 49f
  psychosocial typology matrix and, 29, 30t–31t
  recurrences, 23–24, 25, 44
Relationships. *See also* Couple functioning; Marital functioning, parental
  childhood and adolescent conditions and, 201, 209
  engagement and, 242–243
  repair or healing, case example of, 182–183
  siblings and, 213–217
  terminal phase of illness and, 179, 180–183, 189–190
Relationship imbalances or skews, 258–271
Religion, 110, 134–136, 150–151, 179–181, 291. *See also* Spirituality
Remission, 24–25, 31. *See also* Course
Residential care settings, 239, 357. *See also* Facility placement
Resiliency
  experiences with crisis and adversity and, 98
  family functioning and, 6–7, 76, 77–88, 78t, 89
  Family Systems Illness (FSI) model and, 5
  parental illness and disability and, 221
  uncertainty and, 29
Resources
  anticipatory loss and, 164
  course of disorders and, 22
  engaging the family system and, 64
  family functioning and, 78t, 84–85
  Family Systems Illness (FSI) model and, 13–14
  onset and, 21
  principles of intervention and, 61
Respiratory condition, 22–23, 28
Responsibilities, 183–184, 225–226, 242, 282–283
Risk screening, 272–273, 290. *See also* Screening
Rituals, 151–153, 191, 312–313, 338
Role functioning, 50, 225–227
Roles within the family. *See also* Family factors
  aging parents and caregiving and, 231–232, 233–234
  clinicians and, 331–332
  couple functioning and, 247, 248–251, 261–265
  disability and, 28–29
  health beliefs and, 134, 136–137
  initial crisis phase of illness and, 38–39
  life-cycle issues and, 115, 125
  multigenerational factors and, 96, 97–98
  neurocognitive conditions and, 312
  onset and, 21
  overview, 79

Index 399

siblings and, 215
treatment regimes and, 35
triangulation and, 83–84

Schizophrenia, 302, 333
Screening, 59–60, 90, 272–273, 297, 353–354. *See also* Assessment
Secrecy, 68, 282–283
Seizure disorders, 147–148, 242, 302
Self-awareness, 320–321, 330–332
Self-disclosure, 337–338
Separation, 44–45, 180–181, 183
Service delivery applications, 53–54. *See also* Collaborative health care or practice; Specialty care systems
Severity of crises, 33–34, 139, 306–307, 311
Sexual abuse, 183
Sexual orientation, 62, 84, 110, 259
Sexual relations, 243, 251–256, 321–322. *See also* Couple functioning
Shame
  anticipatory loss and, 164–165
  clinicians and, 331
  family system and, 63
  genetic factors and, 289–290
  health beliefs and, 142–143
  labeling language and, 147–148
  modalities of treatment and, 68
  neurocognitive conditions and, 315
  principles of intervention and, 61
  psychosomatic label and, 8
  terminal phase of illness and, 183
Shared "we" perspective, 244–245
Shared experience of illness. *See* Clinician personal themes
Shortened life span outcome, 25, 29, 30t–31t, 49f. *See also* Outcome
Siblings
  anticipatory loss and, 175–176
  case examples of, 215–217
  challenges for, 213–217
  communication and, 205
  family functioning and, 79, 81
  guilt and, 212
  modalities of treatment and, 69–70
Sick role, 83–84, 134, 261–265. *See also* Roles within the family
Sickle-cell disease, 149–150, 200, 290
Single-parent households, 68, 227–228
Social support, 50, 78t, 84–85
Socialization, 86, 145, 249–250, 264–265
Socioeconomic factors, 62, 110, 242, 290, 291
Specialty care systems, 84–85, 350–351, 352–357. *See also* Health care
Spinal cord injury, 23, 24–25, 31, 52

Spirituality. *See also* Belief systems
  assessment and, 61
  collaborative care and, 366
  Family Systems Illness (FSI) model and, 12f
  genetic factors and, 291
  genograms and, 91, 92–93
  health beliefs and, 134–136, 143–144
  life-cycle stages and, 110
  principles of intervention and, 62
  psychosocial map and, 15
  terminal phase of illness and, 179–181
Stability, 79–81
Stamina, 28, 76, 313–314
Stigma
  anticipatory loss and, 176
  disability and, 28
  genetic factors and, 290
  health beliefs and, 150–151
  labeling language and, 147–148
  LGBTQ couples and, 256
  neurocognitive conditions and, 308, 310
Stroke
  case examples of, 317–318, 339–340
  crisis management skills and, 34
  disability and, 28
  onset and, 21
  outcome and, 25
  psychosocial typology matrix and, 29
  uncertainty and, 31, 32
Substance abuse, 74, 92
Suffering, 135, 180, 182, 266–267, 312
Sundowning, 306–307
Support. *See also* Caregiving system
  collaborative care and, 359
  extramarital affairs as, 254–256
  family functioning and, 81
  family psychoeducation and, 70
  genograms and, 92
  group-oriented services and, 72
  levels of systems-based involvement and, 58t
  neurocognitive conditions and, 312
  terminal phase of illness and, 178
Support groups, 72, 163, 211. *See also* Group-oriented services
Survivor guilt, 164, 286, 345–346
Symptoms
  anticipatory loss and, 169–170
  behavior and, 76
  childhood and adolescent conditions and, 216–217
  genetic factors and, 287–288
  illness characteristics and, 32–33
  initial crisis phase of illness and, 38
  neurocognitive conditions, 302–303
  visibility of, 32–33

Systems theory, 9–10
Systems-based approach with families, 57–60, 58t–59t, 67–75, 70

Terminal phase of illness. *See also* Illness time phases
  aging parents and caregiving and, 238
  arrival period of, 186–189
  case examples of, 140–142, 177–178, 182–183, 185–186, 191, 193, 199, 344–345
  couple functioning and, 241–242
  departure period, 192–194
  developmental tasks associated with, 46t
  ethical and legal issues and, 194–199
  genetic factors and, 294f
  here-for-now period, 189–191
  illness phase transitions and, 45–48, 46t
  living during, 178–186
  overview, 37f, 44–45, 177–178
  psychosocial developmental model and, 48–50, 49f
Testing and posttesting phase, 278f, 279t, 284–286, 294f
Therapeutic relationship, 76–77, 139
Therapeutic triangle, 51–53, 52f
Time line, family, 89, 93
Time phases of illness. *See* Illness time phases
Traditions, 152, 232–233
Transitions
  anticipatory loss and, 171–172
  caregiving and, 62
  case examples of, 118–119, 171, 187, 210–211, 269–270, 295–296
  childhood and adolescent conditions and, 209–213
  collaborative care and, 366–367
  couple functioning and, 263–264, 269–270
  course of disorders and, 24
  determining chronicity and, 43
  examples of, 46–47
  family functioning and, 79
  genetic factors and, 291–293
  life structures and, 110–111
  life-cycle issues and, 111, 118–119, 125
  neurocognitive conditions and, 316–318
  overlapping, 118–119
  phases of illness and, 45–48, 46t
  psychosocial map and, 15
  terminal phase of illness and, 177, 186–188, 189
Trauma, 74, 100–103, 101f, 170–171
Traumatic brain injury
  anticipatory loss and, 170
  caregiving and, 62
  case examples of, 100–103, 101f, 112–114, 266

couple functioning and, 258
course of disorders and, 23
Family Systems Illness (FSI) model and, 17
normative illness experience, 132
onset and, 21
overview, 301, 304, 310–311
psychosocial typology matrix and, 29
Treatment. *See also* Intervention
  adherence to, 139
  family psychoeducation and, 70
  genetic factors and, 276–277
  initial crisis phase of illness and, 39
  issues with, 17
  levels of systems-based involvement and, 57–60, 58t–59t
  modalities of, 67–75
  overview, 34–35
  phases of illness and, 50–53, 52f
  planning, 155–156
  service delivery applications, 53–54
  therapeutic triangle and, 51–53
Triangulation
  case examples of, 103–105, 104f
  childhood and adolescent conditions and, 205–206
  clinicians and, 334
  couple functioning and, 260–261
  family functioning and, 83–84
Typology of illness. *See* Psychosocial typology of illness

Uncertainty. *See also* Anticipatory loss; Psychosocial typology of illness
  course of disorders and, 22
  determining chronicity and, 42–43
  following diagnosis, 159
  initial crisis phase of illness and, 38, 39
  levels of systems-based involvement and, 59
  life-cycle issues and, 125
  overview, 20, 21f
  psychosocial typology matrix and, 29, 31–32
  terminal phase of illness and, 177
  threat of future cognitive impairment, 306

Values. *See* Belief systems
  anticipatory loss and, 175–176
  assisted dying and, 198–199
  collaborative care and, 362
  experience of illness and, 132–133
  Family Systems Illness (FSI) model and, 14f
  fit among family members and, 153–154
  initial crisis phase of illness and, 39

"We" perspective, 244–245
Wills, 230